GLOBAL HEALTH AND GLOBAL AGING

JB JOSSEY-BASS

GLOBAL HEALTH AND GLOBAL AGING

MARY ROBINSON
WILLIAM NOVELLI
CLARENCE PEARSON
LAURIE NORRIS

EDITORS

Foreword by Robert N. Butler, M.D.

Published by Jossey-Bass
A Wiley Imprint
989 Market Street, San Francisco, CA 94103-1741—www.josseybass.com

Jossey-Bass books and products are available through most bookstores. To contact Jossey-Bass directly call our Customer Care Department within the U.S. at 800-956-7739, outside the U.S. at 317-572-3986, or fax 317-572-4002.

Jossey-Bass also publishes its books in a variety of electronic formats. Some content that appears in print may not be available in electronic books.

Library of Congress Cataloging-in-Publication Data

    Global health and global aging / [edited by] Mary Robinson . . . [et al.]; foreword by Robert Butler.—1st ed.
      p.; cm.
    Includes bibliographical references and index.
    ISBN 978-1-118-42407-0
      1. World health. 2. Population aging—Health aspects. I. Robinson, Mary, 1944-
[DNLM: 1. Aging. 2. World Health. 3. Health Policy. 4. Health Services for the Aged. 5. Internationality. 6. Population Dynamics. WT 104 G5615 2007]
    RA441.G565 2007
    362.1—dc22

                                                2007026852

CONTENTS

PART THREE: COUNTRIES FACING RAPID POPULATION AGING IN THE NEXT TWENTY TO THIRTY YEARS

ABOUT THE AARP FOUNDATION

Opportunity, justice, and security. These are the words that best describe what the AARP Foundation offers every day to improve the lives of people as they age. The foundation is committed to helping the most vulnerable members of our society: low-income individuals, women, and minorities are primary target audiences. Its work includes the direct delivery of programs and services, legal advocacy, and the fostering of debate around the extent to which public programs are meeting the needs of these individuals and protecting them from fraud and abuse.

The foundation is also committed to helping individuals at risk of falling into poverty in the second half of life. We know that millions of people are a paycheck away from disaster. A major illness, loss of employment, and death of a spouse are all examples of common life events that could move an individual quickly from a relatively secure situation to one fraught with fear and uncertainty. The foundation is engaged in a variety of activities intended to help individuals avert such a crisis. Through the delivery of information, education, programs, advocacy, and services, the foundation helps individuals to help themselves so that they can be better prepared for the second half of life and the inevitable unexpected life events that can disrupt one's life.

In sum, the AARP Foundation serves as a catalyst for social change and as a champion for people age fifty and older, particularly those facing significant challenges in meeting basic needs. It creates opportunities for individuals to improve their lives; it protects their rights and seeks to ensure that they will be financially secure in the second half of life.

THE WORK OF THE FOUNDATION

As the charitable arm of AARP, the AARP Foundation delivers direct community service, information, legal advocacy, and education to improve the experience of aging in America. The foundation raises money to support its efforts through government grants and from individuals, corporations, foundations, and AARP. Tax-deductible donations enable the Foundation to serve more people who need help, protect individuals from discrimination and abuse, and develop new programs and initiatives.

The AARP Foundation engages in a wide variety of activities that directly benefit individuals and society and encourages other organizations to make aging issues a part of their agendas for change. It brings national attention to the issues and challenges facing individuals and offers new and innovative models for enhancing program effectiveness. Through direct service and grant making, the foundation also provides assistance to older adults impacted by disasters such as Hurricane Katrina.

The AARP Foundation programs serve more than 2.2 million people annually. Through its programs, the AARP Foundation addresses the core issues that help older members of our society meet their health and financial needs and reduce the risk that they will fall victim to poverty and fraud. These programs also explore emerging trends that will affect people more and more as they age. For example, the AARP Foundation champions the needs of older workers. Through programs like Work Connections, the Senior Community Service Employment Program (SCSEP), and the Prepare to Care resource, the Foundation is increasing opportunities for workers aged fifty and over to remain in or reenter the workforce by facilitating their navigation of the workforce system and by providing access to training, resources that help them if they are facing caregiving responsibilities, and connections to companies that value their experience.

The AARP Foundation also champions the needs of the approximately 3.4 million older persons who are living below the poverty level and another 2.2 million who are considered "near poor." Our Tax-Aide program helps individuals file basic tax forms, avoid preparation costs, and receive credits, deductions, and benefits to which they are entitled. Research indicates that tax refunds represent an important opportunity for lower-income persons to save and develop assets. Our Money Management Program helps low-income older individuals remain independent by providing daily money management services to those who have difficulty budgeting, paying routine bills, and keeping track of financial matters.

Recent research conducted on behalf of the AARP Foundation exposed women's concerns about achieving and maintaining financial security as they age. Women want and need tools they can use to build a secure future. The AARP Foundation Women's Leadership Circle (WLC) leverages the philanthropic power and passion of women to improve and enhance women's lives as they grow older. The WLC seeks to raise national awareness of issues faced by women as they age and to provide resources— both private and corporate—to support initiatives that result in empowerment, protection, and security for all women.

These programs are a sample of how the AARP Foundation uses philanthropy to enable the delivery of important help and support older adults. We also provide individuals with opportunities to give back to their communities in ways that are fulfilling for them and those they serve. Future plans include building on its past successes to establish the AARP Foundation as a leader in the nation's philanthropic community.

Nelda Barnett   Robin Talbert
Chair, Board of Directors   Executive Director
AARP Foundation   AARP Foundation

FOREWORD

Global Health and Global Aging is a comprehensive report on the great demographic revolution of the twenty-first century: the increase in longevity due to worldwide improvements in public health, from sanitation to vaccines to antibiotics. However, this unprecedented historic and demographic shift is incomplete, for although older persons in the developed nations have an average seventy-five years of life expectancy, those in the developing world live an average of only fifty years. Terrible sanitation in the developing world, poverty, and the massive assaults by malaria, tuberculosis, and resurgent AIDS, in addition to six diseases that are vaccine-preventable, are continuing afflictions.

The dedication of foundations such as the Bill and Melinda Gates Foundation and William Jefferson Clinton Foundation and the generosity of nations, including those composing Scandinavia, are beginning to make a dent. But as successes against the world's terrifying infectious diseases grow, chronic diseases come to the forefront. Already in India, chronic diseases are a greater problem than infectious diseases, at the same time that we are gaining new understanding of the ways that the chronic diseases of old age are generated early in life. For example, osteoporosis and atherosclerosis have their roots in childhood.

There are those who worry that financial liabilities will compromise this extension of life and its quality, but economists of all ideological persuasions and schools of thought are coming to the conclusion that health creates wealth. We have long known that as countries become wealthier, they are better able to provide health and other benefits for their peoples. That health and longevity *per se* bring about wealth is a very different and new consideration.

Imagine a healthy child who remains healthy throughout life. That child becomes better educated and more productive, earns more income, saves and invests more, and works longer. Productive engagement through the years, collectively, produces greater national wealth. And healthy individuals cost society less money. Concurrently, imagine the growth of industries that serve older persons, such as the health and pharmaceutical industries, financial services, living arrangements, travel, and hospitality. These all contribute to the gross national product.

The authors of this volume represent an impressive variety of positions related to this revolution in longevity and offer valuable insights, perspectives, and knowledge.

Robert N. Butler, M.D.
President and CEO,
International Longevity Center-USA
New York
October 2007

PREFACE

When I considered editing a book on global health and aging, I thought of the close connection health and aging have with my strong interests in and commitment to human rights. What could be more important to human rights than our concern for the health of our increasingly older population in the world today? How can we ensure a more secure, healthier, and happier life for all as new technology is discovered that is bringing a longer life to many—but not all? The World Health Organization definition of health—"a state of complete physical, mental, and social well being, not merely the absence of disease or infirmity"—conceived over fifty years ago, still resonates and is the cornerstone of this book.

Today, more than halfway through the first decade of the twenty-first century, inequalities in health status and access to health care for our aging population and for all are still wide and deep. What is worse, by all indications these divides are growing. We should acknowledge that the state of public health and its effects on longevity in many countries improved significantly during the twentieth century. We can also find hope in the fact that we now have the health interventions available to prevent or treat most conditions, and new aging research is constantly surfacing, bringing hope to the world for our ever-aging population. But we also recognize the enormous challenge still to be faced. That challenge is one of implementation—of ensuring access to health for all through all stages of life.

The message in this book is that we will not make sustainable progress toward our objectives without greater attention to capitalizing on the links between health, aging as a continuum of life, and the realization of fundamental human rights. The greater focus on the right to health and on human rights–based strategies can make a practical difference as we age.

Realizing the right to health for all requires shared responsibility, sustained capacity, and strengthened accountability at every level, from the local village to the national health and aging ministries, from meeting rooms in intergovernmental organizations to the boardrooms of multinational corporations. Only through committed leadership and effective partnerships between the global North and South, between the public and private sectors, and between human rights advocates and health professionals, will we see real progress towards the goal of access to health for all in the years to come, particularly for those who have been most marginalized and excluded, such as our aged population.

I am encouraged by the fact that Trinity College, Dublin—my alma mater and the university where I currently serve as chancellor—has developed a consortium on aging, drawing together a diverse range of academic enterprise and clinical practice and experience. I would encourage universities worldwide to consider similar initiatives.

The objective of this book is to highlight the needs and the hope for a better future for our ever-increasing aging population globally. The book illustrates the opportunities and the success of some countries and the despair affecting the health and longevity of people in too many other countries, resulting when economic, social, and cultural rights have been neglected and violated in a massive way.

There is hope but, in the end, nothing could be more important to promoting greater access to the right of health than capacity building. It is best described by this quote from William H. Foege, M.D., M.P.H., senior advisor to the Bill and Melinda Gates Foundation: "As the tools and resources improve in global health, the real barriers now are deficiencies in our leadership abilities, management, logistics, the ethics of business practices, and an infrastructure needed for the practical application of our science and technology." The potential results: strengthening of the health systems around the world, with appropriate emphasis on a nation's aging population as its life force. A country's health and its concern for its aging population are fundamental not only to its wellness, but also to its social cohesion, its prosperity, and perhaps even to its political stability. The strength of every country's health system—and, within each country, its local and community-based capacities—is of paramount importance and is addressed in this book.

HOW THE BOOK IS ORGANIZED

The book has been organized into five major sections. Part One looks at "The World and Its Aging Population" and presents a broad overview of the topic, including international policies affecting aging populations, population data, WHO and global aging, leadership and governance challenges, and perceptions of aging in different cultures.

Part Two, "Countries with High Rates of Longevity," includes chapters written by the presidents, prime ministers, ministers of health or aging, and NGOs or experts in the field of health and aging in selected countries with record high rates of longevity in their populations. (Because of a change in leadership of Australia's Ministry for Ageing that coincided with the manuscript deadline, we were not able to include a chapter on Australia.)

Part Three, "Countries Facing Rapid Population Aging in the Next Twenty to Thirty Years," features experts from major countries and continents of the world writing about their experiences, anticipating the future health and longevity of their citizens, and identifying the needs of their populations to age successfully.

Part Four, "Leaders in Research and Innovative Programs," presents authors discussing their experiences and reporting on research programs being conducted globally. They highlight new and innovative programs and resources in transportation, housing, education, financing, planning for retirement, and services for aging people with disabilities.

Part Five, "Epilogue: The Road Ahead," looks to the future and identifies opportunities for the countries of the world to improve their programs, attitudes, and policies in support of their aging populations.

THE GLOBAL HEALTH BOOK SERIES

This is the third in the series of books on global health conceived by Clarence Pearson, who saw a need for more visibility and linkages among business, government, and the nonprofit sector, based on his years in public health, working in all three sectors in the United States and abroad. The book series began with *Critical Issues in Global Health*, published in 2001 with U.S. Surgeon General C. Everett Koop as principal editor. Using the book as a point of departure to encourage more active international interest in the topic, the W. K. Kellogg Foundation and the Rockefeller Brothers Fund supported major grants to hold a conference in Salzburg, Austria, which involved the book's authors and other distinguished experts. Discussions inspired the next in the series on capacity building, and the second book, *Global Health Leadership and Management*, whose principal editor was Dr. William H. Foege, was published in 2005.

Global Health and Global Aging, the third in the series, took shape as a result of Clarence Pearson's position as an active member of the board of directors of AARP and as vice chairman of the board of the AARP Foundation, the book's sponsoring nonprofit organization, to which all royalties will be contributed. AARP is the largest voluntary membership organization in the world that works for the health and well-being of people age fifty and older.

One remarkable aspect of organizing this book was the willingness of the forty-one international experts who volunteered to write for this book pro bono. They represent such a broad and rich array of expertise and experience. The circumstances and life experiences of people aging around the world and the related challenges, threats, and opportunities should resonate with readers everywhere. There are also indications in parts of the world that the outlook for an aging population globally is improving. Although people are living longer, healthier lives, we still see many disparities. These conditions must be faced by countries that are rich in resources and knowledge they can share with countries that are not so well off.

ACKNOWLEDGMENTS

So many people have contributed their energies to make this book possible that it is difficult to thank everyone individually. I first want to thank my three coeditors—William Novelli, Clarence Pearson, and Laurie Norris—for their support and orchestration of the myriad details, from selecting authors through final book production. Andy Pasternack, Health Editor, and Seth Schwartz, Assistant Editor, for Jossey-Bass/John Wiley & Sons, Publishers, continue to contribute their support and publishing expertise for this third book in the series.

The collective, heartfelt thanks of the editors go to several organizations and many individuals for their strong support. My team members at Realizing Rights: The Ethical

Globalization Initiative, Heather Grady and Mary Baylis, were great communicators and kept the flow of information to the editors moving smoothly. The staff of both AARP and the AARP Foundation collaborated effectively to help the book evolve. For their tireless efforts on many aspects of the book, we are grateful to Josh Collett, Lisa Davis, Teng Fu, Irene Hoskins, Ladan Manteghi, Susan Necessary, Cheraé Robinson, John Rother, Trish Shannon, Robin Talbert, Line Vreven, Edna Kane Williams, and Joan Wise. Our special thanks go to Rick Moody and Boe Workman of AARP for their writing contributions. And the editors are grateful for the technical expertise and assistance of Xin Pei.

We appreciate the general support of the members of the board of AARP and the members of the board of the AARP Foundation. And finally, our heartfelt thanks to the many authors and experts—friends and colleagues and others—who have expressed their ideas and concerns and have represented their respective countries and cultures on the universal issues of global health and global aging.

Mary Robinson
New York
October 2007

THE EDITORS

Mary Robinson is the president of Realizing Rights: The Ethical Globalization Initiative. She served as United Nations High Commissioner for Human Rights from 1997 to 2002 and as president of Ireland from 1990 to 1997. She is chair of the Council of Women World Leaders and vice president of the Club of Madrid. She chairs the International Board of the International Institute for Environment and Development (IIED) and the Fund for Global Human Rights. She is honorary president of Oxfam International and patron of the International Community of Women Living with AIDS (ICW). She is a professor of practice at Columbia University, a member of the Advisory Board of the Earth Institute, and Extraordinary Professor at the University of Pretoria in South Africa. Before her election as president of Ireland, Mrs. Robinson served as a senator for twenty years. In 1969 she became Reid Professor of Constitutional Law at Trinity College, Dublin, and she now serves as chancellor of Dublin University.

Bill Novelli is CEO of AARP, a membership organization of thirty-eight million people age fifty and older. He joined AARP in January 2000 and became CEO in June 2001. Prior to joining AARP, he was president of the Campaign for Tobacco-Free Kids and executive vice president of CARE, the world's largest private relief and development organization. He cofounded and was president of Porter Novelli, one of the world's largest public relations agencies. He retired from the firm in 1990 to pursue a career in public service. He is the author of *50+: Igniting a Revolution to Reinvent America.*

Clarence E. Pearson, M.P.H., is a former senior advisor to the World Health Organization Office at the United Nations. He was formerly president and chief executive officer of the National Center for Health Education and served as vice president of the Peter Drucker Foundation for Nonprofit Management and vice president and director for health and safety for Metropolitan Life Insurance Company. Pearson conceived and is executive editor of a series of books on global health published by Jossey-Bass/John Wiley & Sons. He is a member of the board of AARP and serves as vice chairman of the board of the AARP Foundation.

Laurie Norris is an interdisciplinary, intercultural communications consultant. She wrote a history of the China Medical Board, a pioneering medical education organization, and is managing editor for a global health series published by Jossey-Bass/John Wiley & Sons. Previously she was director of communications for Catalyst, an organization focused on working women's upward mobility and work and family issues, and vice president for communications at the American Heart Association/NYC. She has served as an NGO representative at the UN and is a member of the board of directors of Big Apple Greeter. She earned a bachelor's degree in journalism and a master's degree in intercultural communications from New York University.

CONTRIBUTORS

NANA ARABA APT, M.S.W., Ph.D., is dean of academic affairs, Ashesi University in Ghana. She previously chaired the departments of sociology and social work at the University of Ghana and was the director of the university's Centre for Social Policy Studies. Her research and publications focus on aging and later life, the family as a support system, and gender and gender roles. Currently she is the president of HelpAge Ghana and a board member of the International Federation on Ageing (IFA). She served on the United Nations technical team at the Second World Assembly on Ageing in 2002.

Before his death in November 2006, **PAUL B. BALTES** was director of the Max Planck International Research Network on Aging at the Max Planck Institute for Human Development in Berlin and professor of psychology at the University of Virginia. He chaired the Berlin Aging Study and was coeditor-in-chief of the twenty-six-volume *International Encyclopedia of the Social and Behavioral Sciences* (Elsevier). In addition to receiving many awards, he was a foreign member of the American Academy of Arts and Sciences and the Royal Swedish Academy of Sciences and received the German order Pour le mérite of Science and the Arts.

MARIE-ANNE BRIEU, M.D., is presently scientific director of ILC-France and of the Alliance for Health and the Future. Previously she served as secretary general of the International Longevity Center-France (ILC-France) from 1995 to 2003. For two years she worked as senior registrar in cardiology at the Hospital das Clinicas, Sao Paulo, Brazil. On her return to France, she occupied different executive positions in the pharmaceutical industry. She graduated from the University of Paris, France.

LINCOLN C. CHEN, M.D., is president of the China Medical Board of New York. He founded and directed the Global Equity Initiative in Harvard University's Asia Center (2001–2006). He was formerly director of the Harvard Center for Population and Development Studies and chair of the Population and International Health Department (1987–1996). From 1997 to 2001 he served as executive vice-president for strategy of the Rockefeller Foundation. Since 2001 he has been chair of the board of directors of CARE/USA. He is currently a member of the Global Advisory Board to the UN Fund for International Partnership and chair of the facilitation group of the NGO President's Forum.

MOHAMED H. EL-BANOUBY, M.D., is professor of geriatrics and founder and prior head of the Geriatric Medical Department, Faculty of Medicine, Ain Shams University, in Cairo, Egypt. It is the only academic institute in the region that grants undergraduate and postgraduate degrees. He is currently head of the Geriatric Medical

Department, Misr University for Sciences and Technology and member of the Supreme Committee for Geriatric Care in the Ministry of Social Affairs. He is a short-term consultant to the World Health Organization (WHO) Eastern Mediterranean Region and arbitrator for its journal.

FRANK E. EYETSEMITAN, Ph.D., is professor of psychology and associate dean of the Feinstein College of Arts and Sciences at Roger Williams University in Bristol, Rhode Island. He has held teaching positions at the University of Jos in Nigeria; the State University of New York in Alfred, New York; the University of Michigan in Ann Arbor, Michigan; and McKendree College in Lebanon, Illinois. He is a coauthor of *Aging and Adult Development in the Developing World: Applying Western Theories and Concepts* (Praeger, 2003).

BRIAN FINDSEN, Ed.D., is senior lecturer, adult education, and head of department, adult and continuing education, at the University of Glasgow. Prior to this appointment, he worked in university-based adult education in New Zealand for about twenty years. His research interests are in the field of educational gerontology, international adult education, and the sociology of (adult) education.

A. JAMES FORBES Jr. is an international health care professional experienced in both the for-profit and nonprofit sectors. His career has included such positions as executive vice president and chief financial officer for Lighthouse International in New York City, founding partner of MedYield, Inc., which practices international health-care consulting, and AmeriCares, the international relief organization, where he rose to vice chairman, with both financial and operational responsibilities. He is a director of the AARP Foundation in Washington, D.C., and was also founding chairman of the Biomedical Engineering and Alliance Consortium Foundation in Connecticut.

FRANÇOISE FORETTE, M.D., has been professor of internal medicine and geriatrics, University Paris V, CHU Cochin-Necker, since 1994. She is CEO of the International Longevity Centre-France since 1995 and cochair of the Alliance for Health and the Future since 2003. She has served as director of the French National Foundation of Gerontology since 1982 and president of the board of directors of the Hôpital Broca since 2002. Forette was elected a member of the Council of Paris in 2001. Since 2005, she has served as special adviser on aging to the Minister of Health and the Minister of Social Security, Elderly, Family, and Disabled Persons.

DR. SHARAD D. GOKHALE, eminent international social scientist, administrator, researcher, writer, and editor, is the founder president of the Community Aid & Sponsorship Programme, International Longevity Centre – India and chairman of the International Leprosy Union. He served two terms as president of the International Federation on Ageing. He has also been a consultant to the United Nations, UNDP, UNICEF, WHO, and the government of India and board member of UN InIA, Malta. His awards include the IGA Award for Leprosy, Government of India, and IFA Awards for Ageing, Birla Award for Humanitarian Service, and the WHO-Sasakawa Health Prize.

BARONESS SALLY GREENGROSS is chief executive of the International Longevity Center, UK. She has been appointed a commissioner of the newly formed Commission for Equalities and Human Rights, which comes into force late in 2007. Before entering the UK Parliament in 2000, she was chief executive officer of Age Concern, Britain's nonprofit organization working for older people. She serves as an adviser to a wide range of organizations concerned with aging societies.

GLORIA M. GUTMAN, Ph.D., is director of the Simon Fraser University Gerontology Research Centre-BCIT Dr. Tong Louie Living Laboratory in Vancouver, Canada; professor in the gerontology department; and a coleader of the British Columbia Network for Aging Research. She served two terms as president of the Canadian Association on Gerontology and is a fellow of the Gerontological Society of America, a member of the World Health Organization's Expert Advisory Panel on Health and Ageing, a director of the International Institute on Ageing-UN Malta, and immediate past president of the International Association of Gerontology and Geriatrics (IAGG).

ANGELA HASSIOTIS, Ph.D., F.R.C. Psych, is a clinical academic with a commitment to improving the lives of people with intellectual disabilities and enhancing the evidence-based, service-user care of this population group. Her main interests are in epidemiology and health services research.

BJARNE HASTRUP, M.A. (economics) has been the chief executive of DaneAge in Copenhagen, Denmark since 1984. Under his leadership, the organization has developed from zero to 490,000 members out of a total population of five million. He has written several books on a variety of subjects, ranging from economic history to social welfare in Denmark and other parts of the world. He also lectures at the University of Copenhagen on a range of subjects, including economic history and senior citizens' policies. He studied economics at the University of Copenhagen.

C. ROBERT (ROB) HENRIKSON is chairman of the board of directors, president and chief executive officer of MetLife, Inc. (NYSE: MET), the global insurance and financial services company. Recognizing the implications of increasing longevity over a decade ago, he began positioning the company to meet the retirement needs of the baby boomers and future generations. An industry thought leader, Henrikson is regularly called on to testify before and advise members of Congress on retirement-related issues. He recently provided direction to U.S. senators and other congressional leaders to better inform the Social Security and corporate pension debates.

ALEX KALACHE, M.D., has directed the WHO Global Programme on Ageing and Life Course since 1995. He earned a medical degree at the Federal University of Rio de Janeiro and a master's degree in social medicine at the University of London. He worked as a lecturer at the Department of Public Health, University of Oxford, where he earned a Ph.D. in cancer epidemiology. From 1984 to 1995 he was the head of the London School of Hygiene and Tropical Medicine's Programme on Public Health Implications of Ageing and launched the first-ever master's degree course on health promotion. He is a native of Rio de Janeiro.

VLADIMIR KHAVINSON, M.D., Ph.D., is a founder and director of the St. Petersburg Institute of Bioregulation and Gerontology, vice president of the Gerontological Society of the Russian Academy of Sciences, and associate member of the Russian Academy of Medical Sciences. His interest lies in antiaging technologies; developmental, experimental, and clinical studies of new classes of peptide bioregulators; and bioregulation therapy. He has over six hundred scientific publications, including 108 patents in biotechnology, immunology, biochemistry, pharmacology, oncology, and gerontology. He is an Honored Inventor of the Russian Federation and was recognized as an "Author of Scientific Discovery" and for outstanding achievements in preventive and social medicine.

JOSHUA LEDERBERG, Ph.D., is president emeritus and professor emeritus of molecular genetics and informatics at Rockefeller University and former chair of the Department of Genetics of Stanford University. His honors include senior membership in the National Academy of Sciences, a Nobel Prize for his basic research in bacterial genetics (1958), the National Medal of Science (1989), and the Presidential Medal of Freedom (2006). He has made a major contribution to the support of basic research on the biology of aging via his founding chairmanship of the Scientific Advisory Committee of the Ellison Medical Foundation.

JAIME LERNER is an architect and urban planner and founder of the Instituto Jaime Lerner. Three-time mayor of Curitiba, Brazil, he led the urban revolution that made the city renowned for urban planning in public transportation, environment, and social programs. He served as governor of Parana State twice and conducted an urban and rural economic and social transformation. His international awards include the highest United Nations Environmental Award (1990), the 2001 World Technology Award for Transportation, and the 2002 Sir Robert Matthew Prize for the Improvement of Quality of Human Settlements from the International Union of Architects. He is former president of the International Architects Union (UIA).

GEORGE M. MARTIN, M.D., is professor emeritus of pathology at the University of Washington and scientific director of the American Federation for Aging Research. His honors include senior membership in the Institute of Medicine of the National Academy of Sciences, a Lifetime Achievement Award from the World Alzheimer Congress, the Robert W. Kleemeier Award of the Gerontological Society of America, and the IPSEN Foundation Longevity Prize. He is a past president of the Gerontological Society of America.

HECTOR MEDORA is head of disability services in the Camden National Health Service Primary Care Trust (Provider Services) and the London Borough of Camden, an integrated health and social care service for disabled people in the community. He has worked on a range of projects in the field of disability in England and internationally. For his work in the field of disability, in 2004 he was awarded the Order of the British Empire by Her Majesty Queen Elizabeth II.

OLGA N. MIKHAILOVA, Ph.D., is an executive director and vice-director on International Collaboration of the St. Petersburg Institute of Bioregulation and Gerontology and scientific secretary of the Gerontological Society of the Russian Academy of Sciences. She works in collaboration with international organizations, including the UN, WHO, and IAGG, and served as secretary of the II European Congress on biogerontology (2000, Saint Petersburg) and an executive manager of the VI European Congress of the IAGG (2007, Saint Petersburg). Her interest lies in the organization of health-care systems and the role of international collaboration in the development of gerontology in Russia. Her doctorate is in gerontology.

SHIGEO MORIOKA has been president of the International Longevity Center–Japan since 1999. Previously, he was president and CEO and chairman of the board of Yamanouchi Pharmaceutical Co., Ltd. (current Astellas Pharma Inc.) for about twenty years. He has served in several key positions in the pharmaceutical industry in Japan and abroad, including chairman of the Fair Trade Council of the Ethical Pharmaceutical Drugs Manufacturing Industry and executive vice chairman of the International Federation of Pharmaceutical Manufacturers Associations. He was awarded the Order of the Rising Sun, Gold and Silver Star in 1999.

ERIK OLSEN, D.D.S., became president of AARP on May 2, 2006. Previously, he served as AARP state president in Arizona in 1996 and joined AARP's national board of directors in 2000. A practicing dentist, he was president and CEO of the Delta Dental Plan of California, the nation's oldest and largest dental health insurer. By the end of his fifteen-year tenure, one of every three people in California had Delta benefits. He also chaired Delta's effort to include dental heath in health care reform. He has served as executive director and managing editor of the Academy of General Dentistry.

THOMAS PERLS, M.D., M.P.H., is founder and codirector of the New England Centenarian Study (NECS) and associate professor of medicine at Boston University School of Medicine in Boston, Massachusetts. Since 1995, the NECS has grown to be the largest study of centenarians and their families in the world.

JULIA PREECE, Ph.D., is professor of adult and lifelong education and director of the Centre for Research and Development in Adult and Lifelong Education, University of Glasgow, Scotland, UK. She has also worked in Malawi and Botswana and participated in HIV/AIDS education research in Botswana. She has consistently studied and published on issues of social justice and social exclusion in lifelong learning for the past ten years.

PEKKA PUSKA, M.D., Ph.D., M.Pol.Sc., is currently the director general of the National Public Health Institute of Finland (KTL). He served as director for noncommunicable disease (NCD) prevention and health promotion at WHO in Geneva from 2001 to 2003. Previously, he served KTL as department director. For twenty-five years he was the director of the North Karelia Project. He has worked in numerous international scientific, expert, and public health functions and has also served as a member of the parliament. He is the vice-president of the International Association of National Public Health Institutes and president-elect of the World Heart Federation.

CLEMENTIA IGNATIA JOHANNA MARIA (CLÉMENCE) ROSS-VAN DORP served as state secretary for health, welfare, and sport in the Netherlands from 2002 to 2006. Among her achievements as state secretary was the introduction of the Social Support Act. From 1990 to 1998, she was a policy officer for Mr. Arie Oostlander, a member of the European Parliament representing the Christian Democratic Alliance/ Evangelical People's Party. From 1998 to 2002, she was a member of the House of Representatives of the States General for the Christian Democratic Alliance (CDA). A native of Delft, she did several vocational courses and qualified as a teacher of Dutch and English after completing her secondary education. She subsequently studied sinology at Leiden University.

ULLA SCHMIDT has served as the Federal Minister of Health of Germany since January 2001. From October 2002 to November 2005, she was also assigned responsibility for Social Security. She has been a member of the German Bundestag since 1990. She studied psychology and training as a teacher for primary and lower secondary schools. She graduated from the Open University of Hagen as a teacher of special education and has worked in the field.

ALEXANDRE SIDORENKO, M.D., Ph.D., is the United Nations Focal Point on Ageing. As the chief of the United Nations Programme on Ageing from 1993 to 2002, he coordinated substantive preparations for the Second World Assembly on Ageing in Madrid, Spain, including drafting and negotiating the Madrid International Plan of Action on Ageing. His current principal responsibilities include follow-up to the Second World Assembly on Ageing. His specific areas of professional involvement are the monitoring of the Madrid International Plan of Action on Ageing and the development of evidence-based policy on aging.

JACQUI SMITH is a professor of psychology and research professor at the Institute for Social Research, University of Michigan. She was previously a senior research scientist at the Max Planck Institute for Human Development in Berlin, collaborating with Paul B. Baltes on the Berlin Aging Study and related studies. She is a member of the Academia Europaea, a fellow of the American Psychological Association, a fellow of the Gerontological Society of America, and a member of the advisory boards of several longitudinal studies of aging in Europe.

JEANETTE C. TAKAMURA is dean and professor at the Columbia University School of Social Work, the first established academic social work institution in the nation. She was assistant secretary for aging in the U.S. Department of Health and Human Services during the Clinton Administration (1996–2000). She led the design and proposal of the National Family Caregiver Support Program. She has participated in international expert exchanges and consultations, including those organized by the UN and

WHO and nongovernmental organizations. She has served on numerous boards and commissions and is the recipient of a number of honors and awards.

DELLARA F. TERRY, M.D., M.P.H., is codirector of the New England Centenarian Study and assistant professor of medicine at Boston University School of Medicine. Dr. Terry specifically studies the offspring of centenarians as a prospectively studied model of age-related disease resistance and successful aging.

ENRIQUE VEGA is the PAHO/WHO Regional Advisor on Aging and Health. Before joining PAHO, he was a professor of gerontology and geriatrics in Havana Medical University, chair of the Health and Aging Cathedra in the National School of Public Health, national director for the Elderly Care and Social Assistance Program of the Ministry of Health, and vice director of the Iberoamerican Center for the Third Age, in Cuba. He developed an international advisory service in geriatrics and public heath and aging in several countries of Latin America. He has several publications in national and international journals and books.

MARY BETH WEINBERGER, M.A., is a consultant demographer who worked in the United Nations Population Division until retiring from that post in 2006. From 1995 to 2006 she was chief of the Division's Population and Development Section, concentrating on population aging and relationships between population dynamics and social, economic, and environmental change. Her other research topics have included living arrangements of older persons and global trends in contraceptive use and fertility.

BARBRO WESTERHOLM, M.D., Ph.D., returned in 2006 as a member of the Swedish Parliament and is chairperson of the Parliamentary Committee on Housing for the Elderly. Previously, she had served in Parliament for eleven years, leaving when elected president of the Swedish Association of Senior Citizens. She is professor emerita in drug epidemiology at Karolinska Institute. She has served as medical director of the Swedish National Corporation of Pharmacies, director general of the Swedish National Board of Health and Welfare, and vice president of the WHO Executive Board.

DEREK YACH, M.B.Ch.B., M.P.H., is director of global health policy at PepsiCo. Previously he was head of health at the Rockefeller Foundation. For ten years he served in several capacities at WHO, including executive director of noncommunicable diseases and mental health. He coordinated WHO's global consultation that led to the adoption of a new global policy, Health for All in the 21st Century, by WHO's member states. From 1985 to 1995, he played a leadership role in developing South Africa's epidemiological and health policy capacity. He has published on issues related to globalization and health and provides advice to multinationals, international NGOs, the World Bank, and international research bodies.

JOSÉ LUIS RODRÍGUEZ ZAPATERO was sworn in as president of the government of Spain by His Majesty King Juan Carlos on April 17, 2004, after the general elections of March 14. He earned a law degree at the University of Leon. Since 1979, he has been affiliated with the Spanish Socialist Workers Party (PSOE). He served as secretary-general of the Socialist Federation of Leon from 1988 to 2000. He has served as secretary general of the Spanish Workers Party from 2000 to the present.

LINGLING ZHANG, M.P.A., is a doctoral student at Harvard School of Public Health. She is a research fellow at the Global Equity Initiative in Harvard University's Asia Center and a fellow researcher of Harvard China Initiative. Her interest is promoting health equity and improving quality of care through building the capacity of health systems.

GLOBAL HEALTH AND GLOBAL AGING

PART

THE WORLD AND ITS AGING POPULATION

CHAPTER

WORLD POLICIES ON AGING AND THE UNITED NATIONS

ALEXANDRE SIDORENKO

For those who have been following the international vocabulary on aging during the past decade or two, its transformation is obvious—from negative and pessimistic to positive and forward-looking. Of course, this does not mean that reaching a secure, healthy, and dignified old age has become a universal blessing and ubiquitous achievement. This is definitely not the case in many countries of sub-Saharan Africa, where life expectancy may not exceed thirty-three years (as in Swaziland), or in the countries of the former Soviet Union, where for millions of middle-age people the progression into old age coincided with the hardship of societal transformation. And throughout the world, too often older persons are left on their own to adjust to changes associated with individual aging—at the workplace, at home, and in a rapidly changing society.

Nonetheless, in the United Nations policy documents on aging, the words *aging* and *problem* rarely are placed together. *Aging* is referred to as an issue, an area, and most emphatically as a challenge and opportunity (United Nations, 2002b). This is not just political correctness, but a reflection of new thinking and emerging new policy responses to individual and population aging in the twenty-first century (Kinsella and Phillips, 2005). The Second World Assembly on Ageing, which took place in Madrid, Spain, in April 2002, elaborated these responses. This chapter outlines the major parameters of the new responses to the challenges and opportunities of aging as formulated in the Madrid International Plan of Action on Ageing and promoted through follow-up actions.

INTERNATIONAL CONSENSUS ON AGING 2002

The majority of decisions made by the United Nations are based on the consensus, or universal agreement, of all its member states. The voting procedure is also envisaged and has been exercised, but in the "social domain" of the UN it is rare. Reaching a consensus could be cumbersome and painful and thus requires a great deal of good political will to negotiate and compromise. One can argue that political compromises may dilute the ideas and obstruct actions. Despite these obstacles, consensus unites the international community on the basis of universally agreed values and goals. In aging, the most recent and most significant international consensus document is the Madrid International Plan of Action on Ageing.

To develop the Madrid Plan of Action, the forum for the political process of consensus-building was the Preparatory Committee for the Second World Assembly on Ageing, which had two regular sessions in 2001. The committee focused on negotiations on the content of the future plan of action on aging. This process was completed during the Second World Assembly in Madrid from April 8 to April 12, 2002, by its Main Committee, which finalized the texts of the Madrid Plan of Action and the Political Declaration.

The entire negotiation process was supported by the work of the Technical Committee: fifteen individual experts and several observers representing various organizations of the UN system and international nongovernmental organizations. The governments of Germany, Spain, and Austria provided financial support to all three meetings of the Preparatory Committee, which were hosted by the governments of Germany (June 2000), the Dominican Republic (Santo Domingo, October 2000), and Austria (Vienna, April 2001).

The most important role of the Technical Committee was its contribution to the formulation of proposals regarding the content of the new plan of action. These proposals helped the UN Secretariat to prepare the draft plan of action for subsequent intergovernmental negotiations at the meetings of the Preparatory Committee and the Second World Assembly.

Two major outcomes of the Madrid Assembly include the Political Declaration and the Madrid International Plan of Action on Ageing. The most important content of the Political Declaration is the commitment of governments to address the challenges and opportunities of aging in the twenty-first century. The United Nations member states that gathered at the Madrid Assembly committed themselves to eliminate all forms of discrimination, including age discrimination; to effectively incorporate aging within social and economic strategies, policies, and action; to protect and assist older persons in situations of armed conflict and foreign occupation; and to provide older persons with universal and equal access to health care and services. Governments also expressed their commitment to act at national and international levels on three priority directions: older persons and development; advancing health and well-being into old age; and ensuring enabling and supportive environments.

Priority Direction I for action strives to integrate global aging within the larger context of development. The overall goal is to ensure that older persons are full participants in the development process and also its beneficiaries.

Priority Direction II emphasizes that the health of the population is vital to development and that for the individual, good health is the most important asset and human right. To reach old age in good health requires the combined efforts of government, civil society, and the individual.

Priority Direction III aims to ensure enabling and supportive environments. It promotes positive perceptions of aging and positive, realistic images of older persons to influence public values relating to social, cultural, and economic exchange between generations. The Madrid Plan of Action also calls for greater access to both the physical environment and services and resources, including care and social protection.

The elaboration of the Madrid Plan of Action was informed by the major United Nations conferences, summits, and special sessions of the General Assembly. The decisions of these international gatherings and their follow-up processes helped to formulate the *central themes*, or foundations, of the Madrid Plan of Action. These themes include the issues of human rights and fundamental freedoms; empowerment and participation; individual development, self-fulfillment, and well-being throughout life; gender equality; intergenerational interdependence, solidarity, and reciprocity; health care, support, and social protection; partnership among government, civil society, the private sector, and older persons; scientific research, expertise, and technology; and the situation of aging indigenous peoples.

CENTRAL CONCEPT OF THE MADRID PLAN OF ACTION: ORIGIN AND EVOLUTION

The *central concept* of the Madrid Plan is the concept of a *society for all ages*. This concept was formulated during the preparations for the 1999 International Year of Older Persons and later became the year's theme. The concept of a society for all ages emerged from the concept of *a society for all*, laid out in the Copenhagen Declaration and Programme of Action, which was developed at the World Summit for Social Development in 1995 (United Nations, 1995). In the Programme of Action of the World Summit, a society for all was described as an inclusive society, "in which every individual, each with rights and responsibilities, has an active role to play."

The Report of the Secretary General, "Conceptual Framework for the Preparation and Observance of the International Year of Older Persons in 1999" stated that a society for all ages "would . . . enable the generations to invest in one another and share in the fruits of that investment, guided by the twin principles of reciprocity and equity" (United Nations, 1999).

Four facets were suggested to explore the society for all ages and, consequently, to develop a strategy to achieve such a society. These are *situation of older persons, lifelong individual development, multigenerational relationships, and development and aging of populations*.

The situation of older persons, the first facet of the Conceptual Framework, emphasizes a "traditional" approach of policy action on aging. This approach incorporates "policies designed to enhance the lives [of older persons] as individuals and to allow them to enjoy in mind and in body, fully and freely, their advancing years in peace, health and security" (United Nations, 1982, p. 9). The Vienna International Plan of Action on Ageing—adopted by the first World Assembly on Ageing in 1982 in Vienna, Austria—identified the following areas of primary concern to older persons: health and nutrition, protection of elderly consumers, housing and the environment, the family, social welfare, income security and employment, and education. The recommendations of the Vienna Plan of Action are viewed as specific measures for supporting the *independence, participation, care, self-fulfillment*, and *dignity* of older persons as outlined in the United Nations Principles for Older Persons (United Nations, 1991).

The second facet of the Conceptual Framework, lifelong individual development, was a relatively new priority within the UN program on aging. It was based on the idea that the interplay of individual behavior and various policies affecting people at different ages will shape the situation of persons in older age. To respond to various needs at different stages of individual development, policy should provide an enabling and supportive environment fostering lifelong education, skills-upgrading, healthy lifestyles, and provision of care when it is required.

Multigenerational relations are the third facet of the Conceptual Framework. The debate during the International Year of Older Persons explored how the relations of interdependence could be maintained in family and society as the proportions of older and younger people change. The implications of aging for family include primarily caregiving, and for society, provision of social services and income security.

The fourth facet, aging and development, focused on harmonization (reconciliation) of population aging with continuing socioeconomic development. This requires multisectoral adjustments, including employment, income security, social welfare, health care, education, and also investment, consumption, and savings patterns. One of the principal directions for such an adjustment is ensuring that older persons have opportunities to participate and contribute and also to receive care when needed.

When first put forth in the late 1990s, the concept of a society for all ages appeared as an innovative approach to aging—and to some as a controversial deviation from earlier commitments to care and support for older people. The controversy was based on a presumption that efforts to achieve a society for all ages could lead to abandoning the policies that address specific and often difficult situations of older persons, shifting already limited resources to other social groups, such as children and youth. In the course of debate during the International Year, the UN Programme on Ageing emphasized that although the concept of a society for all ages took a broad and long-term approach to individual and population aging, improving the situation of older persons would remain a paramount task for future action on aging.

The strategies for a society for all ages could embrace aging issues instead of singling them out and thus isolating and marginalizing older persons. This approach was later incorporated into the implementation strategy for the Madrid Plan of Action, which promoted a two-faceted action: advancing the aging-specific programs while simultaneously mainstreaming aging into national and international development strategies (United Nations, 2003).

Subsequently, the UN General Assembly decided that the concept of a society for all ages would serve as the context for the future plan of action on aging, which later became the Madrid Plan of Action. Eventually, the four facets of the Conceptual Framework evolved into the three priority directions of the Madrid Plan.

ACTION ON AGING IN THE TWENTY-FIRST CENTURY: PURPOSE, GOAL, AND CONTENT

The purpose of the Madrid Plan is to respond to the opportunities and challenges of population aging in the twenty-first century and to promote the development of a society for all ages. All three priority directions of the Madrid Plan are designed to guide policy aimed at reaching the *specific goal of successful adjustment to an aging world*. The success of this adjustment, states the plan, will be measured in terms of social development, improvement in quality of life for older persons, and sustainability of the various systems—formal and informal—that underpin well-being throughout the life course.

The Madrid Plan clearly focuses on developing countries not only because that is where the process of population aging will happen in the twenty-first century, but also—and more important—because these countries will have to respond to the implications of aging from a rather limited economic and social base compared to the developed world. The challenge is to develop policy approaches that keep aging from becoming an additional burden for developing countries and to transform it into an opportunity for development.

Unfortunately, older persons today are largely absent from the international developmental discourse, including in the most prominent document of the United Nations on development, the Millennium Declaration (United Nations, 2000), which fails to address aging among the eight Millennium Development Goals (MDGs)s. Meanwhile, issues related to aging and older persons are being pursued in the context of other global processes, including the International Conference on Financing for Development, held in Monterrey, Mexico, and the World Summit on Sustainable Development, held in Johannesburg, South Africa. For example, the Monterrey Consensus of the International Conference on Financing for Development (United Nations, 2002c) addressed the role of pension schemes as a source of social protection as well as savings and resources for development. The Johannesburg summit outcome—the Johannesburg Plan of Implementation (United Nations, 2002a)—recognized the role of holders of traditional knowledge and practices, who are typically community elders, and called for their effective participation in decision and policy making.

Although these references to aging in Monterrey and Johannesburg were important, one can hardly deny that aging remains at the outskirts of global development efforts and that the developmental potential of older persons remains untapped. Essentially, most policymakers continue to think of aging primarily in humanitarian terms, with concern centered on pensions and caregiving, while ignoring its developmental potential. An inability to recognize and develop the potential of aging will certainly become both unaffordable and inexcusable tomorrow when it becomes a really dominant issue globally—particularly in developing countries.

The major challenge in adjusting to an aging world is to transform aging into a force for progress and development at both societal and individual levels. Such a possibility is real: population aging did not start all at once; in the more developed parts of the world, the phenomenon has been present for more than a century. That period witnessed unprecedented advancement of science, technology, and quality of life, including the increase in individual longevity. Significantly, individual longevity has been growing together with societal development. The reasonable assumption is that societal development and population aging are two *parallel* processes. The principal task is to ensure that they are *compatible* and *synergistic*.

Specific policy action should support the multilevel adjustment to an aging world. Two types of policy approaches are necessary: aging-specific and aging-mainstreaming.

The first policy approach, aging-specific, includes policies and programs designed to address the needs of older persons. Following the Vienna International Plan of Action on Ageing and the UN Principles for Older Persons, policies and programs should be formulated within several areas of primary concern to older persons (discussed previously) and ensure their independence, participation, care, self-fulfillment, and dignity.

Empowerment of older persons represents the principal content of aging-specific policies with both immediate and long-term action. Immediate action includes legislative measures to guarantee the basic human rights of older persons and prevent violence and abuse against them. Long-term action should focus on establishing or sustaining positive images of older persons in a society.

The essence of the second key approach to implementation of the Madrid Plan is inclusion, integration, or *mainstreaming* of aging and older persons into national development strategies. This type of policy is significant for both developed and developing countries as it aims to mobilize older persons as additional resources for development and, simultaneously, to improve their well-being. Thus efforts to mainstream aging could ensure a win-win scenario for both older persons and society at large.

At the same time, mainstreaming should not create separate or new programs where implementation becomes hindered by lack of resources. This could be prevented through *focused* or *targeted* mainstreaming. Targeted mainstreaming could link aging to a *recognized* development priority instead of trying to squeeze it into *all* policies and programs. Complementing the traditional and often prevailing approach of focusing national efforts and international assistance on the specific, if not discrete, aging-related activities, targeted mainstreaming could promote an integrated strategy for addressing issues of aging in the development context, as called for in the Madrid Plan of Action.

IMPLEMENTING THE MADRID DECISIONS: FIRST RESULTS

During the first five years following the adoption of the Madrid Plan of Action, the national implementation efforts focused on developing and strengthening capacity on aging (United Nations, 2006). The essential elements of national capacity include institutional infrastructure; human resources; mobilization of financial resources; research, data collection, and analysis; and policy process.

The viable *institutional infrastructure* envisages productive collaboration among all major national stakeholders, including government, organizations *of* and *for* older persons, academia, and the private sector. The scope and strength of national infrastructure depends on such factors as the level of recognition of aging—making it a priority—in the national public arena and is closely linked to the availability of financial and human resources.

Government offices on aging at the ministerial or similar level include the Department of Health and Ageing in Australia, the Division of Aging and Seniors in Canada; the National Committee on Ageing in China; the Federal Ministry for Family Affairs, Senior Citizens, Women and Youth in Germany; and the Administration on Aging in the United States. When resources are insufficient and competing demands are many—often the case in many developing countries—the government office on aging could be a single person focal point in a ministry dealing with social issues.

Interesting examples of collaboration between national stakeholders can be found in various countries. In Austria, for example, an independent council of senior citizens has become an important participant in debates on national policy on aging. The Chilean National Service for Older Persons (SENAMA) includes an advisory committee composed of representatives of older persons' organizations, academia, and institutions working with older persons. In India, the watchdog agency National Council of Older Persons monitors policy on aging.

Human resource development envisions investing in the training of professionals and, simultaneously, providing opportunities for volunteering for and by older persons. Developing countries experience a critical shortage of health workers, including doctors, nurses, and lab technicians (World Health Organization, 2006), owing to insufficient training capacity and the "brain drain" of skilled health professionals from developing to developed countries. Many other countries, both developed and developing, lack enough trained professionals with sufficient knowledge of aging and specific needs of older persons.

Meanwhile, several countries are making efforts to compensate for this deficiency. For instance, the Uganda Reach the Aged Association and the African Regional Development Centre of HelpAge International, with the financial support of the United Nations Population Fund (UNFPA), conducted the training of policymakers and the local UNFPA staff in the area of population aging. In Chile, the government is planning to train health professionals to specialize in geriatrics and also to provide health training to leaders of clubs and community unions of older persons. The State Educational Geriatric Centre established in Ukraine in 2005 offers educational and training programs for medical and social workers, as well as volunteers, in the field of care for older persons.

Generational equity in public spending and clear allocation of *financial resources* are necessary to adequately tackle the often underserved needs of older persons, especially in developing countries and countries with economies in transition. Both developed and developing countries are concerned with inadequate resources for programs addressing the needs of older persons. However, the content and degree of financial resources available for programs on aging vary greatly: while in Europe and the United States, for instance, much attention is drawn to the costs of *maintaining and adjusting the existing* pension and health plans for older persons, in many developing countries the lack of financial resources is seen as the main stumbling block to *establishing* programs to support older persons.

The costs of social pension programs may not be as prohibitive as initially anticipated. According to HelpAge International, as of October 2006, seventy-two countries had a social pension; forty-six of these were low- or middle-income countries (Pension Watch, 2006). Moreover, of eighteen low- and middle-income countries that introduced social pensions, 67 percent deliver a social pension for less than 1 percent of GDP. It is also significant that the social pensions could be an effective tool for directing the aid to the poorest older persons and their families and reducing the number of people living in extreme poverty.

The quality and quantity of policy *research* on aging and availability of age-disaggregated data need improvement practically everywhere (United Nations, 2002). Predictably, the lack of "domestic" research on aging—both fundamental and applied studies—is particularly felt in developing countries. Yet despite their limited capacity for research and data collection, in developing countries there are signs of progress as well. In Thailand, for example, the Second National Long-Term Plan for Older Persons

(2002–2021) has included research strategies to support policy design, monitoring, and evaluation. In Argentina, the Programme of Ageing and Society of the Latin American Faculty of Social Sciences (FLASCO-Argentina) has begun studying the issue of the aging workforce, and the Group of Socio-Anthropology of Older Persons and Community Planning of Ageing at the University of Mar del Plata has developed extensive research on social support networks for older persons.

In countries of the former Soviet Union, in addition to the world-renowned Kiev Institute of Gerontology of Ukraine, new research centers have been established in the Russian Federation in Moscow, Samara, and St. Petersburg. However, in other countries of the former Soviet Union, particularly in the Central Asian region, research capacity on aging remains severely limited.

Advanced population aging has prompted significant progress in aging research in developed countries. In the European Union, the European Research Area in Aging (ERA-AGE), a four-year project funded by the European Commission, was established to promote the development of a European strategy for research on aging. In Australia, the Department of Health and Ageing of the Australian Government has funded various research and publications aimed at guiding future policy directions in the area of aging. The National Health and Medical Research Council (NHMRC) also provides funding to support medical research and training on health issues for people of all ages throughout Australia.

The United States has an advanced network of research entities on aging, including the government, academia, foundations, and nonprofit organizations. Among the most famous are the National Institute on Aging, the National Academy on an Aging Society, and the Gerontology Society of America. Every ten years, the White House Conference on Aging, last held in 2005, is convened to develop recommendations for the U.S. government on policy and research in the field of aging.

All of the components of national capacity just described should ideally act in synergy supporting the *policy process* aimed at implementing the Madrid Plan of Action. Leaving aside inter- and intraregional differences in priorities on aging, income security actions feature most prominently in national implementation efforts, along with the efforts to develop high-quality, affordable, and sustainable health and care services, particularly long-term care.

In developing countries, income support programs for older persons include a regular, noncontributory cash payment in the form of a social pension (mentioned earlier); cash payment programs targeting a small number of poor older persons, such as the cash assistance provided by the government in Indonesia; and government-sponsored savings plans, such as a pension-linked savings scheme in India.

Besides designing specific policies on aging, some developing countries and countries with economies in transition have also attempted to mainstream aging issues in national development plans, including poverty reduction strategies. For instance, Tanzania recently incorporated several issues pertaining to older persons in its National Strategy for Growth and Reduction of Poverty for the period 2005–2010, and several countries with economies in transition, such as Azerbaijan and Bosnia and Herzegovina, have included older persons in their Poverty Reduction Strategy Papers.

In developed countries, public debate and, increasingly, policy actions have focused on reforming pension and health care and social care programs and adjusting to the decreasing labor force participation. It is encouraging that the introduced adjustments have so far avoided large-scale cutbacks in benefits or strong measures to postpone retirement. Instead, reforms in pension and health care programs have attempted to secure financial stability and ensure the continuing delivery of benefits without jeopardizing the welfare of future generations.

REVIEWING THE PROGRESS

The examples of national actions on aging presented in the preceding section offer a very preliminary snapshot of major trends in the implementation of the Madrid Plan of Action in the first five years since its adoption. It is expected that the first cycle (2007–2008) of the review and appraisal of the Madrid Plan will bring a much more comprehensive picture of implementation efforts.

The Madrid Plan of Action designated the Commission for Social Development to be responsible for follow-up and appraisal of the implementation process. In accordance with the decisions of the commission, review and appraisal will be undertaken every five years and include two dimensions: aging-specific policies and aging-mainstreaming efforts. Each review and appraisal cycle will focus on a theme based on the priority directions of the Madrid Plan, and the bottom-up participatory approach will be the major format of the review and appraisal exercise.

The bottom-up participatory approach has a dual function in the process of implementing the Madrid Plan of Action. The first function is "technical," as the participatory methodology will be used for an in-depth evaluation of national implementation efforts. Participatory evaluation of policy and programs is generally associated with qualitative methods of information gathering, including participatory listening and observation, visual tools such as maps and various diagrams, semistructured interviews, and focus group discussions.

The second function of the bottom-up participatory approach is promotional. Although the immediate purpose of the participatory approach is to ensure that older persons have an opportunity to express their views on the impact of national policy actions affecting their lives, the overall goal is to ensure that older persons are involved in all phases of policy actions on aging, including policy design, implementation, monitoring, and evaluation. Therefore, the participatory approach to review and appraisal of the Madrid Plan could become an *entry point* for engaging older persons in the entire process of the plan's implementation. This is in full agreement with the aim of the International Plan of Action *to ensure that persons everywhere are able to age with security and dignity and to continue to participate in their societies as citizens with full rights.*

The participatory approach should not be seen as a panacea aimed at replacing all other methods of monitoring, review, and appraisal. Rather, it attempts to supplement the "traditional" quantitative methods with a wider use of qualitative tools. The quantitative monitoring of social situations—such as through censuses, surveys, and civil registration—can play a very important role by revealing principal trends and helping to identify local and national priorities on aging for more targeted participatory inquiry.

To ensure the success of the bottom-up participatory process requires a catalyst and a facilitator. Government should be seen as the principal catalyst and end user of policy-relevant information, involving facilitators with sufficient experience in conducting participatory research. Such facilitators should be found among community workers or members of nongovernmental organizations active at the local level, as well as academia and research institutions.

The first global cycle of review and appraisal of the Madrid Plan of Action is anticipated to be a year-long process, starting in 2007 and finishing in 2008. The theme of this first review and appraisal is "Addressing the challenges and opportunities of ageing." The major activities and events of the review and appraisal will occur at the national and even local levels—at the site of real implementation action—and ascend through regional levels to the global stage.

Overall, it is expected that the future review and appraisal exercise will involve all major stakeholders, ensure broad participation of older persons, and promote the implementation of the Madrid Plan of Action.

ACKNOWLEDGMENTS

The author wishes to acknowledge the continuing contribution of his colleagues in the UN Programme on Ageing to the concepts and formulations underlying this chapter: Brigid Donelan (retired), Margaret L. Kelly, Rosemary Lane, Diane Loughran, and Robert Venne.

REFERENCES

Kinsella, K., and Phillips, D. R. "Global Aging: The Challenge of Success." *Population Bulletin*, March 2005, *60*(1), 3–42.

Pension Watch. HelpAge International, 2006. [http://www.helpage.org/Researchandpolicy/Socialprotection/PensionWatch]. Dec. 1, 2006.

United Nations. Vienna International Plan of Action on Ageing. New York: United Nations, 1982. [http://www.un.org/esa/socdev/ageing/ageing/ageipaa.htm]. Dec. 12, 2006.

United Nations. *United Nations Principles for Older Persons*. New York: United Nations, 1991. [http://www.un.org/esa/socdev/iyop/iyoppop.htm#Principles]. Dec. 12, 2006.

United Nations. *The Copenhagen Declaration and Programme of Action. World Summit for Social Development, 6–12 March 1995*. New York: United Nations, 1995. [http://www.un.org/esa/socdev/wssd/agreements/index.html]. Dec. 12, 2006.

United Nations. Report of the Secretary-General, "Conceptual Framework for the Preparation and Observance of the International Year of Older Persons in 1999" (A/50/114). New York: United Nations, 1999. [http://www.un.org/esa/socdev/iyop/iyopcf0.htm]. Dec. 12, 2006.

United Nations. *United Nations Millennium Declaration, United Nations, 2000.* New York: United Nations, 2000. [http://www.un.org/millennium/]. Dec. 12, 2006.

United Nations. Johannesburg Plan of Implementation. New York: United Nations, 2002. [http://www.un.org/esa/sustdev/documents/WSSD_POI_PD/English/POIToc.htm]. Dec. 12, 2006.

United Nations. *Madrid International Plan of Action on Ageing. Report of the Second World Assembly on Ageing. Madrid. 8–12 April 2002.* New York: United Nations, 2002. [http://daccessdds.un.org/doc/UNDOC/GEN/N02/397/51/PDF/N0239751.pdf?OpenElement]. Dec. 12, 2006.

United Nations. *Monterrey Consensus of the International Conference on Financing for Development.* New York: United Nations, 2002. [http://www.un.org/esa/ffd/]. Dec. 12, 2006.

United Nations. *Report of the Secretary-General "Follow-up to the Second World Assembly on Ageing"* (A/58/160). New York: United Nations, 2003.

United Nations. *Report of the Secretary-General "Follow-up to the Second World Assembly on Ageing"* (A/61/167). New York: United Nations, 2006. [http://daccessdds.un.org/doc/UNDOC/GEN/N06/436/37/PDF/N0643637.pdf?OpenElement]. Dec. 12, 2006.

United Nations and International Association of Gerontology and Geriatrics. *Research Agenda on Ageing for the Twenty-First Century.* United Nations and International Association of Gerontology and Geriatrics, 2002. [http://www.un.org/esa/socdev/ageing/ageing/ageraa.htm]. Dec. 5, 2006.

World Health Organization. *The World Health Report 2006: Working Together for Health.* Geneva: World Health Organization, 2006.

CHAPTER

2

POPULATION AGING: A GLOBAL OVERVIEW

MARY BETH WEINBERGER

The world today is in the midst of a profound demographic transformation which includes population growth and population aging. Population growth has been the defining feature of this transformation through the twentieth century . . . Population aging will be the essential characteristic during the twenty-first century.

—Mrs. Brigita Schmögnerová, UNECE Executive Secretary, Address to the Ministerial Conference on Ageing, Berlin, Germany, 2002

In 2006, 11 percent of the world's population—approximately 690 million people—were aged sixty or over. By 2050, that number is expected to be almost three times as large—nearly two billion persons, making up 22 percent of the total population. Additions to the older population are projected to account for half of all population increase between 2006 and 2050. The scale, the pace, and the worldwide extent of population aging are unprecedented in human history.

Population aging is the result of two great human achievements: lower mortality and the improved ability of couples and individuals to choose their number of children, which, combined with declines in desired family size, has resulted in lower fertility. The large declines in mortality and fertility during the second half of the twentieth century will produce rapid aging in most parts of the world during the first half of the twenty-first century and especially between 2005 and 2030.

This chapter provides a global synopsis of these demographic trends as a background to the discussions of health and policy issues in this volume. Following the practice adopted at the 1982 and 2002 United Nations World Assemblies on Ageing, "older persons" are considered to be those aged sixty and over. Except as separately indicated, the data presented in the following sections are drawn from the estimates and medium-fertility variant of the United Nations estimates and projections of population (United Nations Population Division, 2005b).

POPULATION AGING AND GROWTH OF THE OLDER POPULATION

In all regions, and in the large majority of countries, the population is growing older. In the more developed regions, 20 percent of the population is currently aged sixty or over, and this is projected to increase to 27 percent in 2025 and 32 percent by 2050 (see Table 2.1). In the developing world, the proportion averages only 8 percent in 2006, but by 2050 this is projected to rise to 20 percent, the same as in the more developed regions today.

Throughout human history, the number of children in the population has greatly outnumbered that of older persons. In 1950, the world contained over four children aged under fifteen for every person aged sixty or over (see Figure 2.1). Today, in many developed countries, the number of older persons already exceeds the number of children. By 2050, this is likely to be true for the world as a whole.

Population aging also means that the ratio of working-age to older persons will decline sharply, posing challenges to current arrangements for funding retirement and health care. Globally, between 2006 and 2050, the number of persons aged fifteen to sixty-four for each person aged sixty-five or older is projected to decline from nine to four. In the more developed regions, the ratio will decrease from four to two.

And the older population itself is aging (see Figure 2.1). By 2050, the oldest-old—those aged eighty or over—are expected to make up 20 percent of the over-sixty population, up from 13 percent today. The number of the oldest-old is projected to be 4.4 times as large in 2050 as in 2006, and their share of the total world population will increase from 1.4 percent in 2006 to 4.3 per cent in 2050 (and up to 15 percent in Italy and Japan).

TABLE 2.1. **Number of Persons Age Sixty or Over and Their Percentage of the Total Population, World and Major Areas, 1950–2050.**

| | Population Aged 60 Years Or Over | | | | | | | |
| | Number *(millions)* | | | | Percentage of total population | | | |
Region	1950	2006	2025	2050	1950	2006	2025	2050
World	205	688	1,193	1,968	8	11	15	22
More developed	95	248	343	400	11	20	27	32
Less developed	110	440	849	1,568	6	8	13	20
Africa	12	49	85	193	5	5	6	10
Asia	94	375	706	1,231	7	9	15	24
Europe	66	152	198	225	12	21	28	34
Latin America	10	51	101	189	6	9	14	24
Northern America	21	57	94	118	12	17	24	27
Oceania	1	5	8	12	11	14	20	25

Note: More developed regions include Australia/New Zealand, Europe, Japan, and Northern America. Less developed regions include all other areas. Latin America includes the Caribbean.

Source: United Nations Population Division (2005b), estimates and medium-variant projections.

However, countries vary greatly in the timing and speed of the aging process, and there will remain for a long time large differences by region (see Table 2.1) and between countries. In 2050, in some developing countries, including China, older persons are projected to make up 30 percent or more of the total population, while in many African countries that proportion will still be only 5 to 10 percent. Among developed countries, in 2006 the proportion had already reached 26 percent in Italy and 27 percent in Japan. By 2050 those countries, among others, are projected to have over 40 percent of their populations aged sixty or over.

In the United States, the proportion of older persons is currently 17 percent, which is projected to rise to 24 percent by 2025 and 26 percent in 2050—much higher than today,

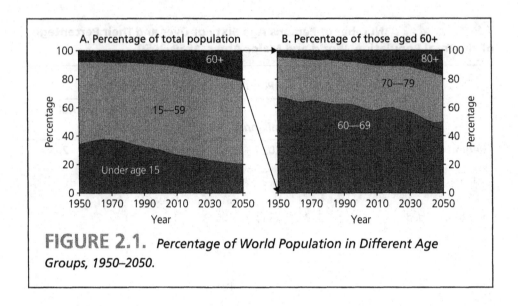

FIGURE 2.1. *Percentage of World Population in Different Age Groups, 1950–2050.*

but lower than in most other developed countries. That difference is mainly because of higher fertility in the United States, which is discussed in the following section.

SPEED OF POPULATION AGING

Rapid changes in age structure are more difficult for societies to accommodate than changes that occur over a longer period. Even though developed countries are further along in the aging process, developing countries will go through the process more quickly and, in many cases, at lower economic levels than the developed countries had achieved when they reached comparable degrees of aging. Developing countries face the prospect of "becoming old before becoming rich."

Figure 2.2 shows, for selected countries, the dates when the population reached, or is expected to reach, the point when 10, 20, and 30 percent of the population is aged sixty or over. Typically, the transition from 10 to 20 percent took longer for countries that reached the 10-percent level at an earlier date. For example, France and Sweden, which reached the 10-percent point before 1900, took 142 years and 89 years, respectively, to reach 20 percent, but that transition required only 28 years in Japan (from 1967 to 1995). Many developing countries—including the demographic giants, China and India—will also make a rapid transition from 10 to 20 percent aged sixty or over. And it will often take substantially less time for the next 10 percent to be added. In Japan, the transition from 20 to 30 percent is expected to take only sixteen years. Many developing countries will also go through that transition very quickly.

The world's older population will increase especially rapidly during the next twenty-five years. Between 1950 and 2005, the number aged sixty or over increased at an average rate of 2.2 percent per year, but that already rapid pace is now speeding up. Between 2010 and 2030, the number of older persons will grow at nearly 3 percent per

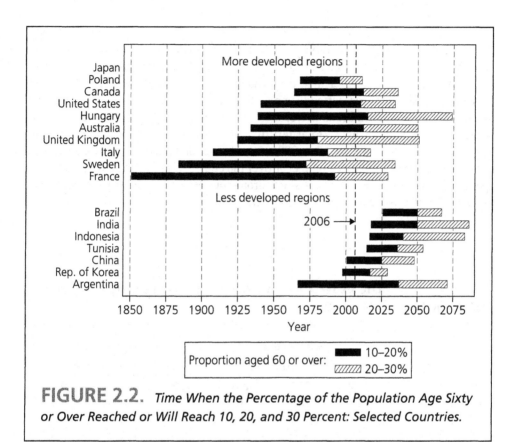

FIGURE 2.2. *Time When the Percentage of the Population Age Sixty or Over Reached or Will Reach 10, 20, and 30 Percent: Selected Countries.*

Source: United Nations (1956, 2004); United Nations Population Division (2005b).

year, doubling the number between 2005 and 2030. After that, the rate of increase will slow, although the older population will still be experiencing substantial growth in 2050 and beyond.

The absolute number of older persons is increasing especially rapidly in the less developed regions, where the number aged sixty or over will grow by over 250 percent between 2006 and 2050, compared with 60 percent in the more developed regions. Currently, about two-thirds of the older population live in the less developed regions, but by 2050, 80 percent will live there.

DEMOGRAPHIC SOURCES OF POPULATION AGING: TRENDS IN MORTALITY AND FERTILITY

Trends in mortality and fertility affect population age structures over a period of generations. The demographic transition during the second half of the twentieth century has set the stage for rapid global population aging during the twenty-first century.

Global life expectancy at birth increased by nineteen years between 1950 and 1955 and 2000 and 2005 (see Table 2.2). As mortality declined, the rate of population growth sped up, and by the late 1960s the global population was growing at slightly over 2 percent per year. After that, even though mortality continued to fall in most countries, fertility declines started to spread throughout the developing world, and the rate of population growth began decreasing. In the less developed regions, the average number of births per woman (total fertility rate or TFR) was halved, falling from 6.0 children in 1965–1970 to 2.9 in 2000–2005. (The total fertility rate is the average number of children a woman would bear over the course of her lifetime if current age-specific fertility rates remained constant throughout her childbearing years; this also assumes that the woman survives to age fifty.)

TABLE 2.2. **Life Expectancy and Birth and Total Fertility Rate, World and Major Areas, 1950–2050.**

Region	Life Expectancy at Birth (years)			Total Fertility Rate (children per woman)		
	1950–1955	2000–2005	2045–2050	1950–1955	2000–2005	2045–2050
World	46.6	65.4	75.1	5.0	2.7	2.0
More developed	66.1	75.6	82.1	2.8	1.6	1.8
Less developed	41.1	63.4	74.0	6.2	2.9	2.1
Africa	38.4	49.1	65.4	6.7	5.0	2.5
Asia	41.4	67.3	77.2	5.9	2.5	1.9
Europe	65.6	73.8	80.6	2.7	1.4	1.8
Latin America	51.4	71.5	79.5	5.9	2.5	1.9
Northern America	68.8	77.6	82.7	3.5	2.0	1.9
Oceania	60.4	74.0	81.2	3.9	2.3	1.9

Source: United Nations Population Division (2005b), estimates and medium-variant projections.

As fertility declined, the world's proportion of children started to fall and the relative proportions of working-age adults and older persons both rose (see Figure 2.1). The proportion of children is projected to continue to fall as fertility levels in the less developed regions continue declining. The proportion in the working ages will also start to decline after 2010 in the more developed regions and after 2030 in the less developed regions. World population is still growing by about seventy-six million persons per year—at an annual growth rate of 1.2 percent during 2000–2005—but the growth rate is expected to drop steadily as fertility falls further in the developing world (see Table 2.2). Global population doubled during the forty-two-year period between 1964 and 2006, but it is not expected to double again.

Fertility in the more developed regions has also declined significantly since the 1960s, in most cases to levels well below the 2.1 children needed for replacement of the population from one generation to the next. As of 2000–2005, the TFR in Europe stood at 1.4 children per woman; it had been below 2.1 since the mid-1970s. In some Eastern and Southern European countries, as well as in Japan (and recently, also in the Republic of Korea and Singapore), the TFR has fallen to 1.1 to 1.3 children per woman. Such low fertility has produced an age structure with a narrow "base" of children (see Figure 2.3). In the more developed regions, only at ages above the late fifties is *any* net

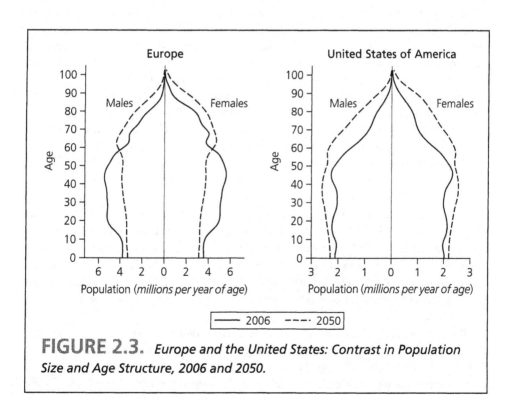

FIGURE 2.3. *Europe and the United States: Contrast in Population Size and Age Structure, 2006 and 2050.*

Source: United Nations Population Division (2005b).

growth projected to occur between 2006 and 2050. Most developed countries are expected to experience declines—in many cases substantial declines—in the working-age population. The United States is an exception to this pattern (see Figure 2.3), primarily because the TFR in the United States has remained near 2.0 children per woman and, to a lesser extent, because of immigration.

Past trends in fertility and mortality account for the especially rapid growth in the older population that will occur during the next twenty-five years. First, many countries experienced a "baby boom" following the Second World War; the baby boom in the United States was among the largest. These baby boomers are now starting to turn sixty. Second, in developing countries during 1950–1970, improved control of infectious disease saved so many young lives that the age structures of most developing countries became younger during the period before their fertility began to decline. The children who were saved from early death during those years will make a large contribution to growth of the older population in coming years. For instance, in some Latin American countries, about half of the projected increase in the number of older persons in the coming decades can be attributed to earlier improvements in mortality that have allowed more people to survive to age sixty (Palloni and others, 2005).

The United Nations projects that global life expectancy will increase by ten years between 2000–2005 and 2045–2050, from sixty-five to seventy-five years (see Table 2.2). The large gap between world regions is expected to narrow, but it will still be substantial in 2050. Japanese women currently have the world's highest life expectancy—eighty-five years during 2000–2005—and it is projected to increase to ninety-two years by 2050. The projected increases cannot be taken for granted, however. The last few decades provide examples of significant mortality setbacks—notably in African countries heavily impacted by HIV/AIDS. In many parts of the former USSR and Eastern Europe, mortality rose substantially between 1975 and the early 1990s, especially for men. Even by 2000–2005, in several European countries, including the Russian Federation, male life expectancy was below the level of the early 1970s.

Success at preventing deaths among infants and children means that increases in life expectancy depend more and more on lowering mortality rates at older ages. In high-mortality populations, a large proportion of deaths occur in the few years after birth; in sub-Saharan Africa today, approximately 40 percent of all deaths still occur at ages under five and only 15 per cent at ages sixty or over. But in the more developed regions during 2000–2005, 80 percent of deaths took place at ages over sixty, and only 1 percent at ages under five. In many developing countries, the distribution of deaths is also shifting to older ages. For instance, in China during 2000–2005, nearly 70 percent of deaths occurred at ages sixty or over and in Latin America and the Caribbean, over 50 percent.

It is only recently that a majority of those born could expect to reach age sixty, and this is still not the case in many developing countries. Given the mortality rates of 2000–2005, 76 percent of the world's newborn girls and 70 percent of boys can expect to reach age sixty (see Table 2.3). In the more developed regions, current rates imply that 91 percent of girls and 81 percent of boys will reach age sixty. But in Africa, less than half can expect to reach age sixty at current mortality rates.

Women have a survival advantage nearly everywhere, and this advantage continues into old age. Given the mortality rates of 2000–2005, women reaching age sixty in the more developed regions can expect to live an additional twenty-three years; for men reaching age sixty, it is nineteen years. In the less developed regions the averages are lower, especially in Africa (seventeen years for women and sixteen years for men).

Over recent decades, there have been significant improvements in mortality within the older population, including the oldest-old. The marked mortality decline at high ages has confounded earlier expectations. During the first part of the twentieth century, while there were major advances in lowering mortality at young ages, the declines in old-age mortality were relatively modest, leading many experts to conclude that a

TABLE 2.3. **Probability of Reaching Age Sixty and Life Expectancy at Age Sixty, Given Mortality in 2000–2005, by Sex, World and Major Areas.**

Region	Percentage reaching age 60		Life expectancy at age 60 (*years*)	
	Men	Women	Men	Women
World	70	76	17	21
More developed	81	91	19	23
Less developed	68	73	17	19
Africa	45	47	16	17
Asia	74	80	17	20
Europe	77	90	18	22
Latin America	74	84	19	22
Northern America	86	91	20	24
Oceania	82	85	20	24

Source: United Nations Population Division (2005b).

natural limit was being approached. Subsequent advances in prevention and treatment of some of the main killers of older adults (particularly cardiovascular disease and stroke) led to large, and still ongoing, mortality declines in countries where death rates were already low (National Institute on Aging, 2006; Rau and others, 2006). The recent declines in old-age mortality have renewed attention not just to the question of how long life can be extended, but also to a range of issues regarding the quality of that longer life.

Projections of future requirements for health services and long-term care are sensitive to assumptions about the trends in disability and health as well as in mortality. Most of the available evidence indicates that the number of years free of severe disability has been increasing along with added years of life, but levels and trends of disability are difficult to compare internationally, and estimates for the future are speculative (Jacobzone, Cambois and Robine, 2000). One review estimated that in developed countries, life expectancy without "moderate" disability represented 50 to 80 percent of life expectancy at age sixty-five (Jacobzone, 2000). Although women who reach older ages can expect to live more disability-free years than men, the proportion of remaining years that are free of disability is lower for older women than for men.

IS POPULATION AGING INEVITABLE?

Because the future course of fertility and mortality cannot be predicted exactly, there is uncertainty regarding the numbers and proportions of older persons projected for the future. Fertility change has been the main force contributing to changing population age structures in the past in both more- and less-developed regions up to the present (United Nations Population Division, 2005a). The implications of different paths of future fertility change can be assessed by comparing the high-, medium-, and low-fertility variants of the United Nations population projections, which are believed to encompass the likely range of fertility change up to 2050. These assumptions make a large difference to the projected size of the world population in 2050, which would range from a shrinking population of 7.7 billion under the low variant to an expanding population of 11.7 billion under the high variant. How much effect would such divergent trends have on population aging?

At the world level, the low variant implies a population in which the proportion of the population aged sixty or over in 2050 would be 26 percent. Under the high variant, the proportion of older persons would be significantly lower—18 percent. However, this would still be a substantial increase from the current 11 percent. So even under the assumption of higher fertility and continued population growth, substantial population aging appears inevitable.

How about the effects of mortality? Once child mortality drops to low levels, further mortality decline contributes to population aging. The effect of the projected mortality improvements on age structure can be assessed by comparing the United Nations medium-variant projections to an alternative that assumes that mortality in each region would remain at the levels of 2000–2005 while fertility and migration followed the assumptions of the medium variant. This comparison shows that, even in the absence of further mortality decline, the proportion aged sixty or over would rise by 2050 to 28 percent in the more developed regions and to 18 percent in the less developed regions. Uncertainties about trends in mortality and health certainly matter for pension and health-care costs, and also for individual well-being, but substantial population aging will occur in any case.

Sustained migration flows can also affect the age structure, as young adults and their children typically predominate among migrants. Today, the more developed regions are net receivers of international migrants from the less developed regions. The United Nations medium-variant projections assume that future migration flows will be similar to those observed recently—that is, a net migration gain for the more developed regions of 2.2 million persons annually during 2010–2050. If there were no migration, an alternative projection shows that the proportion aged sixty or over in 2050 would be 3 percentage points higher than implied by the medium variant. So migration is expected to retard population aging in the more developed regions, but the effect is likely to be modest.

Much of the expected future aging of today's population is already inscribed in the current population age structure. Although future trends in fertility, mortality, and migration will help determine population age distributions at mid-century, there is a powerful momentum built into current age structures by past demographic trends.

CHARACTERISTICS OF THE OLDER POPULATION

Gender

Especially among the oldest old, who are the most likely to need social and financial support, the older population is predominantly female (see Table 2.4). As of 2006, there were 378 million women and 310 million men aged sixty or over, or 1.2 women for each man. The ratio increases from 1.1 women for each man at ages sixty to sixty-nine years to 1.7 for those in their eighties, 2.7 for those in their nineties, and 3.8 women for each man among centenarians. The preponderance of women at older ages is greater in the more developed than in the less developed regions, reflecting the greater gender gap in mortality rates in the former group. The female majority at high ages contrasts with the pattern at younger ages, where males predominate. This is because more boys are born than girls—on average 105 boys for every 100 girls. But because mortality rates are higher for males, women predominate at the older ages.

Marital Status

At older ages, men are much more likely than women to be married. Four out of five older men, but less than half of older women, are currently married (see Table 2.4).

TABLE 2.4. **Ratio of Women to Men at Older Ages and Percentages of Older Men and Women Currently Married, Living Alone and in the Labor Force, for the World and Major Areas.**

| | Ratio of women to men at ages: | | Among people aged 60 or over, percentage: | | | | | |
Region	60+	80+	Currently married M	F	Live alone M	F	In the labor force M	F
World	1.2	1.8	80	48	8	19	42	17
More developed	1.4	2.2	79	48	13	32	22	12
Less developed	1.1	1.5	81	47	5	9	51	20
Africa	1.2	1.5	85	39	6	11	65	32
Asia	1.1	1.6	81	50	5	9	48	18
Europe	1.5	2.3	80	47	13	35	15	7
Latin America	1.2	1.5	75	42	7	10	47	19
Northern America	1.3	1.9	75	48	15	34	30	19
Oceania	1.2	1.7	76	50	16	34	27	14

Note: M = males, F = females.

Sources: United Nations (2006); International Labour Office (2006).

The percentages are nearly the same in different world regions. Particularly among women, most of those without a spouse have been widowed, although the "unmarried" group also includes those who never married and those whose union ended in divorce or separation. The large gender difference in marital status comes about mainly because women are likely to outlive their spouses, because of higher female life expectancy, and because wives, on average, are younger than their husbands. Older women are also less likely than older men to remarry following divorce or widowhood.

Living Arrangements

Although gains in life expectancy imply a greater potential for three- and four-generation households, the numbers and proportions of older persons living with their adult children have been decreasing and the number of those living alone has risen, especially in developed countries (United Nations, 2005). Three-fourths of older persons in developing countries live with children, grandchildren, or both, but only about one-fourth of those in the more developed regions do so.

One-quarter of older persons in more developed regions are estimated to live alone, but only 7 percent of those in developing countries. Even though many of those living alone are in frequent contact with relatives and friends and often have children living nearby, surveys in both developed and developing countries show that those living alone are more likely than others to need outside assistance and less likely to receive adequate help in the case of illness or disability. They also are at greater risk of social isolation and, even in countries with well-developed social security systems, those who live alone—especially older women—are disproportionately likely to be poor. In some developed countries, the proportion living alone is continuing to rise, while in others, including the United States, the proportion living alone has leveled off since 1990. The reasons include longer life, which tends to delay widowhood; declines in the proportion that never married; and an upward trend in the age at which children leave home.

In most countries, older women are more likely than older men to live alone, and in the more developed regions the gender difference is large: in those regions, on average, 32 percent of older women and 14 percent of older men live alone (see Table 2.4). The greater likelihood of women being widowed is the reason for their higher levels of solitary living. Older women are also more likely than older men to live in nursing homes and other institutional settings—again, women's greater likelihood of being widowed accounts for this difference (United Nations, 2005).

Especially in developing countries, large numbers of older persons, particularly women, live in "skipped-generation" households consisting of grandparents and grandchildren. These households also tend to be poor. Over 10 percent of older women live in skipped-generation households in most sub-Saharan African and in some Latin American and Caribbean countries. The prevalence of such households has increased recently in many of the countries heavily affected by HIV and AIDS (United Nations, 2005).

Labor Force Participation and Retirement

At the global level in 2006, 42 percent of older men were economically active, compared with 17 percent of older women (see Table 2.4). The proportions are higher in less developed than in more developed countries, especially for men, even though the official retirement age tends to be lower in developing countries (United Nations, 2006). The official retirement age matters only for those who are covered by social security and pension programs. It is estimated that in sub-Saharan Africa and South Asia only about 10 percent of the population is covered by a social security program (Sigg, 2005).

In many European countries where early retirement became common during the 1970s and 1980s, that trend began to reverse after 1990. In most industrialized countries, average retirement age is below the official age for receiving a full old-age pension. At least part of the explanation lies in eligibility and tax rules that, in some countries, have had the effect of encouraging early retirement (Wise and Gruber, 1999). Effective retirement age for men remains below sixty-five years in most industrialized countries and in a few cases is below age sixty, according to recent data (for 2004; Organization for Economic Cooperation and Development, 2006). Japan and the Republic of Korea are exceptions, with the average retirement age around seventy years. Labor-force participation of women has generally been increasing. At the same time, in developed countries women's effective age at retirement remains about two years below that for men (Organization for Economic Cooperation and Development, 2006). In both developed and developing countries, the official retirement age is often lower for women than men, although many countries have recently moved to lessen or eliminate gender differences in entitlements.

As life expectancy has risen, the average time that people can expect to spend in retirement has also increased. For countries belonging to the Organization for Economic Cooperation and Development, men's expected duration of retirement was under eleven years in 1980 but was nearly eighteen years in 2004. For women, the average duration has increased from 14 years to 22.5 years (Organization for Economic Cooperation and Development, 2006).

Education and Literacy

Education is strongly associated with better health and higher income. Because those who will turn sixty in the future have received more schooling than today's older population, education levels of the older population will rise. For instance, in 2000 an estimated 56 percent of persons age sixty or over were illiterate in developing countries, but this was down from 75 percent in 1980, and the proportion was expected to decline to 43 percent by 2010 (United Nations, 2001). In most developed countries, levels of illiteracy are already low, and the proportion of older persons with secondary and higher levels of schooling will rise substantially in coming years. Older women will remain at a significant educational disadvantage in most countries for at least the next several decades, although the size of the gender gap will diminish.

CONCLUSIONS

The mortality and fertility transitions during the second half of the twentieth century have set the stage for rapid global population aging during the twenty-first century. Though there is a range of uncertainty about future trends, substantial population aging seems inevitable.

The scope and pace of population aging today are unprecedented. Developed countries already have older populations than ever before. By mid-century, persons over sixty are expected to make up about one-third of their population on average and, in some cases, over 40 percent. Developing countries are going through the transition later but more quickly, and most will have lower levels of economic development than did the developed countries at a similar demographic stage. Between 2005 and 2030, both developed and developing countries will experience especially rapid growth in the numbers and proportions of older people.

Older populations of the future will be better educated and are likely to spend more years in good health. But there are many unknowns regarding the determinants of good health and the policies to promote it. In many developing countries, serious gaps remain in even basic information about the health status of older adults.

Rapid population aging will require reassessment of many established economic, political, and social policies, including policies affecting labor-force participation at all adult ages, the levels and nature of retirement and health-care benefits, and the mechanisms to finance those benefits. In developing countries, the difficulty of this task is compounded by low population coverage of pension and social security programs and by the limited reach of modern health care services. These countries also face the prospect of coping with the health and support needs of a rapidly increasing older population while child and maternal mortality are still high and while low levels of economic development severely limit the resources that can be devoted to solving these problems.

In 2002, representatives of 156 countries convened in Madrid, Spain, for the Second World Assembly on Ageing. The decision to hold this event was significant, since it signaled a recognition that aging is not just a concern of the rich countries, but has profound implications for social and economic development all over the world. As described in Chapter One, the Assembly adopted the Madrid International Plan of Action on Ageing, which sets out goals and actions for three priority directions: older persons and development; advancing health and well-being into old age; and ensuring enabling and supportive environments. In reality, the theme of health cuts across the three priority areas, since good health enables people to remain independent, productive, and active in family, community, and national life. So advancing health and well-being into old age is a priority not only for enhancing individual welfare, but also for enabling older persons to contribute to social and economic development of all societies during the twenty-first century.

REFERENCES

International Labour Office (ILO) database on labor statistics—LABORSTA. [http://laborsta.ilo.org]. Nov. 12, 2006.

Jacobzone, S. "Health and Aging: International Perspectives on Long Term Care." ISUMA, 2000, *1*(2). [http://www.isuma.net/v01n02/jacobzone/jacobzone_e.shtml]. Nov. 12, 2006.

Jacobzone, S., Cambois, E., and Robine, J. M. "Is the Health of Older Persons in OECD Countries Improving Fast Enough to Compensate for Population Ageing?" *OECD Economic Studies*, 2000, *30*.

National Institute on Aging, "The Future of Human Life Expectancy: Have We Reached the Ceiling or Is the Sky the Limit?" *Research Highlights in the Demography and Economics of Aging*, March 2006 (8).

Organization for Economic Cooperation and Development. *Live Longer, Work Longer*. Paris: Organization for Economic Cooperation and Development (OECD) 2006.

Palloni, A., and others. "Ageing in Latin America and the Caribbean: Implications of Past Mortality." Paper presented at the United Nations Expert Group Meeting on Social and Economic Implications of Changing Population Age Structures, Mexico City, Mexico, Aug. 31–Sept. 2, 2005.

Rau, R., and others. "10 Years After Kannisto: Further Evidence for Mortality Decline at Advanced Ages in Developed Countries." MPIDR working paper. Rostock, Germany: Max Planck Institute for Demographic Research, 2006.

Sigg, R. "A Global Overview on Social Security in the Age of Longevity." Paper presented at the United Nations Expert Group Meeting on Social and Economic Implications of Changing Population Age Structures, Mexico City, Mexico, Aug. 31–Sept. 2, 2005.

United Nations. *The Aging of Populations and Its Economic and Social Implications*. New York: United Nations, 1956.

United Nations. *World Population Ageing: 1950–2050*. New York: United Nations, 2001.

United Nations. *World Population to 2300*. New York: United Nations, 2004, additional tabulations.

United Nations. *Living Arrangements of Older Persons Around the World*. New York: United Nations, 2005.

United Nations. *Population Ageing 2006*. Wall chart. New York: United Nations, 2006.

United Nations Population Division. "The Diversity of Changing Population Age Structures in the World." Paper presented at the United Nations Expert Group Meeting on Social and Economic Implications of Changing Population Age Structures, Mexico City, Mexico, Aug. 31–Sept. 2, 2005a.

United Nations Population Division. *World Population Prospects: The 2004 Revision*. CD-ROM Edition— Extended Dataset. New York: United Nations, 2005b. Wise, D. A., and Gruber, J. (eds.). *Social Security and Retirement Around the World*. Chicago and Paris: University of Chicago Press, 1999.

CHAPTER

3

THE WORLD HEALTH ORGANIZATION AND GLOBAL AGING

ALEX KALACHE

In 1995, when the World Health Organization (WHO) changed the name of its Health of the Elderly program to Ageing and Health, it signaled an important change in orientation. Rather than compartmentalizing older people, the new name embraced a life-course perspective: we are all aging, and the best way to ensure good health for future cohorts of older people is by preventing disease and promoting health throughout the life course. Conversely, the health of those now in older age can be fully understood only if the life events they have gone through are taken into consideration.

The main aim of the Ageing and Health program has been to develop policies that ensure "the attainment of the best possible quality of life for as long as possible, for the largest possible number of people." To achieve this, WHO is required to advance the knowledge base of gerontology and geriatric medicine through research and training efforts. There must be emphasis on fostering interdisciplinary and intersectoral initiatives, particularly those directed at developing countries faced with unprecedented rapid rates of population aging in a context of prevailing poverty and unsolved infrastructure problems. The program also highlights the importance of these principles:

- Adopting community-based approaches by emphasizing the community as a key setting for interventions

- Respecting cultural contexts and influences

- Recognizing the importance of gender differences

- Strengthening intergenerational solidarity

- Respecting and understanding ethical issues related to health and well-being in old age

The International Year of Older Persons (1999) was a landmark in the evolution of WHO's work on aging and health. That year, the World Health Day theme was "active aging makes the difference," and the Global Movement for Active Ageing was launched by the WHO director-general, who stated on that occasion, "Maintaining health and quality of life across the lifespan will do much towards building fulfilled lives, a harmonious intergenerational community, and a dynamic economy. WHO is committed to promoting active aging as an indispensable component of all development programs." In 2000, the name of the WHO program was changed again to Ageing and Life Course (ALC) to further highlight the importance of the life-course perspective. Since then the program has maintained the multiple focus of the previous program and the emphasis on developing activities with multiple partners from all sectors and several disciplines. Moreover, the active aging concept has been further refined and translated into all the program activities, including research and training, information dissemination, advocacy, and policy development.

In addition to the Ageing and Life Course program at WHO headquarters, each of the six WHO regional offices has its own Regional Adviser on Ageing to address specific issues from a regional perspective.

With the launch of the Madrid International Plan of Action and Ageing, the 2002 World Assembly on Ageing marked a turning point in addressing the challenges and celebrating the triumphs of an aging world. For its effective implementation, cross-national, regional, and global sharing of research and policy options is critical. Increasingly, member states, nongovernmental organizations (NGOs), academic institutions, and the private sector are called on to develop age-sensitive solutions to the challenges of an aging world. They need to consider the consequences of the epidemiological transition, rapid changes in the health sector, globalization, urbanization, changing family patterns, and environmental degradation, as well as persistent inequalities and poverty, particularly in developing countries, where the majority of older persons live already.

The World Health Organization maintains that to advance the movement for active aging, all stakeholders need to clarify and popularize the term *active aging* through dialogue, discussion, and debate in the political arena, the education sector, public forums, and media such as radio and television programming.

To facilitate this process, in 2002 WHO launched the Active Ageing Policy Framework, a framework for action for policymakers. Together with the Madrid International Plan of Action on Ageing, this framework provides a roadmap for designing multisectoral active aging policies that enhance health and participation among aging populations while ensuring that older people have adequate security, protection, and care when they require assistance.

The World Health Organization recognizes that public health involves a wide range of actions to improve the health of the population and that health goes beyond the provision of basic health services. Therefore, it is committed to work in cooperation with other international agencies and with the United Nations to encourage the implementation of active aging policies at global, regional, and national levels. Because of the specialist nature of its work, WHO is committed to provide technical advice and play a catalytic role for health development. But this can be done only as a joint effort. Together, we must provide the evidence and demonstrate the effectiveness of the various proposed courses of action. Ultimately, however, it will be up to nations and local communities to develop culturally sensitive, gender-specific, realistic goals and targets, and to implement policies and programs tailored to their societies' unique circumstances.

This chapter reviews the WHO approach to active aging, discusses its underlying principles and approaches, and describes WHO's main activities in the area of aging and health.

THE WHO PERSPECTIVE ON ACTIVE AGING

Population aging raises many fundamental questions for policymakers: How can they help people remain independent and active as they age? How can they strengthen health promotion and prevention policies, especially those directed to older people? As people are living longer, how can the quality of life in old age be improved? Will large numbers of older people bankrupt the health care and social security systems? What is the best way to balance the role of the family and the state when it comes to caring for people who need assistance as they grow older? How can they best acknowledge and support the major role that people play as they age in caring for others?

The WHO Active Ageing Policy Framework addresses these questions and other concerns about population aging (the full version can be found at http://whqlibdoc. who.int/hq/2002/WHO_NMH_NPH_02.8.pdf). The framework targets government decision makers at all levels, the nongovernmental sector, and the private sector; all are responsible for the formulation of policies and programs on aging. It approaches health from a broad perspective and acknowledges that health can be improved and sustained only through the participation of multiple sectors. It suggests that health providers and professionals must take a lead if we are to achieve the goal of healthy older persons continuing to be a resource to their families, communities, and economies, as stated in the WHO Brasilia Declaration on Ageing and Heath in 1996.

The World Health Organization's underlying assumption is that in all countries, and in developing countries in particular, measures to help older people remain healthy and active are a necessity, not a luxury. Population aging is first and foremost a success story for public health policies and social and economic development. Population aging is one of humanity's greatest triumphs—and one of our greatest challenges. Throughout the twenty-first century, global aging will put increased economic and social demands on all countries. At the same time, older people are a precious, often ignored resource, making an important contribution to the fabric of our societies.

The World Health Organization argues that countries can afford the aging of their populations if governments, international organizations, and civil society enact "active aging" policies and programs that enhance the health, participation, and security of older citizens.

The policies and programs should be based on the rights, needs, preferences, and capacities of older people. They also must embrace a life-course perspective that recognizes the important influence of earlier life experiences on the way individuals age.

A LIFE-COURSE APPROACH

A life-course perspective on aging recognizes that older people are not one homogeneous group and that individual diversity tends to increase with age. Interventions that create supportive environments and foster healthy choices are important at all stages of life.

Aging is a lifelong process that begins before we are born and continues throughout life. The functional capacity of our biological systems (for example, muscular strength, cardiovascular performance, respiratory capacity, and so on) increases during the first years of life, reaches its peak in early adulthood, and naturally declines thereafter. The scope of decline is largely determined by external factors throughout the life course. The natural decline in cardiac or respiratory function, for example, can be accelerated by factors such as smoking and air pollution, leaving an individual with lower functional capacity than would normally be expected at a particular age. Health in older age is, for the most part, a reflection of the living circumstances and actions of an individual during the whole life span, as illustrated in Figure 3.1.

These facts lead to the conclusion that individuals can influence how they age by practicing healthier lifestyles and adapting to age-associated changes. However, some life-course factors may not be modifiable at the individual level. For instance, an individual may have little or no control over economic disadvantages and environmental threats that directly affect the aging process and often predispose to disease in later life.

Growing evidence supports critical periods of growth and development—in utero, early infancy, and childhood—when environmental insults may have lasting effects on disease risk in later life. For example, evidence suggests that poor growth in utero leads to a variety of chronic disorders such as cardiovascular disease, non-insulin-dependent diabetes, and hypertension. Exposure in later life may still influence disease risk in structures and a variety of metabolic systems.

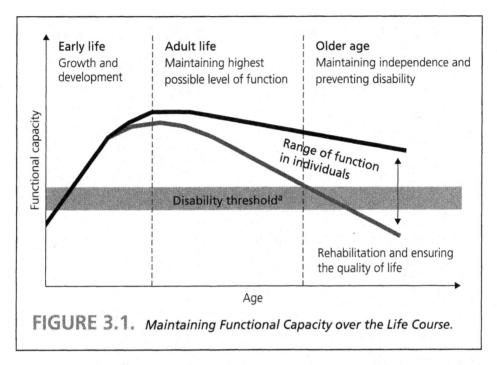

FIGURE 3.1. *Maintaining Functional Capacity over the Life Course.*

aChanges in the environment can lower the disability threshold, thus decreasing the number of disabled people in a given community.

Source: Kalache and Kickbusch, 1997.

A life-course perspective calls on policymakers and civil society to invest in the various phases of life, especially during key transition points when risks to well-being and windows of opportunity are greatest. These include critical periods for both biological and social development, such as in utero, the first six years of life, adolescence, transition from school to the workforce, mid-adulthood, the onset of chronic illnesses, and widowhood. Policies that reduce inequalities protect individuals at these critical times.

THE IMPORTANCE OF NONCOMMUNICABLE DISEASE

As individuals age, noncommunicable diseases (NCDs) become the leading causes of morbidity, disability, and mortality in all regions of the world, including in developing countries. NCDs, which are essentially diseases of later life, are costly to individuals, families, and the public purse. But to a great extent NCDs are preventable or can be postponed. Failing to prevent or manage the growth of NCDs appropriately will result in enormous human and social costs that will absorb a disproportionate amount of resources, which could have been used to address the health problems of other age groups.

MAJOR CHRONIC CONDITIONS AFFECTING OLDER PEOPLE WORLDWIDE

- Cardiovascular diseases (such as coronary heart disease)
- Hypertension
- Stroke
- Diabetes
- Cancer
- Chronic obstructive pulmonary disease
- Musculoskeletal conditions (such as arthritis and osteoporosis)
- Mental health conditions (mostly dementia and depression)
- Blindness and visual impairment

Note: The causes of disability in older age are similar for women and men, although women are more likely to report musculoskeletal problems.

Source: World Health Organization, 1998.

An agenda on health in older age is therefore also an agenda on noncommunicable disease, as indicated in the box.

In the early years of life, communicable disease, maternal and perinatal conditions, and nutritional deficiencies are the major causes of death and disease. In later childhood, adolescence, and young adulthood, injuries and noncommunicable conditions begin to assume a much greater role. By midlife (around age forty-five) and in the later years, NCDs are responsible for the vast majority of deaths and diseases. Research is increasingly showing that the origins of risk for chronic conditions, such as diabetes and heart disease, lie in early childhood or even earlier. This risk is subsequently shaped and modified by other factors, such as socioeconomic status and experiences across the whole life span. The risk of developing NCDs continues to increase as an individual ages. Risk factors for NCDs—such as tobacco use, lack of physical activity, inadequate diet, and other established adult risk factors—are largely responsible for putting individuals at greater risk of developing NCDs at older ages, rather than old age as such (see Figure 3.2). Thus it is important to address the risks of noncommunicable disease from early life to later life—throughout the life course. Comparing two individuals in older age may show that whereas one has accumulated low risk for NCD, the other has a several-fold higher risk for the same conditions.

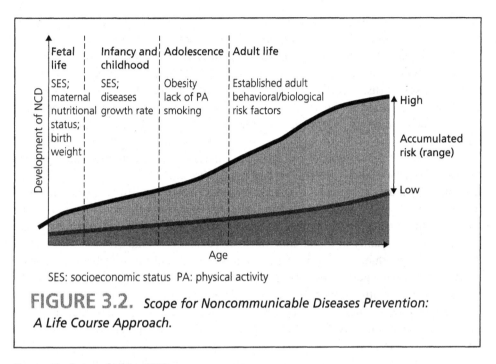

FIGURE 3.2. *Scope for Noncommunicable Diseases Prevention: A Life Course Approach.*

Source: Aboderin and others, 2002.

THE "ACTIVE AGING" CONCEPT AND APPROACHES

Taking into consideration the life-course perspective, the World Health Organization developed its "active aging" concept, defined as "the process of optimizing opportunities for health, participation, and security in order to enhance quality of life as people age." (World Health Organization, 2002a).

Active aging applies to both individuals and population groups. It allows people to realize their potential for physical, social, and mental well-being throughout the life course and to participate in society according to their needs, desires, and capacities, while providing them with adequate protection, security, and care when they require assistance.

The term *active* refers to continuing participation in social, economic, cultural, spiritual, and civic affairs, not just the ability to be physically active or to participate in the labor force. Older people who retire from work and those who are ill or live with disabilities can remain active contributors to their families, peers, communities, and nations. The goal of active aging is to extend healthy life expectancy and quality of life for all people as they age, including those who are frail, disabled, and in need of care.

The term *health* refers to physical, mental, and social well-being, as expressed in the WHO definition of health. Thus, in the active aging framework, policies and programs that promote mental health and social connections are as important as those that improve physical health status.

Maintaining autonomy and independence as one grows older is a key goal for both individuals and policymakers. Although in colloquial language those two terms are often interchangeable, it is important to differentiate them. *Autonomy* is the perceived ability to control, cope with and make personal decisions about how one lives on a day-to-day basis, according to one's own rules and preferences. *Independence* is commonly understood as the ability to perform functions related to daily living; that is, the capacity of living independently in the community with no or little help from others.

The WHO approach to active aging also emphasizes that aging takes place in the context of others—friends, work associates, neighbors, and family members. This is why interdependence as well as intergenerational solidarity (two-way giving and receiving between individuals as well as older and younger generations) are important tenets of active aging. Yesterday's child is today's adult and tomorrow's grandmother or grandfather. The quality of life an individual will enjoy as an older person depends on the risks and opportunities experienced throughout the life course, as well as the manner in which succeeding generations provide mutual aid and support when needed.

The World Health Organization adopted the term *active aging* in the late 1990s. It is meant to convey a more inclusive message than *healthy aging* and to recognize the factors besides health care that affect how individuals and populations age (Kalache and Kickbusch, 1997).

The active aging approach is based on the recognition of the human rights of older people and the United Nations principles of independence, participation, dignity, care, and self-fulfillment. It shifts strategic planning away from a needs-based approach (which assumes that older people are passive targets) to a rights-based approach that recognizes the rights of people to equality of opportunity and treatment in all aspects of life as they grow older. It supports their responsibility to exercise their participation in the political processes and other aspects of community life.

A DETERMINANT OF THE HEALTHY, ACTIVE-AGING APPROACH

There is now clear evidence that health care and biology are just two of the factors influencing health. The social, political, cultural, and physical conditions under which people live and grow older are equally important influences.

Active aging depends on a variety of determinants that surround individuals, families, and actions. These factors directly or indirectly affect well-being, the onset and progression of disease, and how people cope with illness and disability. The determinants of active aging are interconnected in many ways, and the interplay among them is important. For example, individuals who are poor (economic determinant) are more likely to be exposed to inadequate housing (physical environment) and societal violence (social determinants) and to not eat nutritious foods (behavioral determinants).

Figure 3.3 shows the major determinants of active aging. Gender and culture are cross-cutting factors that affect all of the others. For example, gender- and culture-related customs mean that men and women differ significantly when it comes to risk taking and health care–seeking behaviors. Culturally driven expectations affect how

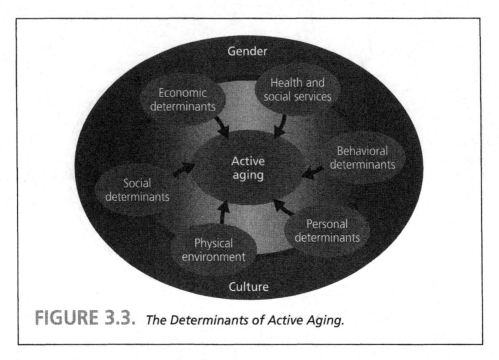

FIGURE 3.3. *The Determinants of Active Aging.*

Source: World Health Organization, 2002.

women experience menopause in different parts of the world. The gendered nature of caregiving and employment means that women are disadvantaged in the economic determinants of active aging. Conversely, in virtually all societies men, beginning early in childhood, are indoctrinated not to expose weakness—the "boys do not cry" message. Later in life, this often translates to a culturally induced behavior of avoiding medical care until a condition is firmly established, impeding either its prevention in the first place or early effective management subsequently.

THREE PILLARS FOR ACTION

The World Health Organization's active aging framework calls on policymakers, services providers, and nongovernmental organizations and civil society to take action in three areas or "pillars": participation, health, and security. The policy framework for active aging is guided by the United Nations Principles for Older People—independence, participation, care, self-fulfillment, and dignity. Decisions are based on an understanding of how the social, physical, personal, and economic determinants of active aging influence the way that individuals and populations age. The framework aims to reduce inequities in health by understanding the gendered nature of the life course. The World Health Organization's main activities on aging are described in the next section.

This chapter follows the rationale provided by the active aging pillars as shown in Figure 3.4.

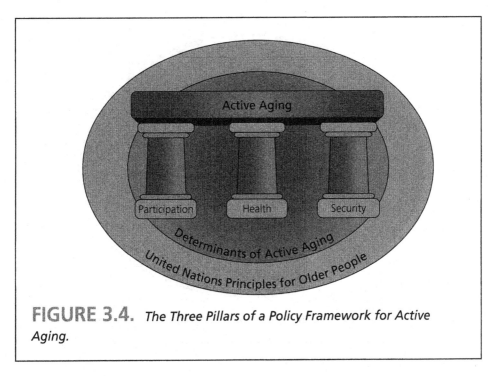

FIGURE 3.4. *The Three Pillars of a Policy Framework for Active Aging.*

Source: World Health Organization, 2002.

ACTIVE AGING POLICIES AND PROGRAMS

An active aging approach to policy and program development has the potential to address many of the challenges of both individuals and population aging. When health, labor market, employment, education, and social policies support active aging, there will potentially be

■ Fewer premature deaths in the highly productive states of life

■ Fewer disabilities associated with chronic diseases in older age

■ More people enjoying a positive quality of life as they grow older

■ More people participating actively as they age in the social, cultural, economic and political aspects of society, in paid and unpaid roles and in domestic, family, and community life

■ Lower costs related to medical treatment and care services

Active aging policies and programs recognize the need to encourage and balance personal responsibility (self-care), age-friendly environments, and intergenerational solidarity. Individuals and families need to plan and prepare for older age and make

personal efforts to adopt positive personal health practices at all states of life. At the same time, a supportive environment is required to make the healthy choices the easy choices.

There are good economic reasons for enacting policies and programs that promote active aging: increased participation and reduced costs for care. People who remain healthy as they age face fewer impediments to continued work. The current trend toward early retirement in industrialized countries is largely the result of public policies that have encouraged early withdrawal from the labor force. As populations age, there will be increasing pressures for such policies to change, particularly if more and more individuals reach old age in good health—that is, "fit for work." This will help to offset the rising costs of pensions and income security schemes as well as medical and social care costs.

Regarding rising public expenditures for medical care, available data increasingly indicate that old age itself is not associated with increased medical spending. Rather, it is disability and poor health—often associated with old age—that are costly. As people age in better health, medical spending may not increase as rapidly.

Policymakers need to look at the full picture and consider the savings achieved by declines in disability rates. In the United States, for example, such declines might lower medical spending by about 20 percent over the next fifty years (Cutler, 2001). Applied to the period between 1982 and 1994, in the United States, the potential savings in nursing home costs alone were estimated to exceed $17 billion (Singer and Manton, 1998). Besides, if increased numbers of healthy older people were to extend their participation in the work force (through either full- or part-time employment), their contribution to public revenues would also increase. Finally, it is often less costly to prevent disease than to treat it. For example, it has been estimated that a $1.00 investment in measures to encourage moderate physical activity leads to a saving of $3.20 in medical costs (U.S. Centers for Disease Control, 1999).

WHO PROJECTS AND ACTIVITIES ON ACTIVE AGING

WHO activities on aging reflect the policy framework described in this chapter, following the rationale provided by the pillars depicted in Figure 3.4. There is inevitably an overlapping, as most of the projects, although mainly concerned with one of the three pillars, also address the others. We now describe one example for each of the pillars in some detail, followed by summaries of other projects.

First Active Aging Pillar: Health; Age-Friendly Primary Health Care Centers

Rationale: Strengthening PHC capacity to deal with older persons' needs is the critical action to be taken in developing and developed countries alike if the greatest possible number of older persons are to remain living in their communities, with their families, enjoying the highest possible level of quality of life for as long as possible.

Aim: To sensitize and educate PHC providers about the specific needs of their older clients.

Pillars: Comprehensive and integrated care, continuum of care, the physical and social environment, administrative procedures, and participatory research with users and providers.

Countries: Australia, Brazil, Canada, Costa Rica, Iran, Jamaica, Singapore, Spain, and Turkey.

Status by end of 2006: Piloting of toolkit focused on core competencies (clinical and health promotion), physical environment, and administrative procedures.

Main outcome: A toolkit to make PHC services more accessible and responsive to older people's needs; completion April 2007.

Second Active Aging Pillar: Participation; Age-Friendly Cities

Rationale: The WHO Active Ageing Policy Framework emphasizes that the determinants of active aging are broad and societal in nature. This implies multisectoral initiatives that will ultimately promote healthy aging and empower older people through the process.

Aim: In an age-friendly community, policies, services, and structures related to the physical and social environment are designed to support and enable older people to age actively—that is, to live in security, enjoy good health, and continue to participate fully in society.

Pillars: Community participation; participatory research; listening to older people's voices; involvement of civil society, academic, private, as well as the government sector; results to be shared and discussed with community leaders, experts, and decision makers; identification and exchange of models of good practice; empowerment tool: older persons to be the monitors of the project and interventions derived from it.

Countries: Argentina, Australia, Brazil, Canada, China, Costa Rica, France, India, Ireland, Jamaica, Kenya, Japan, Lebanon, Mexico, Pakistan, Russia, Spain, Switzerland, Turkey, United Kingdom, and the United States.

Status by end of 2006: Common protocol developed; field work being implemented.

Main outcomes: Age-friendly cities guidelines—possibly an index; global network of cities sharing the same principles.

Third Active Aging Pillar: Security; Integrated Health Systems Response to Rapid Population Aging in Developing Countries (INTRA)

Rationale: Older persons depend on health care systems that can adequately address their needs. This requires a more holistic and integrated approach to health care. The epidemiology has shifted from acute to chronic. Thus, the prevailing acute-care model also must shift toward chronic care.

Aim: To produce a knowledge base that will assist policymakers in formulating integrated health and social systems policies through assessing PHC preparedness and responsiveness to deal with aging issues; strengthening the delivery of age-appropriate health and social services; developing policies and strategies that enhance PHC responsiveness; and strengthening continuum of care.

Pillars: Each INTRA phase builds on the strengths and lessons of the preceding one. Key pillars of INTRA are pairing of countries; south-to-south exchanges, learning from each other; cross-fertilization of ideas and approaches; creation and involvement of multisectoral and interdisciplinary national teams; focus on a combination of quantitative and qualitative methods; bottom-up approach; evidence-based policy development; and active involvement of WHO regional and country offices.

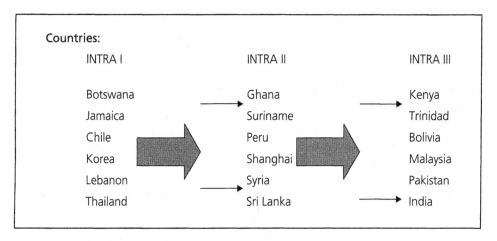

Status by end of 2006: Completion of research phase. Preparing for evidence-based policy development.

Main outcomes: Development of evidence-based national, regional, and global policies that promote and invest in integrated health care services that are cohesive, coherent, and continual in and across settings; encompassing community, social, and family care in the scope of the respective national health care systems.

The three example projects just described are intercomplementary and have adopted a bottom-up approach. In particular, they are centered on older persons who are a main source of information and ideas and intrinsic evaluators and monitors of the projects' outcomes, thus ensuring an empowerment component—older people as active players rather than passive recipients.

The gender and life-course perspectives are built into all projects. Capacity building (national policies, training, research) is an essential component of the projects. They address many Madrid Plan objectives and ultimately will strengthen the Primary Health Care sector and community capacity to deal with population aging as it is in the community and in families, and as the vast majority of the population want to live as they grow older.

OTHER CURRENT MAIN PROJECTS

Other WHO projects on aging and health are described in this section; they are equally linked to the three active aging pillars, as indicated in parentheses.

Women, Aging, and Health from a Gender Perspective (Participation and Health)

In cooperation with the United Nations Population Fund (UNFPA), the World Health Organization has produced a substantial report on women, aging and health from a gender perspective (World Health Organization, 2007). It is particularly aimed at policymakers and draws on the latest evidence to summarize key health issues for aging women, discusses the impact of gender on all other determinants of active aging, raises awareness of the substantial contribution made by older women to their families and communities, and suggests policies to be considered from a multisectoral perspective. The process of producing the report involved an advisory committee of experts from twelve countries representing all regions.

Preventing Falls in Older Age, with a Focus on Developing Countries (Health)

This project focuses on a major risk factor for loss of independence that leads to huge costs, both personal and economic. There is particular focus on successful and feasible initiatives in developing countries and policy development.

Prevention of Elder Abuse at the Community Level (Security)

The World Health Organization has been in the forefront of initiatives calling attention to elder abuse as a common and neglected issue. In 2002, the report *Missing Voices*— the first multicentric international study on this subject—was released, calling attention to the importance of the Primary Health Care setting as critical if elder abuse is to be prevented and cases identified and properly managed (World Health Organization, 2002b). A tool for the detection of suspicion of elder abuse has been qualitatively studied in association with academic and NGO partners from Switzerland, Australia, Costa Rica, Brazil, Spain, Canada, Singapore, Germany, and Kenya. The next phase aims at piloting the resulting reviewed tool.

Older People in Emergency Situations (Security)

Natural disasters are on the increase and the plight of older persons affected by them is badly neglected. For instance, the majority of the victims of Hurricane Katrina in 2005 were individuals aged sixty-five and over. The 2003 heat wave in Europe caused many thousands of deaths that could, by and large, have been avoided through basic surveillance and low-cost interventions. However, available evidence indicates that older persons are resilient, play a critical role in emergency situations, and are precious resources to their communities affected by crises. The World Health Organization is working in partnership with the Public Health Agency of Canada in raising awareness and developing policies focused on older persons in such emergencies. Case studies from ten countries provide the foundation for recommendations for good practice.

Minimum Curriculum: Global Guidelines for Training Health Professionals (Health)

In 2002, the World Health Organization conducted a survey on the teaching of geriatric medicine in medical schools in seventy-two countries around the world in collaboration with the International Federation of Medical Students Associations (IFMSA). This led to a survey on attitudes of medical students toward old age in thirty-four countries, also in collaboration with IFMSA. The World Health Organization is now collaborating with the International Association of Gerontology and Geriatrics (IAGG) as well as academic centers from various countries to establish geriatric medicine teaching guidelines. Finally, in collaboration with the Ministry of Education of Brazil, an interdisciplinary working party was set up in April 2006 to establish a minimum curriculum covering multiple aging issues for all undergraduate health professionals courses. This minimum curriculum will be jointly circulated by the World Health Organization and IAGG worldwide for a critical appraisal and eventually offered for adaptation and adoption worldwide.

Immunization in Older Age (Health)

The World Health Organization is collaborating with the International Council of Nurses to gather information about the cost-effectiveness of immunization in older age (particularly flu and pneumococcal vaccines), focusing on developing countries. Although a substantial amount of data is available from different countries, to date there has been no effort to provide an international overview to support the development of evidence-based recommendations for policy.

Promoting Healthy Aging (Health)

The World Health Organization is one of thirteen partners participating in a pan-European project aimed at promoting healthy aging through the development of an integrated and holistic approach to health in later life. Begun in fall 2004, the initiative is coordinated by the Swedish National Institute of Public Health, with funding from the European Commission. Other partners include health ministries, NGOs, public health institutes, and universities. The project has undertaken a systematic and comprehensive review of health promotion research, policy, and interventions in the European Union and internationally. This review forms the basis for policy recommendations directed to the EU and to member states and for the dissemination of a comprehensive, integrated approach to aging and health. In this partnership, WHO contributes a global policy framework on healthy, active aging and also expertise in aging and in policy development.

Study on Global AGEing and Adult Health (SAGE) (Health)

The WHO Study on Global AGEing and Adult Health (SAGE) is the first ever multidimensional and community-based international survey on aging. It has been designed to develop a range of valid, reliable, and comparable survey modules with the potential to generate cohorts that could then be followed up for a period of five to ten years, funding permitting. It will be conducted in six countries—China, India, Russia, Mexico, Ghana, and South Africa. SAGE's objective is to obtain reliable, valid, and comparable data on levels of health on a range of key domains (health, socioeconomic, measurements of functional capacity, and so on) to examine patterns of health and well-being. The pretest questionnaire, involving over 1,500 respondents in three countries (Ghana, Tanzania, and India), was conducted early in 2006, and the first wave of fieldwork and data collection is expected to be completed by the beginning of 2007. It is expected that the instruments developed by this project will be used increasingly for other similar studies worldwide.

Older Persons as Caregivers in the Context of AIDS Epidemics in Africa

This project proposal builds on a pilot study conducted by WHO in Zimbabwe in 2003–2004. If successful in securing funds, it will focus on the critical role played by older persons in the context of the AIDS epidemics in Africa—as providers of care both to their infected adult children and, on their children's death, to the millions of orphaned grandchildren left behind. Countries to be involved are Botswana, Kenya, Mozambique, Tanzania, and Zimbabwe.

Full details of these activities and projects can be found on the WHO website on aging and health (www.who.int/hpr/ageing).

REFERENCES

Adoderin, I., and others. *Life Course Perspectives on Coronary Heart Disease, Stroke, and Diabetes: Key Issues and Implications for Policy and Research.* Geneva: World Health Organization, 2002.

Cutler, D. "Declining Disability Among the Elderly." *Health Affairs,* 2001, *20*(6), 11–27.

Kalache, A., and Kickbusch, I. "A Global Strategy for Healthy Ageing." *World Health,* July–August 1997 (4), 4–5.

Singer, B., and Manton, K. "The Effects of Health Changes on Projections of Health Service Needs for the Elderly Population of the United States." *Proceedings of the National Academy of Science,* 1998 (23), 321–35.

U.S. Centers for Disease Control. "Lower Direct Medical Costs Associated with Physical Activity." Atlanta: Centers for Disease Control, 1999. [http://www.cdc.gov/nccdphp/dnpa/pr-cost.htm]. Accessed 2006.

World Health Organization. *Life in the 21st Century: A Vision for All* (World Health Report). Geneva: World Health Organization, 1998.

World Health Organization. *Active Ageing: A Policy Framework.* Geneva: World Health Organization, 2002a.

World Health Organization. *Missing Voices: Views of Older Persons on Elder Abuse.* Geneva: World Health Organization, 2002b.

World Health Organization. Women, Ageing and Health: A Framework for Action. Geneva: World Health Organization, 2007. [http://www.who.int/ageing/publications/active/en].

CHAPTER

4

LEADERSHIP AND GOVERNANCE CHALLENGES FOR GLOBAL HEALTH AND AGING

DEREK YACH

We face, whether we like it or not, a "big bang" of oncoming, parallel "unsustainables." That is, [not] unless we wake up in sufficient numbers, on sufficient scale and with joint political leadership, to execute together a list of action "imperatives"... can we progress to a sustainable, not unsustainable, future.... [These] include, of course ... poverty, and global climate change ... water, other eco-systems, global diseases and pandemics, transport systems, mega-cities, pension and health care systems.
—ANTHONY SIMON, FORMER PRESIDENT OF MARKETING, UNILEVER, 2006

Although many new players have joined the ranks of the well-established international health organizations in addressing global health, concepts surrounding leadership in this field have changed little. Despite the expanding global health community, ideals about good governance in health do not yet include nonstate players, practices have not adopted useful corporate management techniques or tapped the energies of the business world, and important demographic and epidemiological trends have not been appropriately considered to ensure that healthy aging becomes a reality for all countries. Although issues of institutional leadership are critical, they are not as important as individual leaders able to inspire us to address the "unsustainables," especially in health.

HEALTH GOVERNANCE IN THE 1990S

In 1996, I attended a meeting at the Pocantico Conference Center outside of New York City, aimed at enhancing the performance of some of the institutions responsible for international health (Pocantico Retreat, 1996). The Rockefeller Foundation sponsored the meeting, as it has so many others over the last nine decades. The meeting addressed deep concerns about the effectiveness of Dr. Nakajima's leadership as the director-general of the World Health Organization (WHO) and the consequences for international health. The players present, their concerns, and the evolving events have implications for our ideas about leadership and governance in global health today and the emphasis that major players give to chronic diseases and their relationship to aging.

Participants at the Pocantico meeting included many public health luminaries with diverse styles of leadership in health. Bill Foege, previously head of CDC, is now a senior advisor to Bill and Melinda Gates and is attributed with lighting their passion for global health. D. A. Henderson, previously dean of the Johns Hopkins School of Public Health, was a dominant figure involved in the smallpox eradication effort and currently leads efforts to protect the United States from the threats of bioterrorism. Halfdan Mahler, previous director-general of WHO, was responsible for hosting the 1978 Alma Ata Conference at which the equity-based notion of Health for All was launched. Adetokunbo Lucas was the first director of the most effective WHO research program, the Tropical Disease Research program. Lincoln Chen, then at Harvard, was soon to become vice president of the Rockefeller Foundation, where he launched several new programs aimed at promoting health equity. Gill Walt is one of the few academics who have for many years focused on institutional effectiveness. And Julio Frenk is the Mexican Minister of Health and an executive director in Dr. Gro Harlem Brundtland's WHO cabinet.

Discussion centered heavily on the roles of WHO, the World Bank, and UNICEF, and despite the range of leadership represented by the participants, it was difficult to fully embrace new models. For example, mention of private-public partnerships—a very innovative style of institutional leadership at this time—was restricted to the Merck ivermectin program and Rotary's support for polio eradication. Participants were extremely cautious about further private-public interaction because of their concerns about the private sector's profit motive.

Later in 1996 came the launch of the first of what would become a flood of new private-public partnerships aimed at developing new drugs and vaccines. The senior Rockefeller Foundation officer responsible for the Pocantico meeting, Seth Berkley, became the first executive director of the International AIDS Vaccine Initiative (IAVI)—a position he continues to use to inspire the investments and action required to get an effective AIDS vaccine.

It seems obvious that successful leaders have access to the information needed to perform well. Yet at Pocantico scant attention was given to data. There was no discussion about epidemiological or demographic trends, despite the availability of the first runs of the burden of disease work. There was no reference to gaps in knowledge required to define the most cost-effective interventions required to improve health and reduce suffering. The eight Millennium Development Goals (MDGs) of the 2000 Millennium Declaration had not yet been developed, but when priority diseases and risks were discussed, there was an implicit sense that infectious diseases and undernutrition should be given priority, with a focus on women and children. Despite decades of demographic research, there was no discussion about aging, the timing and impact of chronic diseases throughout the aging process, or the sociological impact of aging on individuals or society.

Rather, the meeting focused mainly on institutional aspects of leadership, with considerable attention devoted to the crucial role of WHO as the "normative conscience" for world health yet, simultaneously, the need for WHO to be more effective in developing and implementing global normative functions. At that point, these related to an out-of-date version of the International Health Regulations, a weak Codex Alimentarius Commission, and many public health, clinical, and statistical norms that we too easily take for granted. There was an assumption that a stronger WHO would be the natural leader of others involved in health, but there was little discussion of the importance of individual leadership, what it meant, or how it might play out in large organizations.

THE CLINTON GLOBAL INITIATIVE

The Clinton [Global] Initiative combines political savvy, business acumen, individual and institutional support from government leaders, religious leaders, international organizations, NGOs, corporations, banks, foundations, private businesses and individuals across society. It then artfully channels this towards concrete commitments to actions to help improve our world.

—ANTHONY SIMON, 2006

In 2006, the crisis in health governance continues. The stakes have never been higher, and, as suggested by the preceding quote, the level of interest and involvement by a wider and wealthier array of players has never been stronger.

Debates about global health in 2006 are no longer confined to the lofty halls of the World Health Assembly in Geneva. For the last few years, health has emerged as an important topic at the World Economic Forum in Davos. Since the G8 Summit in Okinawa, Japan, in 2000, health has become a permanent feature at G8 meetings. Indeed, discussions at the Okinawa Summit led to the development of the Global Fund for AIDS, Malaria, and TB. In 2006, in St. Petersburg, the health theme remained strong in G8 deliberations, with the focus on avian flu preparedness and a broader range of infectious diseases (although, in general, the G8 has a very constrained view of global health priorities, which does not include aging or chronic diseases).

In September 2006 in New York City, the Clinton Global Initiative (CGI) engaged the global community on a variety of health themes (Clinton Global Initiative, 2006). Pharmaceutical and food corporations, NGOs, WHO and academics made commitments to address neglected infectious diseases, chronic diseases, water-related health problems, improved access to essential drugs, malaria, and AIDS.

In 1996 it would have been difficult to imagine that in the course of just ten years such a wide array of new players would emerge. Many have been influenced by the work of Bill and Melinda Gates in global health. The Global Alliance for Vaccines and Immunizations, the Global Alliance for Improved Nutrition, and the Global Fund for AIDS, Malaria, and TB are three examples of new multibillion-dollar initiatives involved in providing drugs, vaccines, and micronutrients to millions of people worldwide. None were even on the development table in 1996. Since then, over eighty additional partnerships had formed to focus on developing new drugs, vaccines, or diagnostics for malaria, dengue, TB, and a wide range of infectious diseases (Widdus, 2005).

The presence of so many new players and so much more interest by political leaders and corporations has brought needed energy, additional dollars, and new opportunities for improving global health. It has also brought further strains to the governance systems for health.

1950S GOVERNANCE STRUCTURES FOR TWENTY-FIRST-CENTURY PROBLEMS

The same institutional arrangements that were developed after the Second World War, primarily to promote collaboration between governments, are still in place. There have been few changes to the mandate of WHO or the UN. They still primarily regard governments as their sole stakeholders, despite the reality that private groups and some NGOs now command larger operational resources in health than WHO.

The bureaucratic and administrative processes of WHO and the UN are mostly unchanged since the Cold War and the precomputer era. Although cutting-edge information technology solutions are being used on the outside to more rapidly detect emerging pandemics, a "quill and ink" mentality pervades the way many decisions are made in WHO and the UN in relation to policy and actions. Internal labor rules do not promote innovation, productivity, or creativity. Big meetings dominate the decision-making process, in which each country, regardless of its population, has one vote. Influence is sought on the basis of regional or other political affiliations, rather than on the basis of commitment to public health approaches. The corporate sector is represented only through stealth participation in NGOs in "official relations" or through lobbying. The number of NGOs involved in programs has increased and some have been able to effectively partner with the WHO secretariat on selected issues. But most have not been able to reformulate the terms of their engagement with WHO despite several years of trying.

At one point, there were some hopeful prospects of institutional change. During Bruntdland's tenure as director-general of WHO (1998–2003), several efforts were made to convene meetings regularly with pharmaceutical company CEOs and, separately, with NGOs focused on improving access to essential drugs. These meetings promoted modest progress in improving access to several drugs required in developing countries. Also, the first meetings with the food and alcohol industries and with their counterpart NGOs were held in the hope of building bridges to new ways of working. These meetings were tough because they required building trust between groups who had never worked together and regarded each other with suspicion. The fledgling initiatives were not sustained after Brundtland's term. The will to interact has since waned, and there remains both a high degree of distrust among leading NGOs about the motives of corporations and a sense of frustration among corporate players about WHO's overly bureaucratic ways. The losers are populations who could benefit from enhanced private-public interaction.

The absence of visible institutional and individual leadership for global health means that existing resources deployed for health are not having their maximum impact. Duplication of effort and a failure to cooperate at the international level have been best described in relation to AIDS funding. There are now many separate initiatives aimed at bridging the treatment gap. They include the Global Fund, President Bush's Emergency Plan for AIDS Relief (PEPFAR), separate Gates and Clinton Foundation initiatives, and multi-institutional partnerships with a welcome array of pharmaceutical companies, many NGOs, and the expected crowd of academics and researchers.

All come with noble intentions. Unfortunately, though, all tend to have their own reporting requirements, separate approaches to financial management, and different expectations of the real transaction costs for understaffed health departments in developing countries responding to donor needs. Weak governments are struggling to address the multiple demands they must meet to access funding. Further, a recent McKinsey report commissioned by the Gates Foundation showed that additional AIDS funds had exposed underlying weaknesses in health systems in developing countries (McKinsey and Company, 2005).

Who has the responsibility to resolve these complex institutional issues? In the old days, WHO would have been looked at to do so. They could for smallpox, where a relatively simple command-and-control approach worked. The bifurcated needle and a single scratch to about 60 percent of the population were sufficient to eradicate the disease.

But for AIDS—with many players, many leaders, many niches, and many approaches—it will take a special blend of individual leaders who are able to work together more effectively. And it will take a real shakeup of the roles and mandates of the myriad organizations that have recently formed to address the global AIDS problem.

And we must remember that AIDS is just one disease.

WHOSE WHO IS IT?

The director-general of WHO is elected to serve all people in all countries. She is expected to be a leader for the very poor and the rich, for the old and the young, for the disabled and the able, for smokers and for the hungry. A commitment to health and human rights demands nothing less. In reality, though, resources are finite. Priorities must be set in such a way that all governments feel that they are served by their investment in WHO, yet with the biggest impact in poor countries. That is not easy, and it has meant that priorities of WHO and Overseas Development Agencies have changed little since the 1950s.

The current agenda for major development agencies and donors in the health sector is mostly restricted to maternal and child health and selected infectious diseases, driven by concerns about equity and poverty reduction in the very poorest countries. This is and should be the focus of the MDGs, which have their main relevance among countries where the poorest billion in the world reside. Despite there being many more dollars available for global health, in recent years the agenda has narrowed, not broadened. Chronic diseases and healthy aging, of relevance to the four billion people who are neither the poorest nor richest in the world, are not addressed by any major development agency or foundation. When the increased funding that goes to HIV/AIDS is deducted from the total amount of Overseas Development Aid for health, the total available for other areas of health has declined (MacKellar, 2005). Treatment of chronic diseases is so poorly funded that it falls within the rounding error of official ODA funding estimates!

GLOBAL HEALTH IN TRANSITION

Funding priorities set by major foundations and donors have an impact on policy priorities in most low- to middle-income countries, despite the existence of data showing that the major causes of death and disease in these countries are increasingly similar to the causes in developed countries.

Earlier it was mentioned that, in 1996 in Pocantico, the burden of disease data were not considered. By 2006, the availability of these data had dramatically increased and showed that chronic diseases are the dominant contributors to the burden of disease in all countries except those in sub-Saharan Africa (Lopez and others, 2006). We now also have more solid estimates of the likely increase in the aging populations in developing countries. Emerging evidence suggests that not only are developing countries getting older before they are rich, but they are carrying a greater and broader burden of ill health into older age than counterparts in developed countries.

This contrasts with trends under way in the USA suggesting that disability rates among those over sixty-five years of age are coming down faster then death rates, leading to the hoped-for compression of morbidity with increased longevity (Fries, 2005). This is still way off for people growing up in developing countries. Their continued high burden of infections and stunting in early childhood, combined with early exposure to the core risks for chronic diseases—such as tobacco, unhealthy diets, and a lack of physical activity throughout childhood and early adulthood—place them at risk of experiencing higher disease burdens with aging. If current trends persist, they will be poorer and unhealthier as they age compared to their developed-country cohorts. Debates, policy development, and resource allocation in WHO and many international health and donor agencies still largely neglect this emerging reality.

There are varied reasons for the neglect of chronic diseases and aging. Institutional inertia, policymakers' perceptions of the needs of developing countries, and active lobbying by selected corporate groups (such as the tobacco industry) all play a role. Lack of data is no longer an excuse. The recently completed initiative of the Fogarty International Center of the NIH, the World Bank, and WHO has provided current estimates of the burden of disease and risk and has used these data together with economic studies to define the most cost-effective interventions in health for developing countries (Jamison and others, 2006). It provides a challenging approach to future priority setting. The thousand-page report involved five hundred experts over several years. Several challenges to current dogma emerged.

The new burden estimates show that chronic diseases dominate the burden of disease in most countries and that if healthy aging is to be achieved, far greater effort must be given to addressing the major risks for chronic diseases and to doing so from birth.

Many of the most commonly used interventions in public health (for example, mass-based treatment of people with antiretrovirals) were not found to be the most cost-effective. Conversely, many highly cost-effective interventions already in use in some countries are not widely regarded as crucial interventions elsewhere. These include steeply raising the tobacco tax, providing immediate and long-term treatment for people who have had a stroke or heart attack, and investing in speed bumps to reduce traffic injuries and deaths. All are affordable in developing countries.

Globalizing access to this kind of knowledge is essential. Most schools of public health avoid discussing the policy and practical implications of addressing the rising tide of chronic diseases and the emergence of a large and growing group of people who are over sixty years of age. If future public health leaders continue to be taught about a public health agenda applicable several decades back, the prospects for change will remain bleak.

HEALTH IN A GLOBALIZED WORLD

In a globalized world, it is no longer sufficient to consider health concerns of nations as if they did not influence each other. *Global health* is emerging as a term that encompasses both the positive and negative transnational aspects of health. The cross-border movement of goods, people, practices, and services (including infections, the marketing of unhealthy products on the Internet or satellite TV, and the illicit trade in tobacco or pharmaceuticals) all fall under the general rubric of global health. The policy responses to these complex and shifting issues necessarily differ from each other and from past policy efforts. They require international norms, global surveillance, multi-country responses, and the engagement of many players. Progress has been made in developing a new set of international rules to address infectious diseases (for example, through the acceptance of the 2005 version of the International Health Regulations) and also in tackling tobacco use—a core risk factor for chronic diseases. The WHO Framework Convention on Tobacco Control represents the only time that WHO has used its treaty-making authority to challenge a threat to health. The fact that over 140 countries have adopted the treaty augurs well for its ultimate implementation and impact on tobacco use (Yach and Wipfli, 2006).

The neglect of chronic diseases is the neglect of four billion people living in low middle-income countries. For them, the MDGs have been largely met. These countries' continued economic growth depends on a healthy workforce and the creation of wealth before their populations age. Further, it is increasingly clear that the economic health of social security and pension systems in developed countries, particularly in Europe, depend on continued high levels of productivity in low- and middle-income countries. Thus, healthy aging is becoming an issue of mutual interest to developed and developing countries in much the same way that infectious disease has. Chronic diseases and healthy aging are transnational issues requiring global responses.

WHAT THE CLINTON GLOBAL INITIATIVE MEANS FOR GLOBAL HEALTH LEADERSHIP

The most powerful outcome of the 2006 CGI meeting was that health became a major theme at an event where fifty heads of states addressed other pressing global issues. These included debates between President Hamid Karzai of Afghanistan, Queen Rania of Jordan, and Archbishop Desmond Tutu of South Africa about managing diversity in the world, and between former U.S. Vice President Al Gore and leading industrialists about climate change. Health was seen as integral to debates about the future well-being and prosperity of the world. President Bill Clinton, as the overall moderator, frequently referred to health issues in plenary sessions attended by more than one thousand people. And in a special plenary session entitled "Effective Action—Lasting Results," Bill Gates led by stressing his commitment to tackling inequities in global health. The two Bills are likely to be dominant forces for global health over many years. Their decisions and the partnerships they build could profoundly influence the agenda for global health and also the quantity and impact of funding. President Clinton has indicated his support for innovative approaches to address obesity in the United States, and Gates has started to explore how to address tobacco in developing countries. They are both committed to science-based solutions and respond to solid data. Thus it is likely that in time they will include a focus on broader aspects of chronic disease and its relationship to healthy aging.

The content of the global health track highlighted issues beyond the usual focus on specific diseases. The critical need to address the physical and human infrastructural aspects of health emerged in all panel discussions. This will be crucial as health systems adapt to both an epidemiological and a demographic transition. Together, these transitions require us to seriously reconsider who should be the frontline health-care providers and how they will be supported. The shift to a world of more chronic diseases among older people will demand a shift toward more home-based care, more self-management, and more continuous care. Nurses—supported in the field by the best information technology and better diagnostic equipment and methods—as well as generalist technicians are likely to emerge as the major care and management providers; doctors will become less visible on the frontlines but better placed on tap and in referral centers. The debates on future needs for health professionals have yet to consider these shifts and to plan accordingly.

Participants in the CGI health sessions were not typical of participants at the World Health Assembly or around the table at Pocantico ten years ago. Panels included well-known health advocates and experts like Paul Farmer, Srinath Reddy, and Julie Gerbeding, as well as ministers of health from Ethiopia, Nicaragua, and Kenya. However, CEOs or senior representatives from PepsiCo, UnitedHealth Care, De Beers, Procter & Gamble, and TNT International also contributed innovative ideas about their roles in global health. Their insights are rarely heard in traditional health meetings. Of course, many representatives from pharmaceutical companies were present, but unlike in most health settings, they were not seen as the only corporate partners needed to improve global health.

The CGI differed from WHO meetings in another important respect. It required people and institutions to make commitments to improving global health, and that commitment needed to be novel, specific, and measurable. This often came with a large check, but some were solely focused on new partnerships and specific nonmonetized actions. The list of health commitments was impressive. Lois Quam of Ovations, a UnitedHealth Care company, announced support for the creation of global centers of excellence to tackle chronic diseases in developing countries. They intend to build on their expertise in the United States in addressing the health needs of people over the age of fifty. Other commitments related to chronic diseases included pledges by the World Diabetes Foundation, local universities, and service providers to address diabetes in Cape Town, South Africa; the World Heart Federation, to develop a "polypill" to address CVD and diabetes; and PepsiCo, to address the aspects of chronic diseases that are influenced by nutrition and physical activity.

These commitments have the potential to do more than simply provide funds. Some, like the commitments to address chronic diseases, will help contribute to setting a broader agenda for global health and will help chart a path of hope where inaction has dominated.

Many commitments represented new ways of working—and overcame the concerns of skeptics in governments and NGOs about working with business. Of course, the new money was seen as important, but the new ways of partnering were seen as the emergence of different roles for government, NGOs, business, and international agencies. In an extraordinary panel on the future role of business, Colin Powell commented how, since the collapse of the Berlin wall and the end of the Maoist era in China, in broad political terms the action had moved from "the battlefields to the playing fields." Opportunities for new ways of working, unthinkable before, are being tried and tested. The CGI is a critical experiment in how well these evolving ways of working achieve real impact.

Clearly, the economic leadership for global health has now moved beyond the World Bank and the traditional development agencies to include major corporations and the world's largest foundations. For these new players, the role of government is crucial. Many stressed the need for facilitative laws that will create incentives for positive corporate action and penalize the laggards. Further, the importance of a more effective WHO emerged throughout the sessions. Although corporations and NGOs are able to develop projects with impact, their budgets are limited. They need guidance about where the largest needs and opportunities exist. They need government and WHO support with respect to the best approaches to use.

TWENTY-FIRST-CENTURY GOVERNANCE FOR HEALTH

Our health and political institutions have not adapted to the dramatic changes under way throughout the world as a whole and in the health field in particular. The recent elections of a new head of the Global Fund for AIDS, Malaria, and TB, and of the new director-general of WHO, both in late 2006, create opportunities for a serious international debate about comparative advantage and how one could improve the effectiveness of major institutions involved in health. Tough questions should be asked about

- WHO's role and mandate, in the light of so many new players being active in global health

- How governance of health could be expanded to include nonstate players

- How the best of corporate management expertise could be used within the UN and governments in a way that could strengthen the need to address iniquities

- How the rapidly emerging demographic and epidemiological realities can be tackled so that healthy aging becomes a reality for all countries

Although issues of institutional leadership are critical to resolving these questions, they should not displace attention from identifying and strengthening the source and key to sustainable improvements in institutions, thereby inspiring individual leaders.

REFERENCES

Clinton Global Initiative, 2006. [http://www.clintonglobalinitiative.org].

Fries, J. F. "Frailty, Heart Disease, and Stroke: The Compression of Morbidity Paradigm." *American Journal of Preventive Medicine*, Dec. 2005, *29*(5 Suppl. 1), 164–8.

Jamison, D., and others. *Disease Control Priorities in Developing Countries*. New York: Oxford University Press, 2006.

Lopez, A. D., and others. "Global and Regional Burden of Disease and Risk Factors, 2001: Systematic Analysis of Population Health Data." *The Lancet*, May 27, 2006, *367*(9524), 1747–57.

MacKellar, L. "Priorities in Global Assistance for Health, AIDS, and Population." OECD Development Centre, Working Paper No. 244, June 2005.

McKinsey and Company. "Global Health Partnerships: Assessing Country Consequences." Bill and Melinda Gates Foundation, 2005.

Pocantico Retreat. "Enhancing the Performance of International Health Institutions." Social Science Research Council and Harvard School of Public Health, February 1–3, 1996.

Widdus, R. "Public-Private Partnerships: An Overview." *Transactions of the Royal Society of Tropical Medicine and Hygiene*, Oct. 2005, *99*(Suppl. 1), S1–8.

Yach, D., and Wipfli, H. "A Century of Smoke." *Annals of Tropical Medicine and Parasitology*, July–Sept. 2006, *100*(5–6), 465–7.

CHAPTER

5

PERCEPTION OF AGING IN DIFFERENT CULTURES

FRANK E. EYETSEMITAN

During the two decades from 1986 to 2006, around the world the under-age-five population has been shrinking and the adult population has been swelling. Globally, between 2006 and 2031 the elderly population is projected to more than double. If this trend continues, the greatest relative increase will occur in developing countries. Compared to the United States and other developed nations—where the increase will be just over 50 percent—this growth will range from 106 to 174 percent in the developing nations. By 2025, a high proportion of those sixty-five years and over will be living in the developing world (U.S. Census Bureau, 2002).

With the demographic changes currently under way and anticipated in both the developed and developing worlds, it is timely to review perceptions of aging and the elderly in those places. Are they the same or are there differences?

These perceptions influence how others relate to the elderly and how the elderly themselves relate to their own aging. This chapter will discuss the developed and developing worlds as contexts for perceptions of aging and the elderly, exploring the following subthemes:

- Aging, declines, and health

- Differences between developed and developing societies

- Acculturation influences of the developed world in developing societies

- Generational perceptions of aging in developed and developing societies

- Conclusion

AGING, DECLINES, AND HEALTH

Aging, or senescence, begins when we are born and becomes gradual and more pronounced later in life. The different systems and organs in our bodies will experience this change at different rates, as will different individuals, with a wide variation in how quickly this process unfolds. This change is not just biological; the individual's sociocultural environment also contributes to the aging process. It is important to distinguish between *primary aging*, which represents the inevitable physical changes that are universally shared as a result of aging, and *secondary aging*, which results from environmental events that may not be widely shared.

According to Whitbourne (1985), the impact of physiological change cannot be truly understood separated from its context, as physiological changes do not necessarily result in functional changes. An individual's bodily system may undergo considerable physical change, but that person's functioning may not be affected noticeably. A person who believes that he is losing his eyesight and interprets this to mean that he is helpless will be more incapacitated by the decline in eyesight than someone in a similar physical condition who does not feel incapacitated. In a society in which independence is highly valued, this situation would be more devastating to the individual than it would be to another recipient living in a society where high value is placed on interdependence.

Both physical and social elements of culture play a significant role in defining psychological contexts; this has been noted by Westerhof, Katzko, Dittmann-Kohli, and Hayslip (2001), who suggested that the prevalent "deficit model" in gerontological discourse lacks the incorporation of cultural interpretation of health and functionality in later life.

Theories of Aging

Over three hundred theories propose that primary aging or senescence is universal. According to Strehler (1986), for any biological theory on aging to be upheld as universal, the following criteria must apply:

- All members of the species must experience the phenomenon.

- The process must result in physiological decline.

- The process must be progressive; that is, losses must be gradual over time.

- The loss must be intrinsic; that is, it cannot be corrected by the organism.

These guidelines help to distinguish between declines that come from normal aging and those that result from diseases like arthritis and Alzheimer's.

A few popular biological theories that meet Strehler's (1986) criteria are reviewed in this section.

Wear-and-Tear Theory   This theory contends that as organisms age, their organ systems accumulate damage from the frequent abuse they face in the course of daily functioning. So the body is like a machine that eventually wears out after extensive use and deteriorates over time. Because organs and systems in the body are not subject to the same rate of usage and abuse, both the onset and the magnitude of deterioration varies from one organ system to another in the aging process. Environmental contexts such as air and noise pollution may exacerbate the regular wear and tear on the organ systems, contributing to secondary aging.

Autoimmune Theory   As an important defense, the immune system acts against foreign substances that may invade the body. With aging, this system not only becomes less efficient in producing antibodies to fight foreign invaders, but also develops a propensity to attack the body's own proteins. This theory hinges on two main findings. First, as we age, the immune system is no longer able to produce antibodies in sufficient quantities; because of this decline in its ability, we are more likely to acquire and manifest diseases of old age that an efficient immune system might have kept in check in our youth. Second, the declining immune system may become defective and produce antibodies that not only attack foreign bodies but also mistakenly attack and damage the body's own proteins. One culpable part of the system is the thymus gland (located in the upper part of the chest), which produces disease-fighting white blood cells (T cells), a vital component of the immune system. After adolescence and by middle to late adulthood, the thymus gland begins to wither. The shrinkage is considerable: by age fifty, humans retain only 5 to 10 percent of the thymus gland's original mass (Hayflick, 1994). This deterioration is suggested as a trigger for the eventual decline of the entire immune system.

Cross-Linkage Theory   The cross-linkage theory focuses on age-related changes that occur in the protein called collagen. Collagen, an important connective tissue found in most organ systems, makes up almost one-third of all the protein in the human body. Cross-links are essential in joining parallel molecules of collagen together. Supporters of this theory argue that with age, cross-links form a scaffold that connects a larger number of neighboring molecules—a process that may impede the metabolic process, obstructing the passage of nutrients and wastes in and out of cells. Thus the tissue becomes less pliable and may indeed shrink. A clear example of changes in our collagen is wrinkling of the skin. But collagen changes also occur in the lens of the eyes, the blood vessels, the muscle tissues, and other internal organs not as outwardly apparent as the skin.

Cellular Aging Theory   This theory suggests a limit to the number of times cells can divide, thereby limiting the life span of complex organisms. Reports from laboratory studies suggest that cells undergo a finite number of replications, indicating that cells appear to be programmed to follow a biological clock, and the number of possible divisions depends on the age of the donor organism—a process known as the Hayflick phenomenon. Researchers initially believed that the Hayflick limit could account for why cells eventually die, but contradictory evidence points to cells from some older adults that sometimes double as often as those of younger adults. Although at least in humans the Hayflick limit in senescence remains inconclusive, this theory still points to aging as being genetically programmed.

The preceding theories suggest that declines come with age and with declines come attendant health problems. Biological weakening resulting from aging makes the role of culture as an intervening variable very important, as evidenced by cognitive training and support to maintain previous levels of performance into old age. According to Baltes, Staudinger, and Lindenberger (1999), the increase in average life expectancy witnessed in industrialized and technologically advanced societies in the second half of the twentieth century stemmed not from changes in genetic makeup, but from advances in culture, especially biomedical technology. However, the extent to which culture is able to augment or reduce losses that come from biological declines will be limited by the amount of physiological decline that has already taken place. Beyond an asymptote level, it becomes difficult to maintain the same level of performance, even with more training (Baltes, 1997). To adapt to those declines, older people need to reallocate resources either for growth, for maintenance and resilience, or for the regulation of loss. Reallocating resources for growth obviously will decline with aging, but this will increase for the maintenance and regulation of losses (Staudinger, Marsiske, and Baltes, 1995). Growth behaviors include increasing perceptual speed, whereas maintenance behaviors are those intended to keep the same levels of functioning going.

When maintenance or recovery of losses is not possible, dependency can creep in. This is when friends and family support networks are important and institutional support systems (such as adult day care and nursing homes) become useful. However, dependency as described here is Western in orientation. Interdependency in non-Western cultures is the norm, a lifestyle based on intergenerational helping relationships that occur throughout the life course.

DIFFERENCES BETWEEN DEVELOPED AND DEVELOPING SOCIETIES

Two major factors help to delineate the difference between developed and developing societies: (1) industrial and technological advancement and (2) values.

Industrial and Technological Advancement

Industrialization brings about improved living conditions, and with paid employment and work careers, the poverty rate is reduced. Paid employment provides the ability to be well fed, for access to and use of good health care services, and the possibility of income security—thus helping to extend lives.

Vaccines, antitoxins, and toxoids combat many deadly communicable diseases such as typhoid fever, diphtheria, tetanus, spotted fever, whooping cough, polio, cholera, bubonic plague, and measles. Biomedical advances have also included the invention of the electrocardiograph (which detects and records heart irregularities), the kidney dialysis machine, and surgical implantation of the liver, kidney, and heart. With computerized axial topography (CAT), positron omission tomography (PET), and ultrasound and magnetic resonance imaging (MRI) techniques, medical personnel can now examine organ dysfunctions noninvasively. In the span of a hundred years, life expectancy in developed societies has increased from about fifty years to seventy-four for men and eighty for women (Hooyman and Kiyak, 2005). For many developing societies, however, poor advances in industrialization and biomedical technology continue to keep life expectancy low.

Values

In terms of values, Hofstede's (1980) "individualism and collectivism" construct, described in his book *Culture's Consequences: International Differences in Work–Related Values*, has been well cited to delineate the difference between Western (developed) and non-Western (mostly developing) societies. Hofstede surveyed IBM employees from fifty countries and three multicountry regions and constructed an index of individualism and collectivism along with three other pairs of factors: power and distance, uncertainty and avoidance, and masculinity and femininity. Interest in individualism and collectivism preceded Hofstede's work; however, his contribution has led to a resurgence of attention on this construct and in similar areas (see Triandis, 1995 for details).

Societies that tend toward individualism emphasize independence, self-containment, and autonomy—characteristics said to largely represent Western values. In societies that tend toward collectivism, the emphasis is on interdependence, relatedness, and social obligations, and these mostly represent non-Western values. Individualists value equality, freedom, and an exciting life, whereas collectivists value social order, honoring of parents and elders, and self-discipline.

From diverse works on this construct, Triandis (1995) and also Triandis and Bhawuk (1997) have identified four universal dimensions of individualism and collectivism:

1. **Definition of Self.** Collectivists view self in relation to others with interdependency in resource-sharing. Individualists view self as autonomous from groups and are not obligated to share resources; rather, such decisions are made individually.

2. **Structure of Goals.** In collectivist cultures, the individual's goals are subsumed within the in-group's goals; in individualist cultures, the individual's goals are not often related to those of the in-group. The in-group is composed of sets of individuals a person feels similar to, and that similarity may come from common fate or some other attributes (Triandis, 1995). In general, collectivist in-groups are *ascribed* (for example, caste, kin, race, tribe, religion, village, and nation), whereas individualist in-groups are *achieved* (for example, by similar beliefs, attitudes,

values, actions, programs, and occupation). But in cases such as nationality, some attributes are both achieved and ascribed.

3. **Emphasis on Norms versus Attitudes.** Norms, duties, and obligations determine social behavior in collectivist cultures. Attitudes, personal needs, perceived rights, and contracts determine social behavior in individualist cultures.

4. **Emphasis on Relatedness versus Rationality.** In collectivist cultures, relatedness is emphasized; in individualist cultures, the emphasis is on rationality. With relatedness, the individual gives priority to relationships even if this is not to his or her advantage; with rationality, the emphasis is on the costs and benefits of relationships.

It has been noted that researchers indirectly assume differences in participants based on their national and ethnic status, without establishing a causal relationship. Kagitcibasi (1997) has suggested the need to study background variables like education, income, rural-urban standing, and type of employment in individualism and collectivism measures. The levels of technological and economic advancement, of secularity and openness, and of citizen participation should be additional dimensions to consider (see, for comparison, Triandis, 1995). The acculturation influences discussed next are mainly responsible for these suggestions.

ACCULTURATION INFLUENCES OF THE DEVELOPED WORLD IN DEVELOPING SOCIETIES

The environment of developing societies is no longer as monolithic as some still believe. Eyetsemitan (2002a) argued that because of the dominant influence of the Western value system, the developing world has three environmental dimensions, operating either independently or in interactive ways.

1. **The *Global* Dimension.** The *global* environmental dimension, created by experiences (mostly biological) that people around the world share in common—including aging and death—is likely to promote pancultural attitudes and behaviors.

2. **The *Developed* Dimension.** With industrialization—Western education and Western medicine being examples—the dominance of Western value systems is likely to affect how developing world people perceive aging and the elderly.

3. **The *Developing* Dimension.** The *developing* environmental dimension includes cultural elements and practices native to the inhabitants of developing societies. These include native medicine and spiritualism, local languages, a non-Western educational system, simple technology, and collectivism (see Eyetsemitan, 2002a for details).

These three environmental dimensions can influence, either independently or in an interactive way, the attitude and behaviors of an individual. In an interactive way, *accommodation behavior* results, described among Indians and seen among natives of other developing societies. In one study of health-seeking behavior and attitudes among 212 tuberculosis (TB) patients in Botswana, for example, Steen and Mazonde (1999) reported that patients who believed that TB was caused by the breaking of taboos (Tswana) used modern medicine for symptom relief (*developed* dimension) but also sought traditional treatment for the perceived cause of the disease (*developing* dimension). In another study in the South Pacific reflecting accommodation behavior, Harmon (1996) reported that traditional paganism (*developing* dimension) continued to flourish in the islands of the South Pacific despite the people's supposed conversion to Christianity (*developed* dimension).

Studies on individuals described as "bicultural" have provided insight into why accommodation behaviors occur. In what Hong, Morris, Chiu, and Benet-Martinez (2000) refer to as "frame-switching," bicultural individuals (people exposed to more than one culture) are able to shift between cognitive frameworks rooted in different cultural experiences in response to environmental cues. The authors suggest that culture's influence on cognition is neither continuous nor constant, but that a bicultural individual has a repertoire of possible cultural responses that may or may not be complementary (for example, seeking Western medical help and traditional healing at the same time). The internalized cultural frames are not blended but separate and can be tapped in turn to respond as the situation demands, and the extent to which a particular cultural frame is put to more frequent or recent use will make it more accessible or more primed to respond to environmental cues. This has been confirmed in studies whose subjects were primed by exposure to a construct; the influence of the primed construct on their interpretations of some stimulus was measured (such as Chiu and others, 1998).

According to the influence of these three dimensions, the cognitive frame of rural dwellers would be different from that of urban dwellers because rural dwellers are more likely to be influenced by the ready availability of traditional healers in the villages, whereas urban dwellers more likely would be influenced by exposure to Western medical practitioners. Cultural frame-switching, however, is not always subject to environmental cues; values also play an important role (see Eyetsemitan and Gire, 2003). Irrespective of location, an individual who places a high value on traditional healing may travel from the city to the rural area to seek help from a native healer.

GENERATIONAL PERCEPTIONS OF AGING IN DEVELOPED AND DEVELOPING SOCIETIES

Perception of aging is influenced by both cultural factors and the age of the perceiver. We now review two studies of how young people perceive the elderly and how the elderly perceive their own aging, in both developed and developing societies.

How young people perceive the elderly in their respective societies is the focus of Eyetsemitan's (2002b) study. The countries involved in this study are two developed societies (United States and Ireland) and two developing nations (Nigeria and Brazil), with a total of 732 respondents made up of 221 from the United States (mean age = 21.4 years; SD = 6.91) and 194 from Ireland (mean age = 19.50; SD = 3.76), 86 from

Nigeria (mean age = 25.58; SD = 4.86) and 231 from Brazil (mean age = 24.11; SD = 6.60). Respondents (all university undergraduates) were requested to list in order of importance elderly traits they believed to be "attractive" and "unattractive" (see Eyetsemitan, 2002b for details).

The study's results indicate a convergence of traits that respondents from all the countries identified as "attractive" and "unattractive." They fit into broad categories of positive/negative Personal; positive/negative Interpersonal; and positive/negative Need. The positive Personal traits included physical strength, experience, and wisdom; the positive Interpersonal included caring, friendly, give advice, and tell stories; and the positive Need included helplessness, loneliness, and physical/mental difficulties. The negative Personal traits included crabby, grumpy, hygiene, and bitterness; the negative Interpersonal included arrogant, bossy, impolite, and despise modern ways; and the negative Need included demanding, have disease, dependent, and helpless.

The pancultural perception of aging and the elderly noted in this study may have been triggered by an aging process, which is universal. However, among young people in developing societies, Western influences are quite prominent, and this may have contributed to a convergence in perception with their counterparts in the developed world.

The other study on how the elderly perceive their own aging, by Westerhof, Katzko, Dittmann-Kohli, and Hayslip (2001), notes a bilevel approach to the consideration of aging and health issues. The micro level is composed of molecular, cellular, and organ systems of the individual (which are universal); the macro level includes the social structures for curing disease and taking care of the ill (which are not universal). Their research conducted in the United States, India, and Congo/Zaire reflects three societies with different levels of industrialization and technological advancement. The number of respondents from the United States was one hundred and two (mean age seventy-three); from India, one hundred (mean age sixty-five); and from Congo/Zaire, fifty (mean age fifty-five).

Analyzing the study results, Westerhof, Katzko, Dittmann-Kohli, and Hayslip (2001) note cultural differences in the meaning attributed to health in old age, based on levels of technological advancement. In America, health was perceived as important, with respondents expressing fears of becoming ill and dependent, but hoping to maintain autonomy, health, and cognitive functioning into old age and with intentions to pursue good health practices. In Congo/Zaire, respondents expressed fears of death and expected to decline in mobility and strength, but held out hopes for support from their children and for a good death. The Indian respondents fell in between.

Attributing reasons for the disparities, Westerhoff, Katzko, Dittmann-Kohli, and Hayslip (2001) note that compared to the United States, the chances of reaching old age in India are less and in Congo/Zaire, still less, because of illness types and the social structures available for curing the ill and caring for the ill. In India and, to a greater extent, Congo/Zaire, communicable diseases (such as HIV/AIDS, diarrhea, malaria) are the predominant illness type, whereas in the United States and most developed countries the more common illness type is noncommunicable disease (such as diabetes, cancer, cardiovascular diseases).

In the United States, Western medical care is more widely available and acceptable than in India and in Congo/Zaire, and efficient old age pension and social security systems greatly enhance functional independence among American elderly. In the United States, a largely individualistic society, functional independence into old age is a desired outcome. In India and Congo/Zaire, both largely collectivistic societies, interdependency is the desired outcome. Children in collectivist cultures are expected to take care of their parents in old age as a reciprocal gesture for the care they have received from them.

Not surprisingly, the Congolese older person's perception of the health-related self does not include striving for good health as an important value, but instead sees interdependence as a desired outcome. The lack of advanced biomedical technology and a poor financial security system help to encourage this mind set. Similar results have been reported in other non-Western, developing societies. The U.S. respondents also expressed fears of losing their health, but they also had hopes of remaining healthy because functional independence is a desired value. With available biomedical technology and a social security system that works this value system is likely to be reinforced. Studies from other developed countries have provided similar findings. The Indians, although expressing fear of declining health, like their U.S. counterparts, also had expectations for good health, but for a different reason. They saw meditation (which they practice), not technology, as a means to good health. Similar to the Congolese elderly, they also desired a peaceful death.

CONCLUSION

The following factors will influence perception of aging in different cultures:

1. **The Global Experience of Aging.** Universal changes in the aging process could trigger pancultural perceptions about aging. Eyetsemitan's (2002b) study on elderly traits, identified by young people in both the developed and the developing world, could have been triggered by global changes associated with aging, identified in the theories of aging reviewed in this chapter.

2. **The Dominant Influence of Western Culture.** Western culture—including advanced technology, industrialization, and Western-style education—is dominant across the world and likely to influence perceptions about aging and the elderly across societies. Young people in developing societies exposed to Western-style education are likely to perceive aging and the elderly the way their counterparts in developed societies do. (In the Eyetsemitan 2002b study cited earlier, respondents were all university students.)

3. **Generational Differences.** Young and older people are likely to perceive aging and the elderly differently, given where they are in the life course. Young people will likely perceive aging as outsiders looking in, whereas older people's perceptions are influenced by an insider's view.

4. **Indigenous Value System.** Values that are indigenous to a people's group (for example, individualism and collectivism, religion, technology) are likely to influence how aging and the elderly are perceived, especially among the older generation. Individualists value functional independence in old age, whereas collectivists desire interdependence and support from their children over functional independence in later life.

REFERENCES

Baltes, P. B. "On the Incomplete Architecture of Human Ontogeny: Selection, Optimization, and Compensation as Foundation of Developmental Theory." *American Psychologist*, 1997, *52*, 366–380.

Baltes, P. B., Staudinger, U. M., and Lindenberger, U. "Lifespan Psychology: Theory and Application to Intellectual Functioning. *Annual Review of Psychology*, 1999, *50*, 41–507.

Chui, C.-Y., and others. "Stereotyping and Self-presentation: Effects of Gender Stereotype Activation." *Group Process and Intergroup Relations*, 1998, *1*, 81–96.

Eyetsemitan, F. "Suggestions Regarding Cross-Cultural Environment as Context for Human Development and Aging in Non-Western Cultures." *Psychological Reports*, 2002a, *90*, 823–833.

Eyetsemitan, F. "Perceived Elderly Traits and Young People's Perception of Helping Tendencies in the U.S., Ireland, Nigeria, and Brazil." *Journal of Cross-Cultural Gerontology*, 2002b, *17*, 57–69.

Eyetsemitan, F. and Gire, J. T. *Aging and Adult Development in the Developing World: Applying Western Theories and Concepts.* Westport, Connecticut: Praeger, 2003.

Harmon, A. B. "Ignoring the Missionary Position (Retention of Pre-Christian Beliefs in the South Sea Islands)." *New Statesman*, 1996, *12*, 20–21.

Hayflick, L. *How and Why We Age.* New York: Ballantine Books, 1994.

Hofstede, G. *Culture's Consequences: International Differences in Work-Related Values.* Thousand Oaks, Calif.: Sage, 1980.

Hong, Y.-Y., Morris, M., Chui, C.-Y., and Benet-Martinez, V. *Applicability of Assessable Cultural Knowledge.* Unpublished manuscript, Hong Kong University of Science and Technology, 2000.

Hooyman, N., and Kiyak, H. A. *Social Gerontology: An Interdisciplinary Perspective.* Boston: Allyn & Bacon, 2005.

Kagitcibasi, C. "Individualism and Collectivism." In J. W. Berry, M. H. Segall, and C. Kagitcibasi (eds.), *Handbook of Cross-Cultural Psychology*, Vol. 3: *Social Behavior and Applications*, 1–51. Boston: Allyn & Bacon, 1997.

Staudinger, U. M., Marsiske, M., and Baltes, P. B. "Resilience and Reserve Capacity in Later Adulthood: Potentials and Limits of Development Across the Life Span." In D. Cicchetti and D. Cohen (eds.), *Vol. 2: Developmental Psychopathology: Risk, Disorder, and Adaptation*, 801–847. New York: Wiley, 1995.

Steen, T. W., and Mazonde, G. N. "Ngaka ya setswana, ngaka ya sekgoa, or Both? Health Seeking Behavior in Batswana with Pulmonary Tuberculosis." *Social Sciences and Medicine*, 1999, *48*, 163–172.

Strehler, B. L. "Genetic Instability as the Primary Cause of Human Aging." *Experimental Gerontology*, 1986, *21*, 283.

Triandis, H. C. *Individualism and Collectivism.* Boulder, Colo.: Westview, 1995.

Triandis, H. C., and Bhawuk, D. P.S. "Culture Theory and the Meaning of Relatedness." In P. C. Earley and M. Erez (eds.), *New Perspectives on International Industrial/Organizational Psychology*, 13–52. San Francisco, Calif.: The New Lexington Press, 1997.

U.S. Census Bureau. *World Population Profile:*2002 [http://www.census.gov/] 2007.

Westerhof, G. J., Katzko, M. W., Dittmann-Kohli, F., and Hayslip, B. "Life Contexts and Health-related Selves in Old Age." *Journal of Aging Studies*, 2001, *15*, 105–127.

Whitbourne, S. K. *The Aging Body.* New York: Springer, 1985.

PART

2

COUNTRIES WITH HIGH RATES OF LONGEVITY

CHAPTER

HEALTHY AGING IN DENMARK?

BJARNE HASTRUP

Adult Danes commonly believe that the elderly in Denmark today have better functional capacity and more scope for development than before. We say that seventy-year-olds today have the health and strength of the sixty-year-olds of twenty-five years ago. Most people in this age group believe that they are in better health and have more energy and better opportunities than was the case for their parents and grandparents. This general belief is supported by the fact that the Danish life expectancy has increased, but in fact it has not increased as much as in the countries with which Denmark is normally compared.

DENMARK AND THE DANES

Denmark covers an area of forty-three thousand square kilometers and has a population of 5.4 million people, of which 15 percent are aged sixty-five or over and 4 percent are aged eighty or over. Of those sixty-five and over, women account for 57 percent. With increasing age, there is an increasing overrepresentation of women.

The number of people in the sixty-five and over age group doubled in Denmark between 1900 to 1975, but in the twenty-five years between 1982 and 2006 the proportion of elderly people remained almost constant. The proportion of people aged sixty-five years and over is, however, increasing again, and in the decade from 2010 the population of elderly is projected to grow by more than 20 percent when the baby boom generation reaches the age of retirement. By 2035, the sixty-five and over age group will account for a little more than 25 percent of the population.

The proportion of those over eighty will also see a sharp increase, but this growth will manifest itself following the growth in the number of sixty-five- to seventy-nine-year-olds. Though the growth in the proportion of sixty-five to seventy-nine-year-olds will occur from 2006 to 2021, the proportion of people aged eighty years and over will not see any significant increase before 2020. In 2006, the eighty and over age group accounted for only 4 percent of the population. This proportion will increase to approximately 5 percent in 2020, and by 2050 the eighty and over age group is forecasted to account for 10 percent of the population.

WELFARE SOCIETY: THE BASIS FOR HEALTH

During the twentieth century, Denmark and the other Scandinavian countries developed a so-called welfare society. In Denmark, there has been a general political consensus that there should be free access to a number of fundamental social benefits. This includes, for example, the right to financial support for those who for social, health, or other reasons cannot provide for themselves; a public health service with easy and equal access for all; and—generally—free and equal access to education.

The general objective of Danish aging policy—and social politics as such—is to ease the individual's existence and improve the quality of life. It is based on the general principles of continuity in the individual's life, the use of personal resources, and autonomy and influence over one's own circumstances—including the various options that are open to the individual. The foundation of the welfare society is that tax-financed social benefits are made more or less freely available for the citizens and that a financial redistribution is taking place in the form of transferrals via the tax system to the weakest.

PENSIONS

The Danish pensions system generally consists of a tax-financed old-age pension paid to people of sixty-five years and over, a supplementary pension for people formerly engaged in active employment (the Labor Market Supplementary Pension Fund—ATP), labor market pensions based on collective agreements, and private pension schemes. The old-age pension is independent of previous income, and for 40 to 45 percent of pensioners the old-age pension is the only or the most important source of income.

Pensioners whose financial circumstances are particularly difficult may be entitled to health allowances, heating allowances, and a personal allowance.

HOUSING

It is the needs of the individual, rather than the type of accommodation, that determine the type of assistance provided. The great majority of elderly people in Denmark live in ordinary housing. Only a small proportion live in nursing homes: 2 percent of people aged sixty-five to seventy-nine and 14 percent aged eighty and over. Housing benefits for pensioners—pensioners' rent allowance—are available for rented, cooperative, and owner-occupied dwellings and are offered as a subsidy, or partly or fully as a loan, based on household income, capital, the rent, flat size, and the number of household members.

DISABLED PEOPLE

In Denmark, the local authority

- Provides free advisory and counseling services

- Offers domestic help and personal care to people who are unable to carry out daily tasks as a result of permanently reduced physical or mental functional capacity

- Provides technical aids when such devices may considerably relieve the problems faced by people with reduced functional capacity in their daily lives

- Pays for the homes of people with disabilities to be adapted to make the home better suited for the person concerned

- Offers every person who has reached the age of seventy-five a home call at least twice a year

- Provides nursing homes

- Provides retraining and maintenance training (rehabilitation)

Transportation improvements are needed for people with disabilities. DaneAge has carried out a survey showing that quality of life is closely linked to the ability to get around—to maintain an active life even though one has physical problems.

Transport is crucial for leading an active life and preventing social isolation and loneliness. Denmark has one of the highest employment rates in the world, which makes it very difficult for relatives to contribute significantly to the care of the elderly. Older people, like everyone else, need to get out; they want to take care of themselves for as long as possible, and they are afraid of being dependent on others.

THE HEALTH SERVICE

Denmark has a health service that is primarily (83 percent) publicly run and financed. By law, there must be easy and equal access to the health service. A number of services—for example, treatment in public hospitals and at the clinics of general practitioners—are free for the patient. The key element of the health service is the general practitioner (GP), also called the family doctor, because he or she is the family's primary health professional. The GP is the gatekeeper for access to examinations and treatment in hospitals and at specialist practices.

The local authorities offer a number of free health services, in terms of both prevention and treatment. These services include regular supervision carried out by specially trained nurses, regular medical examinations and vaccination of small children, and health services at schools and workplaces. Elderly people also have the option of house calls and treatment in their homes by nurses, such as wound care, dosing and injection of medicine, and so on, and assistance with personal needs and practical daily activities.

In Danish society, a large number of preventive measures are incorporated into the everyday lives of its citizens. These preventive measures stand out in particular in the "technical field" (where the individual citizen does not need to make any decision). The following areas are covered by regulations and public supervision: ensuring that toys are not harmful to children, inspecting electrical installations, traffic and vehicles, buildings and housing, the water and food supply, and so on. For the elderly, preventing falls inside and outside buildings is one of the most important preventive measures.

Some of the social and health measures consist of public supervision; for example, of nursing homes for the elderly. The legislation and the public supervision of workplaces and working conditions are critical for maintaining public health. The purpose of the legislation is to create a "safe and healthy work environment that at all times matches the technical and social development in society." The legislation is accompanied by government supervision of workplaces. The Danish Working Environment Authority can close down a workplace that is considered to be dangerous—and it will be closed down!

There has, on the other hand, been political reluctance to regulate conditions and factors relating to each individual person's lifestyle and options. In spite of the fact that the Danish population ranks among those countries with the highest smoking rate, smoking restrictions in public places have been introduced too late and too hesitantly. People are, for example, still allowed to smoke in restaurants. The primary purpose of food inspections is to protect the population against acute illnesses caused by food. There are no restrictions on food of poor nutritional quality. The only restriction on the sale of alcohol—and tobacco—is that it may not be sold to children under sixteen. Apart from general public information, exercise is by and large a private matter.

LIFE EXPECTANCY: DENMARK IS LAGGING BEHIND

Life expectancy can be seen as a rough measure of the state of health of a population. In the first half of the twentieth century, Danish men and women had a life expectancy among the highest of all the countries with which Denmark is normally compared—as well as one of the highest in the world. Since the 1970s, life expectancy in Denmark has, however, not seen the same increase as that seen in many other countries. In the 1971–1975 period, Denmark ranked fourth and sixth for men and women, respectively, among twenty comparable countries. In the 1996–2001 period, the Danish ranking fell to sixteenth and twentieth, respectively.

To politicians and administrators in almost every field who were used to seeing Denmark as one of the world's leading countries, it came as a great shock to have to acknowledge that Denmark, in terms of life expectancy, had in a short period moved from the top to the bottom. The initial response was to launch an investigation to identify the cause for this situation.

The subsequent report confirmed that the Danish life expectancy had stagnated or not seen the same increase as in other countries. The main reason for this was a higher mortality in the thirty-five to sixty-four age group, most pronounced for women compared to other countries. There was hardly any excess mortality among the elderly. The excess mortality was due not to one single or a few diseases, but to a wide range of causes, particularly lung cancer, chronic bronchitis, suicide, liver cirrhosis (men), heart disease, and breast cancer (women). An analysis of the excess mortality showed that the social differences in mortality had increased since the 1970s, probably because of the marginalization of small segments of the population. In addition, no relationship was found between living conditions and the stagnating life expectancy. Regarding lifestyle, a possible relationship was found between the stagnating life expectancy and smoking. Danish women entered the labor market early and in large numbers and have thus, to a large extent, adopted the lifestyle of men, which includes, for example, smoking. This is considered to be the reason why the lung cancer rate among women is increasing, but the rate for men shows a slight decrease. It has been determined that there is no relationship or only a small one between health expenditure and life expectancy in relatively rich countries like Denmark. The Life Expectancy Committee found significant social differences in mortality, in particular among men, and there was a tendency toward an increase in social differences. The mortality rate was highest among recipients of early retirement pension, recipients of cash benefits, unemployed people, poorly educated people, and unskilled workers.

For the elderly (sixty-five and over), the mortality rate for women had fallen in the first half of the preceding fifty years and has remained at the same level since then. The mortality rate for elderly men has not changed much during the fifty-year period. The results of an investigation of Danish women born in the 1915–1945 period indicate a high prevalence of smoking to be the main explanation for the relatively low life expectancy of this group.

In the ten-year period from 1995, the Danish life expectancy increased by 0.3 years annually for men and 0.2 years for women. However, Danish life expectancy is still below that of the OECD average and much lower than in the other Scandinavian countries. An investigation of mortality in the 1995–1999 period shows that women with little education experienced the lowest increase in life expectancy; the increase was highest for men with intermediate level and higher education. Between 2000–2004, life expectancy in Denmark went up by 0.7 years, whereas in neighboring Sweden— which already had a higher life expectancy—it increased by 1.4 years.

DIFFERENT GOVERNMENTS' APPROACH TO PUBLIC HEALTH

The problems concerning Danish life expectancy were already known in 1989, but at that time there was no political will to address these issues. The government was confident that its 1989 prevention program could solve everything through more information, more coordination between ministries and private organizations combating diseases, more collaboration at the local level, and so on. These initiatives did not cost anything and required no political will or organizational changes, so nothing changed in the 1990s.

However, a more detailed investigation of Denmark's problems with a stagnating life expectancy in the mid-1990s spurred the government to establish a public health program in 1999, inspired by the World Health Organization's Health for All by the Year 2000 strategy. The Social Democratic-Social Liberal coalition government focused on health policy goals such as equality in health, long life expectancy, high quality of life, and prevention rather than treatment. Against this background, a number of short-term targets were set up as well as indicators for assessing whether target were being fulfilled. The elderly were covered by the Public Health Program with the following overall objective: the elderly should be provided with services that aim to maintain their social, physical, and psychological abilities for as long as possible. A number of relatively specific targets were set up vis-à-vis the initiatives directed at the elderly; for example, training of GPs to introduce more preventive measures for the elderly, improved rehabilitation following diseases, more opportunities for sport and exercise for the elderly, prevention of falls, and influenza vaccinations for those over sixty-five.

The 1999 Public Health Program was discontinued following the change of government in 2001, and the new Conservative-Liberal government prepared a new public health program. A significant difference was that inequality as a basic problem in the state of the population's health was now reduced to a minor problem. The elderly are included in the program when discussing "common challenges" such as physical activity, nutrition, loneliness, and the preventive initiatives on the part of GPs. In addition to this, other problems are discussed in the program, such as the prevention of falls. The objectives set up are less binding than was the case in the previous public health program; another difference is that the new program focuses on eight widespread diseases.

One overall conclusion is that the three prevention and public health plans have had limited effect in terms of implemented and evaluated preventive measures. Prevention—for all ages—is still implemented without the necessary political commitment, both at national and local government level.

STATE OF HEALTH OF THE ELDERLY AT THE TURN OF THE MILLENNIUM

Every five years, Denmark's national research institute for public health (under the Danish National Institute of Social Research) carries out a survey of the health of the population using questionnaires and interviews. The survey for 2000 has been published and the health of the elderly is briefly described in this section.

A person's own assessment of his or her health is a very good predictor for mortality and morbidity. Sixty-five percent of Danish men age sixty-seven to seventy-nine state that they are in good or very good health. This proportion is a little lower for women (59.4 percent). For the eighty and over age group, the corresponding percentages are 58.8 and 49 percent. The period from 1987 to 2000 shows a slight increase from approximately 59 to approximately 62 percent of people age sixty-seven or over who assess their health to be good or very good.

The institute's surveys have previously shown a connection between a physically stressful working environment and a poor health self-assessment, and other surveys have shown that working environment conditions are a significant factor in the development of poor health self-assessments over time, a development that is most pronounced in the lowest social classes. In the sixty-seven to seventy-nine and the eighty and over age groups, 67 and 42 percent, respectively, state they are generally well enough to do what they want. For the sixty-seven and over group, the proportion has, however, seen only a slight increase from 1987 to 2000.

From 1987 to 2000, there was a considerable increase in the proportion of those sixty and over with good mobility, from 53 to 64 percent, as well as a considerable improvement in the dental state of the elderly. For those aged sixty-seven and over, the proportion who have at least twenty of their own teeth has gone up from approximately 10 to almost 30 percent.

The same period, however, saw an increase in the number of people suffering from a long-term illness. This also applies to the elderly, among whom approximately 60 percent of people age sixty-seven or over had a long-term illness in 2000. The dominating illnesses among women are musculoskeletal diseases (approximately 29 percent), followed by cardiovascular diseases (approximately 17 percent). Among men, the rates of musculoskeletal diseases and cardiovascular diseases are almost identical, with approximately 17 and 20 percent, respectively.

If it were possible to eliminate cardiovascular diseases in Denmark, this would increase the remaining life expectancy by four years for sixty-five-year-olds. Eliminating forms of cancer would in the same way increase the remaining life expectancy by 2.4 years. Eliminating musculoskeletal diseases would not increase the remaining life expectancy, but for men it would mean, on average, one year of that life free of a long-term stressful disease. For women, it would mean 2.4 years of life free of a long-term stressful disease.

INITIATIVES OF SPECIAL IMPORTANCE FOR THE ELDERLY

The rehabilitation services Denmark offers to sick and weak people are a good example of the slow progress in this area. The obligation to offer rehabilitation services has for many years been divided between local authorities and counties, according to relatively unclear rules. As a result, neither local authorities nor counties felt obliged to offer rehabilitation. Following a clarification of the rules, it was stipulated in 2001 that patients who require rehabilitation after hospitalization should be given a rehabilitation plan that can form the basis for their continued rehabilitation. In 2005 a survey showed that only two out of three patients in medical departments who required rehabilitation were provided with a plan. Another survey showed that rehabilitation plans were registered for only 11 percent of patients treated for hip fractures and for 2 percent of patients treated for chronic obstructive pulmonary disease (COPD). Even though the figures do not agree, they show that the rules on rehabilitation plans are not observed, and the uncertain figures alone indicate that the infrastructure for issuing rehabilitation plans—that is, ensuring that they are prepared and registered—is not in place. At the same time, there is a need for enhanced rehabilitation efforts on the part of local authorities.

THE ELDERLY AND PREVENTION

The elderly present a tremendous opportunity for prevention and health promotion, with positive results quickly apparent. It is important that local authorities identify elderly citizens with special needs for physical training and other support before they become too frail. Society should focus on the following tasks:

- Providing rapid rehabilitation, so that elderly people regain their mobility as soon as possible after an illness

- Stimulating continuous activity and breaking the vicious circle of inactivity

- Providing information for citizens, GPs, and health professionals about rehabilitation options for the elderly

- Communicating information about fitness training and on lending material, such as videos and DVDs with training programs, which are easy to follow at home

- Communicating information about training that can be carried out during hospitalization and prevent the deterioration of physical fitness and strength during hospitalization

It is also important to motivate the elderly to eat a healthier diet. Healthy food plans for the oldest and weakest citizens may contribute to preventing deterioration of their health and to a higher quality of life, better mobility, and thus more independence. There is a need for

- A food policy for the municipal food service for the elderly

- Training of social and health assistants and professionals in the importance of food

- Offering of group meals for weak elderly people

- Nutritional therapy

It is never too late to start good habits and improve one's living conditions. It is possible to retain relative independence at a very old age despite various impairments. A number of training studies have also shown that it is never too late to improve one's physical condition.

Preventive and health promoting efforts must be placed on the political agenda, and more funds must be allocated to this area.

SOCIAL INEQUALITY IN HEALTH

Denmark is one of the countries in the world with the least social inequality. The Danish welfare society aims to create more equality in terms of the living standards of its citizens. There are, however, still large health differences between the different social groups. As a general rule, people with less formal education and lower incomes have poorer health. This applies to both morbidity and mortality.

Living conditions, lifestyle, and psychosocial factors influence the social inequality in health. European studies show that there is considerable social inequality in health in Europe, and that social differences are not being reduced, but rather are increasing, and that this is also the case in Denmark. Those with the least resources in a country have poorer health than those with the most resources.

One of the goals of the Danish government's public health program "Healthy Throughout Life" is to increase the number of years with a good quality of life (QALY = quality-adjusted life years). A new Danish survey shows significant social differences in remaining life expectancy and quality-adjusted life years for thirty-year-old men and women when considering educational level; this is most pronounced when measuring the health quality of the remaining life expectancy. It is thus still relevant to improve the living conditions and habits of those in the worst social position.

Social inequality in health in Denmark also manifests itself in population surveys in terms of self-assessed health and in the lifestyle areas of smoking, physical activity, diet, and alcohol.

IMMIGRATION

In the forty years between 1966 and 2006, Denmark received immigrants and refugees from a number of different countries with cultural patterns different from those of the Danes. There is general agreement that the integration of these new Danish citizens into society has been less than successful. The health of the ethnic groups in Denmark is generally poorer than that of the native-born Danes. There are particular higher morbidity rates for diabetes, cardiovascular diseases, mental disorders, and dental diseases. Ethnic minorities use the services of the health service more often than native-born Danes. With the high morbidity among immigrants, there is a considerable and growing need for health and care services for which Danish society is badly prepared.

NEED FOR DOCUMENTATION

Though it may seem obvious, it is a relatively new concept in Denmark that planning in the health service be based on knowledge of the health situation, and the work performed be based on documented knowledge. In light of this, it is no surprise that necessary knowledge is still lacking in a number of areas. Denmark does have a good statistical basis in most areas, but in the health area the purpose of the statistics has been first and foremost to shed light on production issues such as admissions, bed-days, and staff. It is no coincidence that the recording of causes of death for the Danish population is backlogged by several years, in a period of intense discussion in Denmark about the stagnating or only slowly increasing life expectancy. Data on the health of the population have been used to a greater extent for research purposes than for political action.

Starting in 2007, after an administrative reform, there have been signs that many of the country's municipalities will prepare health profiles for their area. This will provide a good starting point for continued work with health aspects, including prevention, and will place health problems on the agenda. It would be advantageous if the health profiles were made using a shared template that allows comparison of health-related aspects between municipalities and over time.

FUTURE CHALLENGES

If life expectancy is used as a rough measure of the state of health in society, Denmark will, at its current rate of development, lag more and more behind the other European countries. Denmark is the last but one on the OECD's list of growth in life expectancy from 2000 to 2004. In other words, something has to be done in Denmark, both in the health service and—perhaps especially so—in society and in the private lives of its citizens.

The health service is facing a major challenge in terms of caring for the large and growing group of elderly people. The growth in the number of elderly people will result in a marked growth in the number of citizens with chronic diseases. For example, the number of people with type 2 diabetes is increasing dramatically; with a growing proportion of the population suffering from this illness, the coming years will see many more suffering its effects and complications—conditions that demand a great deal of the national health service.

A Danish survey has attempted to simulate the projected increase in the number of elderly people and the costs for their treatment and care to the year 2040 under different assumptions—including one in which the sixty-five and over group will increase by 100 percent in the period. It is estimated that society in the same period will become only 80 percent wealthier. This means that the costs for treatment and care in the period (only) will grow from 3.85 percent of the gross national product (GNP) to 4.26 percent. In one of several scenarios, attempts have been made to calculate what would happen if there is a change of behavior in the population and people started following the health advice on diet, smoking, alcohol, and exercise. This would result in even more elderly people by 2040—and even more healthy elderly people—than would be the case if there is no change in behavior. It would, however, at the same time result in an increase in treatment and care expenses, from 3.85 percent of GNP to 4.38 percent.

Another Danish survey shows that personal mobility is the variable that explains most of the variation in public expenses for different individuals. The more restricted a person's mobility, measured as the ability to carry out a number of everyday activities, the higher the costs.

TREATMENT OF PATIENTS WITH CHRONIC DISEASES

The Danish National Board of Health has prepared a plan for the future treatment of the chronically ill. Its aim is twofold: to strengthen the patient's own care and to place the main focus of the treatment of the chronically ill outside the hospitals. To achieve this, each individual patient with a chronic disease should, through offers of patient training and rehabilitation, be allowed to live with and handle his or her own disease, possibly also taking responsibility for monitoring and adjusting treatment.

The health service must be organized so that across the various areas of expertise it is capable of providing seamless services, whereby caregivers and patients—that is, all parties involved—on country and municipality levels share the same information and agree on a particular action based on that information. This requires a definition of good treatment and a good course of treatment, and clearly defined roles in patient treatment in every single part of the health service. At the same time, we must monitor whether this is working as presumed.

Steps have been taken to implement parts of the plan. Other parts still require the development of strategies for collaboration, treatment, course of treatment, and monitoring. As of this writing, the Danish health service is experiencing significant problems with the development of a shared electronic patient record—a basic tool for ensuring a coherent course of treatment of, for example, the chronically ill. It is doubtful whether the Danish health authorities and the Danish health service are prepared to take the overall treatment of the chronically ill further than the planning stage.

It is not yet possible to evaluate whether the plan for future treatment of the chronically ill by strengthening the patient's own care ("empowerment") will lead to a real improvement of the state of health of the chronically ill or, on the contrary, lead to poorer treatment—and thus poorer health—for this group. The plan assumes that partnerships are established—for example, between sports associations and educational associations—to implement the plan content.

STILL "MACHINE ERROR" THINKING

The Danish health service is still predominantly characterized by "machine error" thinking. There is a lack of focus on the whole person, which would entail a holistic approach and a seamless course of treatment. An example of this is elderly hip fracture patients. At many departments of orthopedic surgery, many elderly patients risk having to wait several days for their operation, during which period they have fasted while waiting to be anesthetized. The surgical departments are not good at preventing, identifying, and treating acute mental disorders that many elderly patients manifest. After the operation, many patients find that they are discharged with minimal rehabilitation. According to the objectives set up, 90 percent of patients must be screened for nutritional risk within two days. In all of Denmark, this was carried out for only 18 percent of patients in 2004–2005. There are also standards covering the assessment of patients' activities of daily living (ADLs) before the fracture and before discharge after treatment. This has been carried out in only 56 and 50 percent of cases, respectively. There is no national monitoring of the patients' pre- and post-fracture functional capacity. Such shortcomings in the overall treatment course affect elderly patients the most because they have a higher risk of complications in general and of complications that lead to a permanent loss of functional capacity.

There is no point in wondering whether surgeons or other specialists are more interested in the "technical" aspects of the operation—repairing the fracture—than in whether the patient's functional capacity will be as good as before the fracture. What is important is that treatments in the entire health service must be optimized from the patient's point of view. It is the responsibility of the health authorities and the professional environments to ensure that everyone understands that the main objective is the patient's optimal outcome after treatment.

MORE PROACTIVE ATTITUDE TO TREATMENT OF THE ELDERLY

The health service should assume a more proactive role in the treatment of the elderly, not least in light of the more gentle treatment methods that are being introduced in all areas. With increasing age, the individual often experiences more illnesses as a consequence of reduced resistance, reduced physical and sensory capacity, and so on. The impairments that most often affect the long-living elderly are reduced mobility, a tendency to falls, dementia, and incontinence.

It is critical that health promotion, prevention, and rehabilitation are included in the ordinary activities of the health service and the social services, not just as projects that are implemented by highly committed individuals and then disappear. It is also important that efforts aimed at the elderly are implemented in collaboration between the relevant parts of the health service and the social services.

THE ELDERLY MEDICAL PATIENT

For decades in Denmark, elderly patients have experienced special problems in medical departments. The most visible problems include overcrowding—some patients are placed in hospital corridors. Overcrowding is normally a winter and summer phenomenon: in winter because many elderly patients are admitted suffering from respiratory diseases, and in summer because the staff is on holiday and some departments are temporarily closed down. Overcrowding is, of course, a strain on the entire system, and treatment of the elderly usually deals only with the specific reason for admission to the hospital and does not include other conditions that the elderly patient could benefit from having treated at the same time. DaneAge and a number of health professional organizations have for a number of years—so far in vain—asked for an overall national action plan for elderly medical patients.

RECRUITMENT PROBLEMS

In the future the social and health sector will face a great recruitment challenge. As of this writing, there is a shortage of doctors and nurses in Denmark, and there are signs that it is becoming difficult to recruit nursing staff for elder care. Elder care is one of the most stressful and exhausting areas of work. Relatively speaking, this group has the highest rate of early retirement pension recipients and staff who leave their profession early.

The recruitment problems show that one can solve problems in society by actively working with health aspects—in this case, the working conditions of the employees. In addition to making the working conditions easier, both physically and in terms of stress, it is important to improve the status of this work in society. This can be achieved through training, better pay, and workers gaining more influence over their own working situations. Training would also provide the nursing home area the required professional level, which would benefit the elderly.

NEED FOR CHANGES IN SOCIETY

Changes are also required outside of the health service and in the private lives of citizens to improve health, increase life expectancy, and reduce the burden on society caused by illness. Danes spend a lot of their time working, and the time spent by a family at work is still increasing. At the same time, the pace of work is fast and also increasing. As a result, many people want to leave the labor market earlier. At the same time, Danes, as a group, have a relatively unconcerned view of their pathogenic lifestyle: unhealthy food, smoking, alcohol, and too little exercise. The Danish Folketing recently passed legislation to counter the burden from the increasing number of elderly and to ensure an adequate labor force in the future. This is being achieved by postponing the option of leaving the labor market at age sixty with a pension-like benefit from the state.

From a health perspective, it is strange that society has not looked into the possibility of improving public health by focusing more aggressively on better living conditions and a better lifestyle. This would potentially lead to a smaller burden caused by ill elderly patients and helped to reduce the number of people leaving the labor market for health reasons.

HEALTH ASPECTS MUST FORM PART OF DECISION MAKING

Healthy aging is a process that starts when a human being is born, or even earlier, and it lasts a lifetime. As one of the richest, best-educated, and best-organized societies, Denmark should be able to have one of the highest life expectancy rates in the world, and its citizens should enjoy many years without a stressful disease. Denmark's lagging behind in terms of life expectancy and its slow progress indicates a lack of success in this endeavor so far.

Danish society is to a large extent driven by economic thinking using economic incentives and barriers. Control tools in the form of current economic key figures in all relevant aspects of society are available on line. Yet as far as health aspects are concerned, relevant statistics are available only after several years' delay and are also inadequate.

As a precondition for healthy aging, the political system needs to be trusted to ensure that Danes can look forward to more healthy years by also taking health-related aspects into consideration when deciding how to run society.

CHAPTER

7

CHALLENGES OF LONGEVITY IN FRANCE: THE INTERNATIONAL LONGEVITY CENTRE-FRANCE PERSPECTIVE

FRANÇOISE FORETTE AND MARIE-ANNE BRIEU

Longevity is a remarkable venture at the individual, social, and national level as long as the aging population remains healthy and active. It is indisputable that tomorrow's population will be old and female. But tomorrow's population will be healthy if we promote prevention of age-related diseases, and it will be wealthy if the aging population is allowed to fully take part in the economic circuit.

Before addressing the French issues, let us consider the world population: it will grow from 6.1 billion in 2000 to 8.1 billion in 2050, mainly in strongly emerging nations (India, Africa, and Asia). In contrast, in the most developed nations, the European,

North American, and Japanese populations will decrease. So will the Chinese population, although it will nonetheless stay one of the largest in the world.

All populations share at least these characteristics: a progressive increase in their dependency ratio, defined by the ratio of those aged sixty-five and over to those aged fifteen to sixty-four.

In France, more than 20 percent of the 62.9 million inhabitants are aged sixty and over. The mean life expectancy at birth is continuously progressing, up to nearly seventy-seven years for men and nearly eighty-four for women. As in other nations, there will be a continuous increase in the populations over sixty-five, seventy-five, and eighty-five until 2020, but the percentage of the population under the age of sixty, though decreasing, will remain rather high, probably thanks to the maintained fertility ratio of 1.9, one of the highest in Europe (see Figure 7.1).

The female advantage over males in life expectancy remains nearly universal, and the gap widened in the twentieth century. A precise explanation of the gender difference is not clear because of the interplay of biological and social factors (Kinsella and Velkoff, 2002). But this difference explains the predominance of women in the elderly world population—237 million females and 182 million males. It must be noted that a majority of elderly women live in developing countries.

The same trend is observed in France: at each age and period, the mean life expectancy is significantly higher in females than in males. But there seems to be a slight stagnation in the increase for women, probably because of the increase in lung cancers in female smokers. Nevertheless, the demographic pyramid clearly shows the predominance of women in the older population.

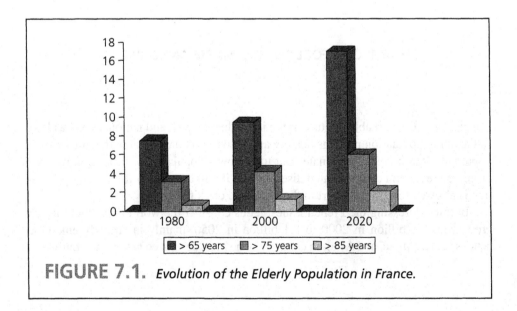

FIGURE 7.1. *Evolution of the Elderly Population in France.*

All people do not equally enjoy this excellent health status: for example, in France, there is a five-year difference in life expectancy at age sixty between white-collar and blue-collar workers. But strikingly, the difference is less marked in the female population—only three years. There are many reasons for the risk of mortality of unemployed men, threefold that of the employed population; it is only twofold in women.

The place where one lives may have an influence: the life expectancy at birth is five years lower for men in the north of France than in the Paris region. For women it is only 2.7 years lower, as if women are protected against a number of extrinsic factors (see Table 7.1).

The absolute number of frail elderly needing assistance or long-term care, either at home or in an institution, seems high—in France, it is probably close to one million individuals—but it must be emphasized that the percentage is low: only 6 percent of the population over sixty-five and 2 percent of the population between ages sixty and sixty-nine suffer from loss of autonomy because of disabling diseases. This percentage increases with age, but it remains rather low until very advanced ages (see Table 7.2).

The rate of loss of autonomy is higher in women than in men at very advanced ages. Only 30 percent of the males are dependent after age ninety versus 46 percent of women.

To increase the rate of autonomy, we must solve a tricky equation:

1. The aging population is increasing worldwide, particularly the female population.

2. Disability increases with age.

3. But disability decreases at each age (people at each age are less dependent than twenty years previous).

4. So the increase in disability because of the aging of the population must be counterbalanced by the decrease of disability at each age, so that the number of disabled elderly is stable or reduced progressively.

TABLE 7.1. **Mean Life Expectancy at Birth in France, Comparison of Two Regions.**

Region	Men	Women	All
North of France	72.7	81.0	76.8
Paris and surroundings	77.1	83.4	80.2

Source: Institut National de la Statistique et des Études Économiques, 2004.

TABLE 7.2. **Senior Population Aged Sixty and Over in France: 6.63 Percent Loss of Autonomy.**

Age	Males	Females	Total
60–69	2.19	1.95	2.06
70–79	4.99	4.35	4.65
80–89	13.40	19.85	17.69
90+	29.31	46.45	42.55
Total	5.00	7.80	6.63

Source: Institut National de la Statistique et des Études Économiques, 2000.

This is an objective that can be reached if prevention is strongly promoted. When considering prevention, it is important to realize that health status is a heterogeneous process at the individual and population levels. Two types of factors, genetic and environmental, may be involved in this heterogeneity (Carnes and Olshanski, 2001).

There are extensive variations at the genetic level. According to a Danish study of twins, the genetic variance component to life span was estimated to account for about 25 percent of total life span variation (Herskind and others, 1996). There is also an accumulation of genetic mutations within the somatic cells over the course of a lifetime, contributing to the wide variation in health status and age at death (Finch and Ruvkun, 2001).

Environmental factors may be more important because they are modifiable. These encompass medical progress, particularly in terms of prevention and access to care, and the socioeconomic factors responsible for within-country and between-country differences. When one looks at the differences in mean life expectancy in different countries and continents, the role of socioeconomic levels is abundantly clear. In some developed countries, life expectancy doubled at the end of the twentieth century. Life expectancy at birth exceeds seventy-eight years in twenty-eight countries. But deep inequalities persist. In 2004, the life expectancy at birth was 82.3 in Japan, 80.6 in Sweden, 79.7 in France, 78.7 in the UK, 77.6 in the United States, 71.9 in China, 70.2 in Brazil, 64.9 in Russia, 62.2 in India, 50.5 in Kenya, 41.4 in Malawi, and 35.7 in Zimbabwe (World Health Organization, 2004).

To increase life expectancy and promote healthy aging, lifestyle, prevention, and medical progress are key determinants. The different components of healthy lifestyles are well known: education throughout life, healthy nutrition, moderate and prolonged physical activity, mental activity, professional and leisure activity, personal commitment, and responsibility. The challenge is to develop in citizens both health literacy and preventive consciousness.

Most age-related diseases can be related to modifiable risk factors and are amenable to prevention—cardiovascular diseases, strokes, osteoporosis and fractures, diminished hearing and vision, cancers, malnutrition, and depression. Medical progress (and chips, cell therapy, biotechnologies) will accelerate the efficacy of prevention approaches. It is never too soon, never too late: osteoporosis can be prevented in teenagers by increasing physical activity and calcium intake in girls. Fighting obesity and smoking in boys may prevent coronary diseases in the forties, fifties, and later. Wearing sunglasses when sailing or skiing may postpone cataracts.

The role of young parents, particularly mothers, is essential, but prevention takes a lifelong perspective and must be continued throughout life. Take the example of hypertension: age-specific relevance of usual blood pressure to vascular mortality was addressed in a meta-analysis of individual data for one million adults in sixty-one prospective studies (Levington and others, 2002). This meta-analysis shows that high blood pressure is still related to cardiovascular complications at higher ages. The randomized trials demonstrated that treatment of hypertension significantly reduces the incidence of strokes and other cardiovascular complications before and after age sixty. In the meta-analysis by Insua (Insua, 1994), the relative risk for strokes is decreased by 35 percent, for cardiovascular complication by 25 percent, and for all causes of mortality by 12 percent. Even if it does not prolong life at more advanced ages, antihypertensive treatment might preserve quality of life by preventing distressing, disabling diseases (Gueyffier and others, 1999).

Prevention of cardiovascular diseases remains the privilege of the most developed countries. A recent WHO report for Europe, *The Health Status of the European Union* (World Health Organization, 2003) shows that the longevity gap between Western and Eastern Europe is increasing. People in Western Europe may expect to live six years longer than people in Central Europe and ten years longer than people of the Newly Independent States born after the dissolution of the Soviet Union. In Eastern Europe, cardiovascular diseases represent 60 percent of the mortality causes, compared to 35 percent in Western Europe. The dramatic difference in cardiovascular mortality between East and West underscores the absolute need for cardiovascular disease prevention in all countries.

Even dementia may be prevented. Given the increase with age of Alzheimer's disease and related disorders and the twofold prevalence in women, prevention has become a striking challenge. A number of risk factors have been identified, including, besides age and sex, the level of education, genetic factors (history and genotypes), and vascular factors. Some of them cannot be modified, but vascular risk factors and—in particular but not only—hypertension may be the target of prevention trials. Two randomized studies (Forette and others, 1998; Forette and others, 2002; Tzourio and others, 2003) demonstrated a reduction in the incidence of dementia by lowering blood pressure. In contrast, prevention using estrogens, anti-inflammatory agents, antioxidants, and cholesterol-lowering agents remains to be confirmed.

Is it possible to go further and act on the cause of Alzheimer's disease? Based on the amyloid hypothesis, two approaches are being tested: (1) the development of beta and secretase inhibitors and (2) beta amyloid immunization. The original work by

Dale Schenk (Shenk and others, 1996) on transgenic ADAPP mice engineered to produce human A beta amyloid protein produced spectacular results. The transgenic mice in the placebo group produce hippocampal amyloid deposition, neuritic plaques, and plaque-associated astrocytosis comparable to one of the two Alzheimer lesions. Mice vaccinated with the human amyloid protein at six weeks do not develop Alzheimer lesions.

The first Phase 2 trial of the amyloid vaccine was stopped because of severe side effects. Seventeen of the three hundred patients developed an immune encephalitis. However, a recent paper by Nicoll in *Nature Medicine* (Nicoll and others, 2003) shows that the immune response generated against the peptide elicited clearance of A beta plaques in the brain of a vaccinated patient, deceased of encephalitis (Gilman and others, 2005). Extensive areas of cortex were devoid of plaques. Other trials, based on fragments of the A beta protein, may prove that it is possible to produce the same effect without the immune inflammation.

All these studies show that finding the key to Alzheimer prevention is possibly not too far off. This is a fantastic hope for the future.

The randomized studies as well as observational statistics show that prevention works: in the period from 1970 to 1997, major health gains evidenced by a significant reduction of premature mortality were observed. Premature mortality by ischemic heart disease was reduced by 42.3 percent, stroke by 57 percent, and bronchitis and emphysema by 73.9 percent (see Table 7.3).

TABLE 7.3. Health Gains over the Past Three Decades.

Health problem (per 100,000 inhabitants)	EU average gain for the period 1970–1997
Life expectancy at birth (years)	+8.4 years
Premature mortality by cancer	−12.0 %
Premature mortality by cancer of the lung	+6.0 %
Premature mortality by cancer of the female breast	+2.2 %
Premature mortality by ischemic heart disease	−42.3 %
Premature mortality by stroke	−57.0 %
Premature mortality by diabetes mellitus	−35.4 %
Premature mortality by asthma, bronchitis, and emphysema	−73.9 %

Source: World Health Organization, 2003.

TABLE 7.4. Source of Mortality Reduction 1960–1990.

| | Percentage contribution of gains in | | |
Reduction	Income	Educational level of adult females	Generation and utilization of new knowledge
Under-5 mortality rate	17	38	45
Female adult mortality rate	20	41	39
Male adult mortality rate	25	27	49
Female life expectancy at birth	19	32	49
Male life expectancy at birth	20	30	50
Total fertility rate	12	58	29

Source: Wang and others, 1999.

It is very interesting to consider which factors contributed to these gains. When one looks, for example, at the life expectancy of males, the economic level is indeed important and accounts for 20 percent of the gain, but the level of education of females accounts for 30 percent and the utilization of new knowledge for 50 percent. This underscores the important role of women in the development of preventive behavior (see Table 7.4).

Promoting health is important not only to reduce disability and suffering in the aging population, but also to promote the wealth of nations and the wellness and happiness of individuals. The positive correlation between health—evidenced by the mean life expectancy—and income per capita is well-known. As emphasized by the economist David Bloom (Bloom and Canning, 2000), this positive correlation is commonly thought to reflect a causal link running from income to health. A higher economic level allows access to goods and services that promote health (nutrition, sanitation, skilled health services, prevention, and so on).

The income-health correlation may be partly explained by a causal link running the other way, from health to income. Health improvement can lead to income growth because of several mechanisms: health improves productivity because of more energy and mental force and fewer lost workdays from illness or the need to care for other members of the family. Healthier populations invest more in education, which in turn promotes greater productivity and income. Higher education is correlated to better cognitive function and long-term preservation of cognition. Higher education is also linked to better compliance with preventive measures. Increased longevity leads to long-term investment and saving that, in turn, stimulate the economy.

The transition from a high to a low rate of mortality is correlated to the progressive reduction in the fertility rate observed in developing countries. Mortality decline in children and youth initiates this transition and progressively increases the proportion of future healthy workers.

A WHO report (World Health Organization, 1999) indicates that health status as measured by life expectancy is a significant predictor of subsequent economic growth.

Health is not enough. The future will be wealthier if the senior population—and particularly the female population—are allowed to fully participate in the economy. Women greatly contribute to the economy of the country: in France, they represent 45 percent of the working population in 2003 compared with 35 percent in the 1960s. But the rate of employment decreases significantly in the senior population. Only 39 percent of those aged fifty-five to sixty-four are working, in spite of a rather good health status, compared with 50 percent in Europe as a whole. The rate of employment after age sixty is particularly discouraging: 7 percent in men and 4 percent in women. In Sweden, 23 percent of men and 14 percent of women are still in the workforce; in the United States, 27 percent and 14 percent; and in Japan, 51 percent and 23 percent (see Table 7.5).

Women's working rate increases progressively while men's decreases slightly, but the difference remains very high. A comparable difference is observed in the purchasing power of women. In the private sector, women earn 25 percent less than men. Also, the so-called "glass ceiling" prevents women from having access to the highest positions. Women hold only 6.5 percent of CEO positions. The figure is similar in the public sector. The problem no longer lies in the education system: women represent 56 percent of the students in the French universities but only 30 percent of professionals in the scientific disciplines.

Time spent in childcare and housekeeping is still significantly higher for women than for men. However, help given to parents by the "crèche" (day care) and the nursery school system allows many young mothers to stay at work. Significant help is given by grandparents, particularly grandmothers. The senior female population represents 80 percent of the caregivers for very old people who have lost autonomy. This unpaid activity plays a very important role in the care of dependent people of all ages.

Discrimination against women was once striking in the French political arena, but progress is being made. Women represented 2 percent of senators in the 1960s and 1970s. The percentage rose to 16 percent at the last election in 2004. Female elected members of the regional councils were 10 percent in the 1980s and were nearly 50 percent as of the 2004 election. The election of the European parliament also demonstrated important progress: in 2004, 30 percent of the members of the European parliament (MEP) were women, compared with 43 percent in 1999 (see Table 7.6).

TABLE 7.5. **Longevity and Activity, Comparison Between Countries 2000–2020.**

Country	Percent 60+ in 2000	Percent 60+ in 2020	Life expectancy at birth in 2000	Percent activity at 60+ in 2000
India	7.6	11	M: 63 W: 64	M: 65 W: 14
China	10.1	16.7	M: 69 W: 73	M: 45 W: 15
USA	16.0	22.8	M: 74 W: 80	M: 27 W: 14
France	20.5	26.8	M: 75 W: 82	M: 7 W: 4
UK	20.6	26.7	M: 75 W: 80	M: 21 W: 8
Italy	22.3	33	M: 75 W: 81	M: 17 W: 4
Japan	23.2	33.7	M: 77 W: 85	M: 51 W: 23

Source: United Nations, 2002.

TABLE 7.6. **Members of the European Parliament.**

	1999–2004 (EU 15)		2004–2009 (EU 25)	
	Number of women/total	Percent of women	Number of women/total	Percent of women
France	26/87	29.9%	34/78	43.6%
Total	166/626	26.5%	222/732	30.3%

In conclusion, the evolution of the French shows the increasingly important part played by the female population in all sectors of activity. Women take an important part in the promotion of health, children's education, economic activity, and policy. Promotion of women is an important challenge.

It is projected that from 2000 to 2050 there will be a 30 percent increase in the working population in the United States. This will remain stable in the OECD countries, but it will decrease by 10 to 15 percent in France and by nearly 30 percent in Japan. It is high time to develop strategies to promote employment of healthy seniors, and particularly of female seniors. The objectives are to encourage changes in attitudes of employers and workers and to promote training for upgrading skills and acquiring new ones. The improvement of working conditions may be a powerful incentive for all generations. The reform of retirement and welfare systems is essential as well.

In conclusion, the challenges of longevity call for a strong promotion of the prevention of age-related diseases. Healthy aging will enable not only a better quality of life but also the possibility of leading an active and productive life until a very advanced age.

The longevity revolution will be an opportunity, not a threat, for women and men if we are able to maintain equity and promote the health, quality of life, livelihoods, and wealth of all generations living together. We must guarantee that the labor market fosters productive engagement and does not compromise the rights of the expanding aging population. A peaceful world also means that all countries may benefit equally from the great promise of longevity.

REFERENCES

Bloom, D. E., and Canning, D. "The Health and Wealth of Nations." *Science*, 2000, 287(5456), 1207–09.

Carnes, B. A., and Olshanski, S. J. "Heterogeneity and Its Biodemographic Implications for Longevity and Mortality." *Experimental Gerontology*, 2001, *36*, 419–430.

Finch, C. E., and Ruvkun, G. *Annual Review of Genomics and Human Genetics*, 2001, 2, 435–62.

Forette, F., and others. "Prevention of Dementia in Randomised Double-Blind Placebo-Controlled Systolic Hypertension in Europe (Syst-Eur) Trial." *The Lancet*, 1998, *352*, 1347–1351.

Forette, F., and others. "The Prevention of Dementia with Antihypertensive Treatment. New Evidence from the Systolic Hypertension in Europe (Syst-Eur) Study." *Archives of Internal Medicine*, 2002, *162*, 2046–52.

Gilman, S., and others. "Clinical Effects of Abeta Immunization (AN1792) in Patients with AD in an Interrupted Trial." *Neurology*, 2005, *34*, 1553–62.

Gueyffier, F., and others. "Antihypertensive Treatment in Very Old People: A Subgroup Meta-Analysis of Randomised Controlled Trials." *The Lancet*, 1999, *353*, 793–6.

Herskind, A. M., and others. "The Heritability of Human Longevity: A Population-Based Study of 2872 Danish Twin Pairs Born 1870–1900." *Human Genetics*, 1996, *97*, 319–323.

Institut National de la Statistique et des Études Économiques (INSEE). *Etudes et Résultats*, Dec. 2000, 94.

Institut National de la Statistique et des Études Économiques (INSEE). [http://www.insee.fr/fr/ffc/chifcle_fiche.asp?ref_id=cmrsos02219&tab_id=473]. 2004.

Insua, J. T. "Drug Treatment of Hypertension in the Elderly: A Meta-Analysis." *Annals of Internal Medicine*, 1994, *121*, 355–362.

Kinsella, K., and Velkoff, V. "Life Expectancy and Changing Mortality." *Aging Clinical and Experimental Research*, 2002, *14*, 322–32.

Levington, S., and others. for the Prospective Studies Collaboration. "Age-Specific Relevance of Usual Blood Pressure to Vascular Mortality: A Meta-Analysis of Individual Data for One Million Adults in 61 Prospective Studies." *The Lancet*, 2002, *360*, 1903–13.

Nicoll, J., and others. "Neuropathology of Human Alzheimer's Disease Following Immunization with Amyloid ß-peptide: A Case Report." *Nature Medicine*, 2003, *9*, 448–52.

Shenk, D., and others. *Journal of Neuroscience*, Sept. 15, 1996, *16*(18), 5795–5811.

Tzourio, C., and others. "Effects of Blood Pressure Lowering with Perindopril and Indapamide Therapy on Dementia and Cognitive Decline in Patients with Cerebrovascular Disease." Archives of Internal Medicine, 2003, 163, 1069–75.

United Nations. *Population Ageing*. Population Division, Department of Economic and Social Affairs. [http://www.un.org/esa/population/publications/ageing/Graph.pdf]. 2002.

Wang, J., and others. *Measuring Country Performance on Health: Selected Indicators for 115 Countries*. The World Bank (Human Development Network, Health, Nutrition and Population Series), 1999.

World Health Organization. Life Tables for WHO Member States. Geneva: World Health Organization, 2004. [http://www3.who.int/whosis/life/life_tables/life_tables_process.cfm?path=whosis,life_tables&language= english]. January 2007.

World Health Organization. *World Health Report 1999: Making a Difference*. Geneva: World Health Organization, 1999.

World Health Organization. *The Health Status of the European Union—Narrowing the Health Gap*. Luxembourg: Office for Official Publications of the European Communities, 2003.

CHAPTER

8

HEALTHY AGING IN FINLAND

PEKKA PUSKA

CHRONIC DISEASES AND AGING

The world is undergoing a rapid epidemiological transition. It means that chronic, noncommunicable diseases (NCD) are rapidly increasing and have also become the main cause of mortality and morbidity in the developing world. People are less vulnerable to infectious diseases and are living longer. This change encompasses global health and aging. The reduction in child and adult mortality, together with reduced fertility, all mean rapid aging of the world's population. The World Health Organization predicts that by 2025, some one billion people will be over sixty years old, and this figure will double by 2050 (World Health Organization, 2002a). The vast majority of these people—some 80 percent of them—will be in the developing world.

Aside from the demographic changes, many transitions in the determinants of health are behind the epidemiological transition. Lifestyles are changing: smoking, unhealthy diets, and physical inactivity are increasing. Aspects of globalization—global marketing, global communications, urbanization, and so on—all have an influence (World Commission on the Social Dimension of Globalization, 2004).

On the one hand, aging of the population is dependent on fertility rates and conversely, on life expectancy. Historically, life expectancy has increased, especially as the result of reduced child mortality and more recently in many developed countries as result of reduced NCD mortality in middle age. This prevention effect is moving to older population groups. Thus successful prevention of chronic NCDs is closely linked with the aging of the population.

Recent World Health Reports and the special WHO report on chronic diseases have reviewed the changing picture of global public health and its determinants (World Health Organization, 2005). Currently some 60 percent of all deaths in the world are from NCDs, and about half of those deaths are from cardiovascular diseases (CVDs). The World Health Report 2002 assessed also the role of the known main risk factors in mortality and the burden of disease (World Health Organization, 2002b). Seven out of the ten main risk factors leading to deaths in the world relate to NCDs. According to these estimates, high blood pressure is the number one risk factor, attributable to over seven million annual deaths. It is followed by tobacco use (five million deaths) and high blood cholesterol (4.5 million deaths).

CHRONIC DISEASE PREVENTION AND HEALTHY AGING

The WHO Global Strategy on NCD Prevention and Control emphasizes three main global behavioral risk factors: unhealthy diet, physical inactivity, and tobacco use (World Health Organization, 2000). These behavioral factors lead to high blood pressure and hypertension, elevated blood cholesterol and hypercholesterolaemia, blood glucose intolerance and diabetes, overweight and obesity. As to unhealthy diet, the main problem is foods that are fatty (from saturated fats and trans fats), salty, and sugary (World Health Organization, 2003).

Thus, in principle, simple changes in these lifestyle can powerfully prevent CVDs and other NCDs and promote health. Much of the preventive effects on several NCDs, like CVDs and diabetes, can take place relatively quickly and also in advanced age. Because of this knowledge, we can say that many major NCDs are preventable diseases to a great extent and to late in life. The main question for NCD prevention is thus not *what* to do, but *how* to do it.

With increased success in NCD prevention in many developed countries, life expectancy has increased greatly, leading to aging of the population. With this development, it has become increasingly obvious how closely prevention of chronic NCDs is linked to aging. The perspective on chronic disease prevention is changing from simple prevention of diseases to the notion of postponing chronic diseases as long as possible and concurrently to make the added years as healthy as possible. The ultimate aim is healthy aging. As often stated, the challenge is to have "more years in life and more life in years."

The World Health Report 2002 also discussed the needed strategies for NCD prevention (World Health Organization, 2002b). There can be very substantial health gains for relatively modest expenditures on interventions. The key is changing population distributions of the risk factors through general lifestyle changes. For CVDs, according to the report, main issues are population-wide changes in dietary fats to lower blood cholesterol levels and salt reduction to lower blood pressure levels. For tobacco control, higher taxes, total advertisement bans, and smoke-free policies are key.

THE FINNISH ACTION: THE NORTH KARELIA PROJECT

In the post-war years of the 1950s and 1960s, Finland was faced with extremely high rates of chronic NCDs, particularly CVDs. This was the cause of exceptionally low life expectancy, particularly among males: at the end of the 1960s, it was only some sixty-five years.

Actions began in Finland to reduce the high CVD rates. The work was begun in Eastern Finland, in the province of North Karelia, which had very high CVD rates. This North Karelia Project was launched as collaboration between health authorities, national experts, and the World Health Organization. After the successful initial years in North Karelia, comprehensive preventive activities were begun all over Finland (Puska and others, 1995).

The primary action targeted dietary habits to lower high blood cholesterol and blood pressure levels, to reduce smoking, and to increase physical activity. Comprehensive activities have involved different sectors of the society, such as health services, schools, NGOs, the private sector, and the media. Health policy and legislation also have been involved. Activities were based on both medical-epidemiological and social-behavioral frameworks and were accompanied by different kinds of monitoring and careful scientific evaluation.

The published results of the North Karelia Project show how, over the twenty-five-year period, there were major changes in the levels of the target risk factors in North Karelia (Puska and others, 1998). Among the male population in North Karelia, smoking was greatly reduced and dietary habits markedly changed. In 1972, 52 percent of middle-aged men in North Karelia smoked; in 1997 this had fallen to 31 percent, and it has continued to decline (see Table 8.1).

In the early 1970s, most of the fat used in Finland was dairy and animal fat, and use of vegetable oil products was very rare; now it is quite common. In 1972, about 90 percent of the population in North Karelia reported that they use mainly butter on bread; today it is less than 5 percent. Use of vegetables was originally very low; it has since increased several-fold.

These dietary changes have led to about a 17-percent reduction in the mean serum cholesterol level of the whole population. Elevated blood pressures have been brought under control and leisure-time physical activity has increased. Among men, the initially high rates of smoking were greatly reduced. However, among women, smoking increased somewhat, but from a low level and already stabilized years earlier at a level below 20 percent.

TABLE 8.1. **Risk Factor Changes in North Karelia, 1972–1997 (30–59 years).**

	Men			Women		
Year	Smoking	S-Cholesterol mmol/l	Blood pressure mmHg	Smoking	S-Cholesterol mmol/l	Blood pressure mmHg
1972	52	6.9	149/92	10	6.8	153/92
1977	44	6.5	143/89	10	6.4	141/86
1982	36	6.3	145/87	15	6.1	141/85
1987	36	6.3	144/88	16	6.0	139/83
1992	32	5.9	142/85	17	5.6	135/80
1997	31	5.7	140/88	16	5.6	133/80

Source: Vartiainen and others, 2000.

By 2002, the annual age-adjusted mortality rate of coronary heart disease in the middle-aged (under age sixty-five) male population in North Karelia had been reduced about 82 percent from the preprogram years 1967–71 (see Figure 8.1). Since the 1980s, favorable changes have spread throughout Finland. By 2002, the annual CHD mortality among men in all Finland had been reduced by approximately 75 percent. Concurrently, lung cancer mortality was also reduced, more than 70 percent in North Karelia and nearly 60 percent in all of Finland (see Table 8.2).

With greatly reduced cardiovascular and cancer mortality the all-cause mortality has reduced more than 50 percent, leading also to greater life expectancy— approximately ten years for men and eight years for women (Koskinen, Aromaa, Huttunen, and Teperi, 2006). Associated with favorable risk factor and lifestyle changes, the general health status of the people has greatly improved.

A separate analysis has shown that most of the decline in CHD mortality was because of reduction in the incidence of the diseases and can be explained by changes to the target risk factors in the population (Vartiainen and others, 1994). The reduction in serum cholesterol level of the population due to general dietary changes has been the strongest contributor.

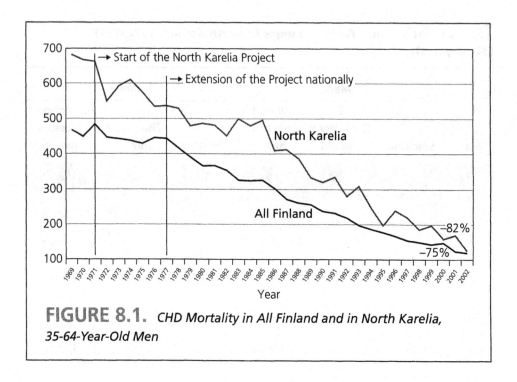

FIGURE 8.1. *CHD Mortality in All Finland and in North Karelia, 35-64-Year-Old Men*

TABLE 8.2. **Mortality Changes in North Karelia in 1970–1995 (per 100,000, age 35–64, men, age-adjusted).**

	Rate in 1970	Change, 1970–1995
All causes	1,509	−49%
All cardiovascular	855	−68%
Coronary heart disease	672	−73%
All cancers	271	−44%
Lung cancers	147	−71%

Source: Puska, Vartiainen, Tuomilehto, Salomaa, and Nissinen, 1998.

TRENDS AMONG THE ELDERLY IN FINLAND

The rapid aging of the Finnish population, along with the baby boomer birth cohorts reaching retirement age, is having major consequences in Finland. The proportion of the working-age population is shrinking—and creating a challenge for the national economy. The number of foreign workers is somewhat increasing to fill the needs of the labor market. The working capacity of the shrinking working-age group is of great importance, putting a new emphasis on worksite health promotion and the health of the working-age population.

The rapidly increasing number of older, retired citizens also concerns national policymakers, in view of increasing pension and health and social-care costs. As a natural consequence, the retirement age is being raised, which reduces pension costs and adds the valuable experience of older people to the labor markets.

Concern over increased healthcare and social-care costs because of the aging of the population has been a topic of intensive national discussion. According to the public health sector, the increasing numbers of older people in Finland should be seen as a great achievement of successful prevention and public health work. Far fewer people die in middle age; far more can enjoy an increasing number of well-deserved years of retirement.

Simultaneously, attention has focused on the issue of health and functional capacity among the elderly because this is the deciding factor for health care use and costs (Aromaa and others, 2006). Studies show consistently that the elderly population is also becoming healthier. The age-specific rates of chronic diseases and their symptoms are being reduced and functional capacity is increasing. With increased years in life, the number of healthy years in life has increased accordingly (Kattainen, 2004; Koskinen and others, 2006; Sulander, 2005). Thus age-related infirmities have been shifted to later in life.

Improvement in the functional capacity of the Finnish elderly population is apparent when comparing the data of the national health survey of 2000–2001 ("HEALTH 2000") with the survey of 1978–1980 ("Mini-Finland"), using similar methods (Martelin, Sainio, and Koskinen, 2004). Figure 8.2 shows how the percentage of older people (aged eighty to eighty-five) that can move (walk up stairs, carry shopping bags, and walk 0.5 kilometer) has greatly increased from about 1978 to 2001 (Figure 8.2).

It is difficult to say whether actual "compression of morbidity"—that is, reduction of years lived with infirmities—has taken place. Regardless, this development has had major positive consequences for the costs of health and social services. A substantial pressure to increase health-care costs is a fact in Finland, as in many other countries. But the main cause of that is not directly related to an increased number of older people, rather to more generally increased demand and increased availability of various, and often more expensive, treatment possibilities.

Obviously, the increased number of older people and their improved health have other major social consequences. More and more, older people want to work longer, but often on a flexible basis. The role of older people in supporting younger families

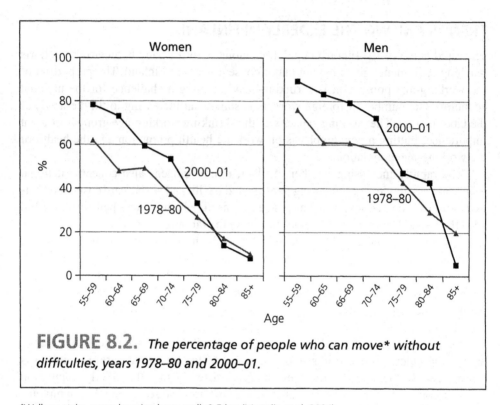

FIGURE 8.2. *The percentage of people who can move* without difficulties, years 1978–80 and 2000–01.*

*Walk up stairs, carry shopping bags, walk 0.5 km (Martelin et al. 2004).

and other structures in the society is important, not to mention the simple human value of longer age.

Numerous studies in Finland also demonstrate how those in the growing older population are taking greater care of their health. The expert message—that reduction of risk factors and adoption of healthy lifestyles from medical point of view pays off even when implemented quite late in life—is well received by these people.

National health monitoring among the population age sixty-five to seventy-nine has shown how, from 1985 to 2003, the proportion of men following certain healthy dietary habits increased from 11 percent to 28 percent and among women from 14 percent to 34 percent. The proportion of daily smokers was reduced among men from 18 percent to 14 percent and among women remained at a low level of 6 percent (Sulander, 2005).

Consumption patterns greatly reflect these healthy changes in lifestyle among both the older and the younger population—and accordingly, in private-sector responses. The profile of food products is rapidly changing to reflect these new consumption patterns. Currently, some three hundred food items already have been given the right to use the "heart symbol" of the Finnish Heart Association, as they comply with the health criteria set by the expert group of the Finnish Heart Association and the

Finnish Diabetes Association. Also in other areas, such as physical activity, the private sector is responding rapidly.

CONCLUSION

The experiences and results in Finland show how well-planned and determined actions can have a major impact on lifestyle and risk factors, and how such a development leads quite rapidly to reduced cardiovascular and other chronic disease rates and increase in life expectancy. And they demonstrate the strength of theory-based and sustained community-based action and respective policy measures in changing lifestyle and chronic disease risk factors, and also provide practical experience concerning such activities.

The experiences also show how a major national demonstration project can be a strong tool for favorable national development. The experiences of the project have actively contributed to a comprehensive national action, with very good results. The decline in heart disease mortality from 1986 to 2006 in Finland has been one of the most rapid in the world, and the overall health of the adult population has greatly improved. Ultimately, the action has greatly contributed to healthy aging of the population.

As of this writing, chronic NCDs are responsible for approximately 60 percent of all deaths in the world. They represent an overwhelming health burden in the industrialized countries and already are a major and rapidly growing problem in the developing countries. But this is an area in which major health gains can be achieved, as shown by the results of the North Karelia Project and Finnish experiences. This kind of intervention is clearly the most effective and sustainable approach to tackling the problem. Thus the Finnish experience has been of great significance and has been internationally cited frequently as a model for prevention of chronic disease and for healthy aging.

In recent years, this experience has made Finnish people more aware that the ultimate aim of chronic disease prevention and health promotion is healthy aging. Adoption of a healthy lifestyle not only leads to reduced disease rates in middle age, but also postpones diseases to a later age and increases health, functional capacity, and well-being in old age.

Thus healthy aging is closely linked with the issue of prevention of chronic diseases. Avoiding risk factors and maintaining healthy lifestyles both prevents diseases and promotes health. In the field of cardiovascular diseases, the emphasis has shifted from "prevention of heart disease" to "promotion of heart health."

There is greater understanding about how the risk factors seem to relate to a whole range of chronic conditions, lending support to so-called "integrated prevention," which is also the basis of the WHO strategy (World Health Organization, 2000). Public service messages to prevent CVDs, diabetes, cancers, oral health problems, COPD, musculoskeletal diseases, depression, and the like show increasing similarities. Thus there has been a shift from disease-specific prevention to this integrated prevention, targeting the common risk factors and promoting healthy aging overall.

A new addition to this concept, concerning aging in particular, arrived recently, with recent studies showing how dementia and Alzheimer's disease seem to share the same risk factors (Kivipelto and others, 2001, 2006). Consequently, the same lifestyle changes recommended for many chronic diseases can also be beneficial for prevention of dementia and Alzheimer's disease in older age.

The Finnish experience has convincingly shown the value of chronic disease prevention and health promotion leading to healthy aging, with all its human, social, and economic societal benefits. In spite of this positive message, both in Finland and elsewhere, the future challenges are great. The challenge is to strengthen the public health infrastructures and health promotion and to tackle the determinants of chronic disease and healthy aging in all sectors of the society—that is, to make the healthy choices easier and the environments more conducive to this development (Puska, 2006; World Health Organization, 1995).

During Finland's recent EU Presidency, emphasis was placed on "Health in All Policies," on both national and international levels (Ståhl and others, 2006). Health and healthy aging are determined in everyday situations in which people live, work, move, and so on. Thus decisions made outside of the health sector have a major influence on our health. A health-friendly society leads not only to successful disease prevention and health promotion, but also to beneficial conditions for the older generation and to favorable overall conditions for healthy aging in the society.

REFERENCES

Aromaa, A., and others. "Functional Capacity and Work Ability." In S. Koskinen, A. Aromaa, J. Huttunen, and J. Teperi (eds.), *Health in Finland*. Helsinki: KTL, STAKES and Ministry of Social Affairs and Health, 2006.

Kattainen, A., and others. "Secular Changes in Disability Among Middle-Aged and Elderly Finns with and without Coronary Heart Disease from 1978–1980 to 2000–2001." *Annals of Epidemiology* 2004, *14*(7), 479–85.

Kivipelto, M., and others. "Midlife Vascular Risk Factors and Alzheimer's Disease in Later Life: A Longitudinal, Population Based Study." *British Medical Journal*, 2001, *322*(7300), 1447–51.

Kivipelto, M., and others. "Risk Score for the Prediction of Dementia in 20 Years Among Middle Aged People: a Longitudinal, Population-Based Study." *Lancet Neurology*, Sept. 2006, *5*(9), 735–41.

Koskinen, S., Aromaa, A., Huttunen, J., and Teperi, J. (eds.). *Health in Finland*. Helsinki: KTL, STAKES and Ministry of Social Affairs and Health, 2006.

Martelin, T., Sainio, P., and Koskinen, S. Ikääntyvän väestön toimintakyvyn kehitys (Development of Functional Capacity in the Elderly Population). In M. Kautto (ed.), Ikääntyminen voimavarana. Tulevaisuusselonteon liiteraportti 5 (Aging as a Resource. Government Report on the Future, Appendix Report 5). Valtioneuvoston kanslian julkaisusarja (Prime Minister's Office: Publications), 2004, *33*, 117–31.

Puska, P. "WHO Director-General Election: Public Health Infrastructures." *The Lancet*, 2006, *368*, 1401–3.

Puska, P., and others. The North Karelia Project: 20-Year Results and Experiences. Helsinki: National Public Health Institute, 1995.

Puska, P., Vartiainen, E., Tuomilehto, J., Salomaa, V., and Nissinen, A. "Changes in Premature Deaths in Finland: Successful Long-term Prevention of Cardiovascular Diseases." *Bulletin of the World Health Organization*, 1998, *76*(4), 419–25.

Ståhl, T., and others. *Health in All Policies: Prospects and Potentials*. Helsinki: Ministry of Social Affairs and Health, 2006.

Sulander, T. *Functional Ability and Health Behaviors: Trends and Associations Among Elderly People, 1985–2003*. Helsinki: National Public Health Institute (KTL) A3/2005, 2005.

Vartiainen, E., and others. "Changes in Risk Factors Explaining Changes in Mortality from Ischaemic Heart Disease in Finland." *British Medical Journal*, 1994, *309*, 23–7.

Vartiainen, E., and others. "Cardiovascular Risk Factor Changes in Finland, 1972–1997." *International Journal of Epidemiology*, 2000, *29*, 49–56.

World Commission on the Social Dimension of Globalization. "A Fair Globalization: Creating Opportunities for All." Geneva: International Labor Organization, 2004.

World Health Organization. *Health Promotion: Ottawa Charter*. WHO/HPR/HEP/95.1. Geneva: World Health Organization, 1995.

World Health Organization. *Global Strategy on Noncommunicable Disease Prevention and Control*. WHA/A53/14. Geneva: World Health Organization, 2000.

World Health Organization. *Active Aging: A Policy Framework*. WHO/NMH/NPH/02.8. Geneva: World Health Organization, 2002a.

World Health Organization. *The World Health Report: Reducing Risks, Promoting Healthy Life*. Geneva: World Health Organization, 2002b.

World Health Organization. *Diet, Nutrition, and the Prevention of Chronic Diseases. Report of a Joint WHO/FAO Expert Consultation*. WHO Technical Reports Series 916. Geneva: World Health Organization, 2003.

World Health Organization. *Preventing Chronic Diseases: A Vital Investment*. Geneva: World Health Organization, 2005.

CHAPTER

9

HEALTHY AGING IN GERMANY

ULLA SCHMIDT

We live in an aging world. Never before have so many people in our world lived so long. Becoming older at the beginning of the twenty-first century is different from becoming older at the beginning or middle of the nineteenth century. In coming years the population group of the very old—those aged eighty and over—will grow faster worldwide than any other population contingent. In the past, life expectancy in the industrialized nations has continually increased. Whereas those born in Germany in 1925 would be happy to reach the age of sixty, a boy born today can statistically expect to reach the age of seventy-six and a girl to become as old as about eighty-one-and-a-half. In Germany today 25 percent of the population is over sixty. The German Federal Statistical Office presumes that the number of those aged sixty and over will increase by seven to eight million by 2050, and at the same time the number of those aged twenty to sixty will decrease by twelve to fifteen million. The rapid demographic change that we must face leaves no doubt that it is important and necessary to act early and throughout our lives to promote healthy aging and remain healthy in old age. However, in spite of the frequent assumption that increasing age goes hand in hand with greater incidence of multiple health problems and illnesses (termed *multimorbidity*) among the elderly, a different picture is emerging in Germany. There are so far no studies proving that the aging German population is becoming more ill as Germans become older.

106

Aging has many faces in Europe, differing from one country or region to another. We find many different forms of aging even within the same country. Performance does not evolve in the same manner as people become older, but differs from one individual to another. The degree of the difference depends on respective health status. Aging is not a biological process pure and simple, but is influenced by social, ecological, and psychological as well as epochal factors. Aging is individual; that is, there are major differences between peers, including within the same country. These differences may be more pronounced in some cases than between individuals who are ten or even twenty years apart. What is more, aging is differential: people do not age equally or at the same rate in all areas. And aging is ultimately multidirectional—the change process can move in various directions. An improvement, deterioration, or unchanged level of the aging process can occur in the same person.

We have experienced a major extension of the life span, brought about by advances in hygiene, progress in medicine and in medical technology, research in pharmacology, improvements in socioeconomic living conditions, and a lifestyle that takes account of our health. We now eat more healthily; we have become aware of the importance of physical and intellectual activity and are more active in prevention. Lifelong learning in the broadest sense of the word—defined as changing conduct as a result of experience—is of vital significance today. However, there have been changes not only in the duration, but also in the nature of learning. Unlike our grandparents and great-grandparents, we are called upon to adapt to increasingly frequent, rapid changes in our social environment. This is also reflected in the vocational sphere. In all sectors, from agriculture to the crafts to industry, the business community, and the administration, technical development has made heavy physical work easier and made it necessary for working people to adopt a fresh orientation.

In general, our life expectancy depends on how we live our lives. *Life expectancy* is meant here in the broadest sense of the term, referring not only to the duration but also to the quality of life. As the saying goes, it is not only a matter of how old we become, but of how we become old. Much more essential than adding years to life is to add life to the years. "More years and more life" should be the goal of health policy activities.

However, demographic change is determined by two processes: on the one hand, the ongoing increases in life expectancy, and on the other, the falling birth rate that can be observed in all European countries. The average birth rate in the EU countries is currently about 1.5 children per childbearing-age woman. With 2.0, Ireland has the highest birth rate, followed by France with 1.9, while the Czech Republic and Slovenia have the lowest, at 1.2, followed, among others, by Italy and Spain and several Eastern European countries at 1.3. Germany's birth rate of about 1.4 is—as is the case for Portugal and Austria—only slightly higher. Unfortunately, significant increases in the fertility rate are not anticipated in the foreseeable future. Only the creation of a framework in which work and family life can be better reconciled could lead to a slight increase. This is a challenge to policymakers, and Germany is taking this path.

Typical of demographic change is the change in the ratio between the generations. Let us start with a quantitative observation: in 1950, there were about

15.7 elderly people (aged sixty-five and over) for every one hundred people aged twenty to sixty-five; as of 2006 this figure had increased to 31.7. The German Federal Statistical Office forecasts that in the year 2050 this figure will double again to approximately 62.0.

In light of this future demographic landscape, the health care system needs to find more ambitious finance concepts. The so-called generational agreement on which the German social system is based must be adjusted. The generational agreement was created by Otto von Bismarck, the first Chancellor of the German Reich, at the end of the nineteenth century. It is based on the premise that those who work for wages will pay taxes and contributions to provide for those who have not yet started work and for those who have already left the workforce. When the generational agreement was introduced, people started work at between age fifteen and sixteen. The retirement age was seventy, so because of the relatively short life expectancy at that time pensions were drawn for a short period only. That has changed: whereas in 1995 men in Germany drew a pension for an average 13.6 years (women 18.2 years), by 2005 men could expect to draw a pension for 14.7 years (women 19.8 years).

It was not until 1916 that the retirement age established by Bismarck was reduced from age seventy to sixty-five. Therefore, at that time, those aged fifteen to seventy financed those individuals who were either not yet fifteen or who were over seventy. The scales have been considerably tipped against those in the workforce. It was therefore decided in November 2006 to gradually increase to sixty-seven the age at which one can start drawing a pension without suffering any deductions; this increase will be effected from 2012 to 2027.

Other types of social insurance in Germany, such as statutory health insurance, are also based in essence on the principle of a "generational agreement." Even though pensioners also pay health insurance contributions, the average health expenditure in old age is much higher than during the working years, whereas regular incomes are lower. For these reasons, other forms of funding must be found for the German health-care system. The question of funding is thus one of the core elements of the ongoing health reform in Germany.

THE STATE OF THE DEBATE WITHIN THE HEALTH SECTOR

The World Health Organization (WHO) presumes that, as much as a growing elderly population presents a major challenge, it also presents an opportunity to make the most of this potential in terms of knowledge and skills benefiting society. It takes the view that societies can certainly afford to age if states, regions, and international organizations develop active aging programs and take steps to improve the health, independence, and productivity of elderly people. Such a policy should build on the needs, preferences, and abilities of elderly people, while taking an approach that deals with all phases of life. If aging is to be a positive experience, longer life must be accompanied by the possibility of remaining independent and healthy, productive and secure in the long term. The World Health Organization uses the term *active aging* to describe the process intended to bring this vision to fruition. Active aging is the process of optimizing the possibilities for lifelong physical, social, and mental well-being, with the goal of expanding healthy life expectancy and expanding productivity and quality of life in old age. The World Health Organization has been using the term since the end of the 1990s. It is intended to deliver a more holistic message than *healthy aging*, given that it recognizes the factors and sectors other than health care that influence the way that individuals and society are aging. The term is also used by other international organizations, such as the OECD, the G8, the EU, and the ILO. The term *active* refers to ongoing participation in social, economic, intellectual, cultural, and civil life, not just the ability to be physically active. Maintaining one's independence—the ability to determine and cope with everyday life oneself—is a fundamental goal for the individual, but also for policy makers. The health that makes such independence possible is key to achieving active aging.

Age is traditionally associated with illness, dependence, and lack of productivity. Policies and programs that are entrenched in these outdated paradigms, however, do not reflect reality. People in all countries remain active and independent into old age, making a major contribution to society through volunteer work.

Chronic diseases such as heart disease, cancer, and depression are rapidly becoming the main causes of death in the developed countries. Chronic diseases are the main causes of disability, invalidism, and a lower quality of life. The independence of an elderly person is at risk if physical or mental disability make it more difficult to carry out the activities of daily living (ADLs) and the instrumental activities of daily living (IADLs); that is, everyday chores and self-care tasks. The three most common physical diseases occurring in Germany as adults age are arteriosclerosis (changes to and stenosis of the arteries, tendency towards clot formation), osteoporosis, and joint arthrosis (also called arthritis). The advance of these diseases can be slowed by avoiding risk factors and living an active life. It is possible to delay the need for assistance and long-term care. A mental disease that is becoming more common is *dementia*, the umbrella term used to designate diseases characterized by memory loss, declining intellect, personality change, and disruptions in self-determined living.

A healthy lifestyle is becoming key to the question of how to promote healthy aging. It has come to be regarded as a given that each individual can take personal responsibility for remaining in good health as long as possible. These are the principal material factors:

- Following a healthy diet

- Not smoking

- Reducing alcohol consumption

- Taking regular physical and mental exercise

- Taking an active role in determining one's everyday life

- Being socially active

A balanced diet helps to maintain our physical and mental performance and makes us less prone to certain diseases. The advance of high blood pressure, heart attack, osteoporosis, or diabetes mellitus can be slowed by a healthy diet. By being aware of the calories contained in the food that we eat, we can help prevent obesity; a slightly higher blood pressure, slightly increased blood sugar and blood fat values can be normalized by making suitable changes in diet. The immune system is strengthened by a healthy lifestyle, so that we become less likely to contract infectious diseases.

Smoking is a serious risk factor when it comes to heart attack, stroke, lung cancer, intestinal cancer, and carcinoma of the mouth and throat. Thus, not smoking is one of the most important preventive measures we can take. If we give up smoking, the blood circulation and the supply of oxygen to the body's organs improve after only a short time; existing diseases such as a chronic bronchitis improve, and the risk of heart attack and cancer is reduced markedly as the years pass.

The body's ability to metabolize alcohol decreases as we age, so older people should consume less alcohol. Special care should be taken when mixing alcohol with medicines, to avoid unfortunate interactive effects. For instance, alcohol can either reduce or amplify the effect of some medicines, and the risk of accidents and falls increases, the latter applying, for instance, to sleeping pills or sedatives.

Regular exercise (hiking, swimming, cycling, garden work, and so on) promotes and maintains physical and mental performance and has a positive impact on all the organ systems. The risk of a heart-circulation disease (arteriosclerosis, heart attack, disruptions in blood circulation) is only half as high among the physically active as among the inactive. Physical activity has a positive impact, for instance, on diabetes and on the course of osteoporosis and prevents weakening of the muscles. Those who practice a sport also reduce their risk of contracting cancer. Regular sports activity promotes not only physical, but also mental and intellectual health. Sufficient movement helps to reduce stress, fear, and anger. What applies to the body applies similarly to intellectual abilities. Regular intellectual activity keeps our memory active and helps us to retain our mental flexibility.

Policies and programs for actions intended to promote active aging offer a response to all challenges, those of both the aging individual and the aging society. They permit elderly people to improve their potential for independence, good health, and productivity, while offering them suitable protection and care should they need it. With support from the health care system, the labor market, employers, the education system, and social policy, active aging can confer considerable advantages:

- More elderly people make a contribution in all areas of society through both paid and volunteer activity

- Fewer elderly people need costly medical treatment and care facilities

- Fewer adults die early in a highly productive phase of their lives

- More elderly people remain independent and enjoy a high quality of life

- Fewer elderly people suffer from pain and disabilities as a result of chronic diseases

The active aging approach is founded on the recognition of elderly people's human rights and on the United Nations' principles of independence, participation, dignity, protection, and self-fulfillment. Active aging encourages us both to take a holistic view of our life span and to foster solidarity between the generations. For a number of years, researchers have been pointing to the significance of networks with regard to individuals' or groups' health conduct when it comes to designing campaigns intended to promote health.

What is Germany's response to these challenges in terms of labor policy? What specific means are being deployed in preventive health policy? This is the subject of the next section.

LABOR MARKET MEASURES

Many labor policy and social policy measures are being undertaken in Germany in reaction to the challenges of demographic change. Labor market policy pursues the goals of considerably improving the professional opportunities open to elderly people and of enhancing the social and macroeconomic potential obtained from society's availing itself of such opportunities. This is necessary because as many as 50 percent of German companies have no employees over age fifty and 55 percent of those over fifty-five no longer work. The priority goal of labor market policy measures is thus that those who become older remain in employment longer and that unemployed elderly people are given an opportunity to reenter employment.

Against this background, the Federal Ministry of Labor and Social Affairs has launched the exemplary "Initiative 50plus" program, which aims to improve the labor market opportunities available to those fifty and over.

First steps have already been taken and false incentives to take early retirement considerably reduced. In particular, by shortening the period that unemployment benefits are paid, by effectively increasing the retirement age, and by virtue of the expiration of the scheme applying to people who have reached the age of fifty-eight (whereby they can have themselves removed from the unemployment statistics and draw up to thirty-two months' unemployment benefits), the Federal Cabinet launched a group of measures on November 29, 2006, to improve employment opportunities for the elderly. These are first steps to extend real working lives and to improve existing labor market tools to keep the elderly at work. To reintegrate elderly unemployment benefit recipients into the labor market as quickly as possible, a combined wage will be introduced for those fifty and over. Elderly unemployed who find employment at net earnings lower than prior to their unemployment will receive partial compensation for their loss of wages.

Furthermore, employers are to be given greater incentives to employ older workers. Anyone appointing older workers can in future receive a new type of integration subsidy. Further training will be stepped up. To this end, the framework for further vocational training will be improved and incentives created to take greater advantage of skill-building measures. Existing programs and initiatives to promote employment of the elderly will be continued. The ideas competition "Perspective 50plus—Employment pacts for older workers in the regions" promotes regional projects for vocational reintegration of older unemployed people over fifty. The "30,000 Additional Jobs for the Elderly" program creates opportunities to gain work experience by compensating employers for the additional effort involved in hiring the long-term unemployed aged over fifty-eight. The "Initiative New Quality of Work" (INQA) places the focus on demographic change. Skill-building and health are key to the ability and willingness of older workers to remain in gainful employment, so INQA offers practical assistance for companies. The Community's EQUAL Initiative provides new possibilities to counter discrimination in the labor market. A "Becoming older at work" toolbox has been developed in a national EQUAL "Age Management" network, offering tools to combat age discrimination, promoting employment for the elderly, and explaining practical implementation. The toolbox will serve as an aid for enterprises, as well as for workers who are becoming older.

In addition to labor market measures, the most important health-policy measures are presented in the next section.

HEALTH POLICY MEASURES

Health policy measures chiefly consist of (1) means of prevention and health promotion and (2) long-term care insurance.

Prevention and Health Promotion

Avoiding illness and improving health are the core areas addressed by health promotion and prevention. Although the German health care system—which remains largely based on remedy, rehabilitation, and care—ensures that all citizens are provided with high-quality health care, prevention must be given much higher priority if we are to meet the challenge of future demographic trends. We can no longer afford to focus our efforts on restoring health. Studies show that not only must we place prevention and health promotion on an equal footing with therapeutic, rehabilitative, and care measures, but all must be integrated. The health care system must not only seek remedies, but also tackle situations that cause the outbreak of a disease.

According to the definition contained in WHO's 1986 Ottawa Charter, health promotion is the process of enabling people to increase control over and improve their health. The term *health promotion* is less about avoiding specific diseases and losses and more about a comprehensive understanding of health. It covers all measures aimed at actively influencing the attitudes, conduct, lifestyles, and working and environmental conditions of individuals, groups, or the population as a whole toward living a healthy life.

The term *prevention* encompasses all measures serving to prevent health deterioration. It can be broken down into *primary*, *secondary*, and *tertiary prevention*.

Primary prevention aims to promote and maintain health and to prevent diseases breaking out. Primary prevention measures can be taken by individuals as well as by groups of individuals. This also includes avoiding risk factors, such as through programs for healthy diet or physical activity, as well as company health promotion.

Secondary prevention is to prevent the onset of a disease in its early stages through early diagnosis and treatment. It includes processes that aim to identify diseases early. Such screening tests, carried out on apparently healthy people for certain asymptomatic manifestations or prodromes, aim to detect diseases at an early stage and to heal them or halt their progress by providing timely treatment. This includes, for instance, statutory cancer screening (see Table 9.1), which may be used by all persons with statutory health insurance in Germany.

Preventing diseases that are already present is referred to as *tertiary prevention*. The aim is to avoid or reduce consequential damage (defects, disabilities) of the disease; for example, patient training programs for obese children and juveniles.

These three prevention components may overlap in some cases.

Prevention has been one of the core tasks of German health policy since 1989. As birth rates fall and retirement ages remain low, health prevention can help to create awareness and to stabilize the social systems by preventing diseases, recognizing them earlier, and coping with them better. At the same time, early retirement and the need for long-term care can be delayed or avoided. To maximize the existing preventive potential, health policy has initiated a German Forum for Prevention and Health Promotion. By amplifying and expanding prevention, the German health care system is being further developed as a modern social system in which prevention, treatment, rehabilitation, and care are placed on an equal footing. To reach as many people as possible, prevention should link directly to people's environments. This means that health promotion must form an integral part of work in kindergartens and schools, in companies, in local authorities. We must also enable the elderly to take responsibility for themselves and for others. To this end, society must undertake supportive and enabling initiatives.

We particularly need to develop incentives for achieving a healthy lifestyle. Further, we need to create conditions in which the elderly can adjust to the loss of abilities caused by aging processes. Education and training can make a special contribution here.

Finally, the success of these measures is determined by the degree to which society is willing to recognize the elderly, to integrate them, and to welcome their participation in the life of society.

As the proportion of the elderly among the population increases, the number of people in need of long-term care will also increase. Targeted prevention and rehabilitation will exert a positive influence on this process. The following section discusses the response of German healthpolicy makers to the growing number of persons in need of long-term care.

TABLE 9.1. Examples of Cancer Screening in Germany.

Test	Age	Sex	Frequency	Remarks	Further information: www.g-ba.de
Genital check-up	Starting at 20	Women	Annual	■ Specific case history interview (e.g., questions about bleeding disorders and discharges) ■ Inspection of the mouth of the uterus ■ Cancer smear and cytological check-up ■ Gynecological palpitation test ■ Consultation on the result	■ Cancer screening guideline
	Starting at 45	Men	Annual	■ Specific case history interview ■ Inspection and palpitation test of the external genitalia ■ Palpitation check-up of the prostate ■ Palpitation check-up of the regional lymph nodes ■ Consultation on the result	■ Cancer screening guideline
Chest and skin check-up	Starting at 30	Women	Annual	■ Specific case history interview (e.g., questions about changes/symptoms) ■ Inspection and palpitation test of the chest and the regional lymph nodes, including instructing patients how to perform the test themselves ■ Consultation on the result	■ Cancer screening guideline
Skin check-up	Starting at 45	Men	Annual	■ In conjunction with the prostate/genital check-up	■ Cancer screening guideline

Colon and rectum check-up	Starting at 50	Women and men	Annual	■ Specific advice ■ Palpitation test of the colon ■ Test for hidden blood in the stool (annual until age 55)	■ Cancer screening guideline
Colonoscopy	Starting at 55	Women and men	Two colonoscopies ten years apart	■ Specific advice ■ Two colonoscopies ten years apart or test for hidden blood in the stool every two years	■ Cancer screening guideline
Mammographic screening (assuming the necessary structures are available)	from 50 to 69	Women	Every two years	■ Invitation to attend a certified screening unit ■ Information ■ Mammographic chest x-ray ■ Consultation on the result	■ Cancer screening guideline
Check-up	Starting at 35	Women and men	Every two years	Screening for common diseases such as heart-circulation diseases, kidney disease, diabetes mellitus. Including the following benefits, among others: ■ Case history interview, in particular recording the risk profile ■ Clinical check-ups (physical tests, including taking blood pressure) ■ Blood and urine tests ■ Consultation on the result	■ Cancer screening guideline

Long-Term Care Insurance

Many people are in need of long-term care at the end of their lives and rely on the help of strangers. Until quite recently this situation frequently forced those in need to claim social assistance, given that even above-average pension incomes were insufficient to pay for accommodation in an institutional long-term care facility. The children were frequently called on to make a financial contribution to those in need of long-term care. The last major gap in the social security system in Germany was closed on January 1, 1995, the inception date of obligatory statutory long-term care insurance. It is operated as an independent branch of social insurance (fifth pillar) and—above all for the self-employed—as private long-term care insurance. This means that Germany's roughly eighty million inhabitants are provided with insurance coverage in the event of their needing long-term care. The principle here is that anyone who has statutory health insurance is enrolled in social long-term care insurance. Anyone who has private health insurance with a right to general hospital benefits has been obliged, since January 1, 1995, to take out a private long-term care insurance policy. Depending on the degree and frequency of the assistance required on a daily basis for personal hygiene, feeding, or mobility, long-term care insurance distinguishes among three grades of long-term care requirements:

1.   Considerable need of long-term care

2.   Serious need of long-term care

3.   Very serious need of long-term care

Whether long-term care is needed and which grade applies are decisions made by the long-term care fund on the basis of a medical report drafted by an independent reporting institution, the Social Medical Service. Anyone wishing to be cared for at home may choose between monetary benefits and benefits in kind up to a value of Euro 1,918 per month or a combination of the two. The risk of needing long-term care increases considerably with age.

More than ten years have now passed since the introduction of long-term care insurance in Germany. More than two million people claim long-term care insurance benefits every month. Roughly 1.4 million people are taken care of in their domestic environments, and approximately 0.7 million in homes. The long-term care insurance pays roughly Euro 900 million annually for almost half a million caring family members.

The introduction of long-term care insurance served to considerably expand the broad range of care infrastructure services, providing significant relief for caring family members, who work hard and deny their own interests, particularly in noninstitutional care. Added to this is the fact that more than 250,000 new jobs have been created in the care sector since the introduction of mandatory long-term care insurance.

Long-term care insurance has proven its value. It performs a major task within our social security system and will continue to become more significant in light of demographic trends. It is anticipated that the number of those in need of long-term care from social long-term care insurance will increase from roughly 1.9 million in 1995 to roughly 3.4 million by 2040. So that long-term care insurance can successfully meet this challenge, it must be continually adjusted in line with changing conditions. The final details of long-term care reform will be agreed between the Coalition partners in 2007.

Apart from looming decisions on the further development and improvement of insured parties' claims under the law on benefits, as well as of the care structures and services on offer, the question of how to ensure that individual contributions are adequate to provide sustainable, reliable funding that does not fall short of individual needs will be central to the coming reform of long-term care insurance.

OUTLOOK

Health and social policy must both address and shape social change. In doing so, it must combine economic dynamics and social security to create synergies for both. The current reform under way in Germany therefore focuses on modernizing the social security systems and guaranteeing their sustainable funding. Health and social policy must flexibly adapt to the changed framework. Future political action will also center on enacting enabling health and social policies that facilitate healthy aging in Germany.

CHAPTER

10

HEALTHY AGING FROM SEVENTY TO OVER ONE HUNDRED IN GERMANY: LESSONS FROM THE BERLIN AGING STUDY

JACQUI SMITH AND PAUL B. BALTES

Depending on country, culture, birth cohort, and idiosyncratic factors, the period of old age in the twenty-first century could extend over twenty to forty years of an individual's life (for example, from age sixty to over one hundred). Although these years are sometimes portrayed in literature as the Golden Age of life, for many individuals the subjective experience of what aging entails is not always positive. For many older Germans, concerns about the consequences of changes in health dampen optimistic hopes about the prospects of a long life. Older people hope to have as many years as possible free from the constraints of poor health, but they fear that physical illness, dementia, and frailty will inevitably have a severe impact on their quality of life.

In some respects, these subjective beliefs about aging reflect reality (P. B. Baltes, 2006). Although for the majority of the over-sixty population the first phase of old age, described as the Third Age, is relatively free of illness, those who survive into very old age face the challenges of frailty and multimorbidity in the Fourth Age (P. B. Baltes and Smith, 2003; Suzman, Willis, and Manton, 1992). These two sides and two phases of old age highlight the dilemmas faced by contemporary societies dealing with population aging. Policies that focus on promoting active, healthy, and independent lifestyles in the Third Age certainly do contribute in a positive way to improved life quality for many individuals aged sixty to eighty. Over time, however, these same policies also contribute to the survival of increasing numbers of individuals beyond age eighty-five into the Fourth Age. A question still to be answered is whether society is sufficiently prepared to foster a culture of aging with dignity in both phases of old age.

From a population demographic perspective, the transition between the Third and the Fourth Age can be defined as the chronological age at which 50 percent of a birth cohort is no longer alive (that is, age seventy-five to eighty, contingent on the age demographics of the country involved) (Suzman, Willis, and Manton, 1992). A more specific definition applies the 50-percent criterion only to the average life expectancy of those people who have attained the age of sixty. For Germany, this strategy places the beginning of the Fourth Age closer to age eighty-five. Of course, individuals differ substantially in the chronological age at which they transit into the Fourth Age. For instance, it could be around sixty for some people or as late as ninety-five or one hundred for others. For this reason, the behavioral sciences consider individual variations in biological aging and patterns of psychological decline and attempts to define a certain amount of time before natural death (for example, five to ten years) as the entry point to the Fourth Age (P. B. Baltes and Smith, 2003).

We review findings about health and its impact on psychological functioning gained from the Berlin Aging Study (BASE) (P. B. Baltes and Mayer, 1999), an extensive multidisciplinary investigation of a heterogeneous sample of men and women aged seventy to over one hundred residing in Berlin. These findings illustrate the characteristics of the Third and Fourth Age and the dynamics between physical and health-related decline and psychological adaptation to a long life. Though the Third Age is a phase of life in which the mind can outwit the body, this is less possible in the Fourth Age. Psychological resources such as knowledge, memory, personality, and self-related beliefs shape one's life and how one deals with illness and an aging body. In very old age, chronic illness and impairments in physical, sensory, and brain functioning test the limits of the adaptive capacity of the psychological system. Multimorbidity has a pervasive impact on the nature and routine of everyday life and, over time, compromises well-being.

THE BERLIN AGING STUDY (BASE): INSIGHTS ABOUT OLD AGE IN GERMANY

The Berlin Aging Study (BASE) (P. B. Baltes and Mayer, 1999; see also Smith and P. B. Baltes, 1997) was established with generous funding from two German federal government ministries (Research and Technology, 1989–1991, and Family Affairs and Seniors, 1992–1997). The study was designed to investigate questions about the different phases of old age from the collaborative perspectives of four disciplines: psychiatry, psychology, sociology, and internal medicine. Distinguishing features of the initial BASE design are (1) a special focus on the very old men and women, (2) sample heterogeneity achieved by local representation of the western suburbs of Berlin, and (3) intensive multidisciplinary data collection involving fourteen sessions and data from each individual collected over three to five months. The initial sample (n = 1908) was obtained from the city registry (in Germany, all residents must be registered). Information about the complete sample is available. Our primary focus, however, has been on the 516 participants (average age = 85; range 70 to 103 years) who completed all of the fourteen two-hour sessions of assessment at the first measurement occasion (1990–1993). This cross-sectional BASE sample of 516 consisted of equal numbers of men and women from three cohort groups in the Third Age (aged 70–74 years, born 1922–1915; aged 75–79 years, born 1917–1910; aged 80–84 years, born 1913–1905) and three cohort groups in the Fourth Age (aged 85–89 years, born 1908–1900; age 90–94 years, born 1902–1896, and age 95–105 years, born 1897–1883). By the end of 2006, seven longitudinal follow-ups of the survivors of this sample had been completed. We also regularly receive information regarding the mortality of the entire BASE sample from the City Register (90 percent of the initial participants were deceased as of October 2006).

At the time of initial assessment, 14 percent of the 516 BASE participants were institutionalized (in homes for seniors, nursing homes, and hospitals). Thirty percent were married, 55 percent widowed, 7 percent divorced, and 8 percent had never married. These demographic characteristics are consistent with city statistics for the Berlin population over the age of seventy. Also representative for these cohorts in Berlin, 65 percent of the sample had primary-level education, 28 percent high school and college level, and 8 percent university level.

Demographically speaking, the elderly population of the western districts of Berlin is more similar to that in other large cities of former West Germany than one might expect from West Berlin's post–World War II history of enclosure. However, there are some differences. Based on 1989 microcensus and 1991 population registry information, 12 percent of West Berlin inhabitants were age seventy and above, compared to 10.5 percent in the former Federal Republic of West Germany. Economically and educationally, the older adults of the western districts of Berlin were somewhat better off than their West German counterparts. On a continuum of social stratification, participants in BASE were distributed as follows: lower class (7 percent), lower middle class

(20 percent), middle class (31 percent), upper middle class (30 percent), and higher class (11 percent).

How about historical and culture-specific cohort effects? BASE participants have lived in the midst of many significant historical events. The oldest participants were born in 1883 and the youngest in 1922. The oldest birth cohorts were aged twenty to thirty at the time of World War I and the youngest were born during or shortly after that war. All participants experienced World War II, although at different stages of their lives. These cohort-specific experiences had an impact on the educational and occupational opportunities, health experiences, and family life course of the individuals (for details see Maas, Borchelt, and Mayer, 1999). The age peers of BASE participants born in other parts of Europe (such as France, England, Russia, Italy, and Poland) had different experiences of these historical events but also much in common on a day-to-day basis. There was a large wave of migration from Germany (and Europe) to the United States, Australia, and Canada from the 1930s to the 1950s. Some of the people who left Germany to begin new lives in the United States have most likely been sampled in studies of old age carried out by researchers there.

HEALTHY AGING: POSSIBLE IN THE THIRD AGE BUT RARE IN THE FOURTH AGE

The definition of *health* during old age is the subject of much debate. There is consensus that health cannot meaningfully be defined as the absence of disease because the prevalence of diagnosable illnesses in elderly populations is high. Beyond illness, a comprehensive assessment of health status in old age must include the indices of physical decline and impairment that contribute to frailty. Though the health status of contemporary age cohorts in the Third Age shows the cumulative benefits of medical advances, nutrition, and lifestyle campaigns initiated since the 1970s, there is still much more to be learned about factors that delay the onset of physical disability and alleviate the impact of frailty on daily life. In particular, because women constitute the large majority of the elderly population in the Fourth Age, a comprehensive view of the health needs and disabilities of very old women ought to be the target of future research.

In BASE, the prevalence of physical illness was found to be very high among individuals aged seventy to over one hundred. Ninety-six percent of the BASE sample had been diagnosed with at least one mild to severe internal, neurological, or orthopedic disease (Steinhagen-Thiessen and Borchelt, 1999). BASE physicians estimated that the illness would be accompanied by moderate to severe symptoms in 71 percent of cases. Life-threatening illnesses, such as congestive heart failure, were observed in 33 percent of the sample. Multimorbidity is also a fact of life for many older persons; 30 percent of BASE participants were diagnosed as having at least five severe physical illnesses. As is often reported in the literature, more older women than older men belonged to the subgroup with multiple chronic illnesses. The most frequent diagnoses were for hyperlipidemia, cerebral atherosclerosis, heart failure, osteoarthritis, degenerative diseases of the spine, and hypertension. Musculoskeletal disorders (for example, osteoarthritis, osteoporosis) were at the top of the list of disorders considered to cause the individual most symptomatic discomfort. Of interest, too, was the finding that the BASE dentists judged that about 75 percent of the participants who had dentures most likely experienced difficulty chewing and speaking because their dentures were in need of renewal or repair.

Age and gender differences were apparent in the majority of functional activities that define limitations in daily life (Smith and Baltes, 1998; Steinhagen-Thiessen and Borchelt, 1999). For example, among those over age eighty-five, 60 percent of women but only 32 percent of men reported that they needed assistance in bathing or showering. Among the very old women (over eighty-five), 81 percent had difficulties shopping and 84 percent could not use public transportation. Though the handgrip strength of seventy-year-old men was, on average 21 ± 6 kilograms (46 ± 13 pounds), for seventy-year-old women it was 8 ± 5 kilograms (18 ± 11 pounds). At age ninety, this was reduced to 12 kilograms (26.5 pounds) for men and 2 kilograms (4.5 pounds) for women. Hand and arm strength are critical for most tasks of daily life, including such things as turning doorknobs, carrying cups, and dressing. Similar gender- and age-related differences were found in measures of physical mobility (such as balance, gait, reaching, and bending).

Visual acuity (even when tested with prescribed glasses) for reading and distance declined from ages seventy to one hundred and was significantly worse for women than for men. At ages seventy to seventy-nine, 22 percent of the BASE sample were classified (by WHO standards) as being moderately or severely visually impaired, compared to 80 percent at the ages ninety to one hundred (P. B. Baltes and Mayer, 1999). Hearing acuity showed similar age differences: 47 percent were classified as having moderate or severe hearing impairment in the speech frequency range at ages seventy to seventy-nine, compared with 93 percent for ages over ninety. Though many seventy-year-olds could discriminate tones at 10 to 30 decibels, no individuals over ninety could hear tones softer than 30 decibels.

The prevalence of specific chronic illnesses, frailty, and incapacity increases as people age from seventy to over one hundred. The percentage of individuals who have to deal with multiple chronic strains associated with physical illness, vision, hearing, strength, and functional activities of daily life also increases dramatically from the Third to Fourth Age: 70 percent for those ages seventy to eighty in BASE had none or only one chronic strain, and 80 percent over age ninety had at least three strains.

MIND OVER MATTER: THERE IS MUCH LATENT PSYCHOLOGICAL VITALITY DURING OLD AGE

The prospects for maintaining good physical health throughout the potentially forty-year period of old age are indeed less than promising. To what extent, then, are older individuals able to rely on their psychological resources to compensate for biology?

Our experimental studies in Berlin, together with longitudinal findings from the Berlin Aging Study, have shown that, especially in the cognitive, emotional, and self-related domains, the functional reserves (plasticity) of the young-old are greater than previously thought (for example, P. B. Baltes, Lindenberger and Staudinger, 2006; P. B. Baltes and Smith, 2003). At least up to age eighty or so, most people function well psychologically and are able to adapt to changes in their life circumstances.

Of course, there are changes in cognitive functioning with increasing age. Few seventy-year-olds can react as quickly to an alarm as a twenty- to thirty-year-old or recall a new telephone number heard only once with the same level of accuracy. Nor can they learn new material as efficiently as they did when younger. However, these losses in the speed of processing information and short-term memory are, for most older people, relatively small and do not interfere with everyday functioning. Despite some loss in efficiency, the aging brain holds sizeable potential for new learning into the Fourth Age, provided that pathology such as stroke or dementia is minimal (see for example Verhaeghan, Borchelt, and Smith, 2003; Yang, Krampe, and Baltes, 2006). Perhaps the best evidence about the potential of the aging mind are findings showing the positive effects of extensive practice in cognitive activities, physical exercise, health modification, or high levels of social participation (see for example Fillit and others, 2002).

Everyday practical knowledge, wisdom, emotional intelligence, and language abilities are facets of the mind that continue to function well during old age as long as they are practiced. Wisdom, as Baltes and colleagues have shown, is a prototypical example of the potential that old age holds in store (P. B. Baltes, 2004). Wisdom deals with life management: it encompasses the meaning and conduct of life. Although the young-old are on average not better than younger adults at laboratory measures of wisdom, they are well-represented in the group of best performers in wisdom tasks.

Other domains in which individuals in the Third Age demonstrate exceedingly high levels of performance are the arts, social intelligence, and intergenerational generativity. Regarding intergenerational solidarity and transfers, in BASE all older generations were willing to reduce their own expenditures and allocate resources to younger generations (P. B. Baltes and Mayer, 1999). Such findings lend support to the notion that older people have specialized forms of knowledge, skills, attitudes, and motivations that can be brought to the task of creating a society with a strong sense of intergenerational connectivity and concern for all stages of life.

Alongside these aspects of cognitive functioning, various other components of the psychological system, such as the motivational aspects of the self (for example, control beliefs, future-oriented goals, and emotion regulation) and processes linked to feeling satisfied and contented with life play a vital role in compensating for declines in functionality (P. B. Baltes and Smith, 2003; Kunzmann, Little, and Smith, 2000). Self-related functioning may be more resilient against decline, especially during the Third Age, than is true for the cognitive system. It is generally expected that regulatory processes operate to protect or "immunize" the self against a loss of efficacy and well-being, even in conditions of poor health and chronic impairment. For example, individuals adjust their aspiration levels and comparison targets to achieve and maintain a sense of control over their lives. These processes contribute to a positive aura of well-being and reflect the psychological vitality of an individual to face the challenges of a long life.

To the extent that an older individual becomes physically dependent on others and experiences accumulated chronic health and life strains, the individual's sense of well-being is compromised. In particular, in BASE we observe a reduction in overall psychological vitality and the potential to experience the positive side of life (P. B. Baltes and Smith, 2003; Smith, Borchelt, Maier, and Jopp, 2002). Although the majority of BASE participants were typically satisfied with their present life conditions, those in the Third Age (aged seventy to eighty-four years) reported significantly higher positive well-being and higher satisfaction with life in general compared with those in the Fourth Age (aged eighty-five to over one hundred).

SUCCESSFUL HEALTHY AGING THROUGH SELECTION, OPTIMIZATION, AND COMPENSATION

The power of the adaptive plasticity of the self is evident in the overall strategies of life management that people use as they conduct their lives and make the journey of aging into advanced old age. The theory of selective optimization with compensation (SOC) that Margret Baltes, Paul Baltes, Alexandra Freund, and their colleagues developed and tested in a series of studies outlines how adaptation is orchestrated (M. M. Baltes, 1996; P. B. Baltes, 1997; P. B. Baltes and M. M. Baltes, 1990; Freund and P. B. Baltes, 2002).

A favorite example of the psychological meaning of selective optimization with compensation comes from interviews with the eighty-year-old pianist Rubinstein. When Rubinstein was asked how he continued to be such an excellent concert pianist, he alluded to three reasons. He played fewer pieces, but practiced them more often, and he used contrasts in tempo to simulate faster playing than he could muster. Rubinstein reduced his repertoire (that is, selection). This gave him the opportunity to practice each piece more (that is, optimization). And finally, he used contrasts in speed to hide his loss in mechanical finger dexterity (compensation).

Rubinstein described a classic scenario of what some of the long-lived BASE survivor report as their strategy of effective aging. People who select, optimize, and compensate are among those who feel better and more in control of their own future. The use of behavioral strategies, such as selective optimization with compensation, increases the level of functioning at all ages and also is particularly effective when resources are scarce (Jopp and Smith, 2006). In this vein, the art of life in old age consists of the creative search for a new, usually smaller territory that is cared for with similar intensity as in the past. The same is true for cultures. The cultures that offer older persons ways of selecting, optimizing, and compensating are the ones that assist best in maximizing the gains of older age.

CONCLUDING STATEMENT AND OUTLOOK

One of the major challenges for gerontology in the twenty-first century is how to combine the opposing findings about functional improvements and potential of the young-old with those findings of dysfunctionality and ultimate limits in the Fourth Age. As the field begins to understand more about the sources and consequences of different trajectories of psychological change, we will be in a better position to intervene in the cultural and social context of these two phases of old age. Revised social judgments about autonomy and dependency in old age and the creation of supportive life environments to compensate for personal frailty may well contribute to more people being able to experience a longer life of quality in the Fourth Age of the future (M. M. Baltes, 1996).

The findings from our Berlin study about health, psychological functioning, and well-being have several theoretical and practical implications. Theoretically, our findings provide evidence that health is critical for the aging brain and well-being in very old age. Various facets of health appear to be differentially important. In particular, aspects of functional health (impairment in vision and hearing, reduced physical mobility, and loss of strength) have a negative impact on cognitive functioning and an older individual's sense of well-being. Indeed, functional impairment explained most variance between individuals in reported frequency of feeling happy and positive about life. On average, the effects of some physical illnesses are minimal by themselves, especially when symptoms are controlled by medical interventions. But physical illness in combination with chronic pain and functional impairments in vision, hearing, strength, and physical mobility eventually rob the individual of a sense of life quality.

We found in BASE that the experience of the positive side of life was especially compromised after age eighty. The transition from the Third Age to the Fourth Age appears to be a significant psychological challenge (P. B. Baltes, 1997; P. B. Baltes and Smith, 2003; Smith and P. B. Baltes, 1997). The capacity of the individual to adapt to conditions of declining health may reach a critical limit. The accumulated chronic strain of dealing with the effects of multiple physical illnesses, frailty, functional impairment, and social losses that characterize the Fourth Age appears to test the limits of adaptive self-related processes. Poor health in very old age may eventually become an overwhelming factor that either dampens the capacity to experience positive emotions or limits opportunities for such experiences. Social participation and social contacts, for example, are prime sources of positive affect. Clearly, older adults who have great difficulty seeing and hearing and rarely move beyond the confines of their place of residence are at risk in terms of reduced opportunity for social contacts. The oldest old typically have to rely on the "social world" to come to them. In today's world, it is telling that in a large city, like Berlin, many old people are lonely and feel socially isolated.

On a practical level, BASE findings point to the important need for further technological and medical advances and social-cultural interventions to improve the quality of life conditions of the Third Age. The multimorbid life contexts of the oldest old highlight the salience of issues of dependency and the personal cost of aging. Many of the functional impairments of old age could, in principle, be compensated for to some extent by efficient aids or specific intervention. Technological advances in cataract surgery, contact lenses, and hip replacement techniques in the 1990s illustrate the potential of medical advances. It is anticipated that future development of efficient hearing aids will improve communication opportunities for many older adults. Advances in rehabilitation methods and interventions, such as exercise and muscular strength training, may delay brain aging and the disablement process and reduce the numbers of older adults who are physically dependent on others. All such advances require that geriatric medicine is well-represented in medical faculties and the training of future physicians. Sadly, in 2007, this is still not the case in Germany.

BASE findings also support proposals about the necessary evolution of a "culture of old age" as a compensatory support for older adults, given their reduced biological capacity to adapt (P. B. Baltes, 1997, 2006). Data from BASE cohorts suggest that social-cultural input should be directed especially to the minimization of the impact of health-related life restrictions and chronic life strains. Older women living alone, who comprise the majority of the population in the Fourth Age, should be targeted for intervention research (Smith and P. B. Baltes, 1998). To some degree, of course, the health constraints observed in BASE and in similar samples from other countries may be cohort-specific. The oldest-old participants in the Berlin Aging Study certainly experienced periods of malnutrition, hardship, and loss in early life and were exposed to epidemics that killed many of their age peers before the general use of antibiotic medications (Maas, Borchelt, and Mayer, 1999). This early life exposure may have had a negative long-term impact for current oldest-old cohorts in terms of chronic health problems, but it also may have contributed to their surviving to an advanced age. Other health and lifestyle factors may prove to be critical for survival and personal well-being in future generations of older Germans. At present, we know relatively little about the biogenetic, life history, and environmental factors predictive of a healthy longevity (Vaupel and others, 1998). Given this lack of knowledge, in the short term, our findings suggest that all efforts be invested to compensate for health-related constraints so that more individuals have the chance to maintain their dignity and a positive sense of well-being into the Fourth Age and at the end of life.

REFERENCES

Baltes, M. M. *The Many Faces of Dependency in Old Age*. New York: Cambridge University Press, 1996.

Baltes, P. B. "On the Incomplete Architecture of Human Ontogeny: Selection, Optimization, and Compensation as Foundation of Developmental Theory." *American Psychologist*, 1997, *52*, 366–380.

Baltes, P. B. *Wisdom as Orchestration of Mind and Virtue*. Book in preparation, 2004. http://www.mpib-berlin. mpg.de/dok/full/baltes/orchestr/index.htm.

Baltes, P. B. "Facing Our Limits: Human Dignity in the Very Old." *Daedalus*, 2006, *135*, 33–39.

Baltes, P. B., and Baltes, M. M. "Psychological Perspectives on Successful Aging: The Model of Selective Optimization with Compensation." In P. B. Baltes and M. M. Baltes (eds.), *Successful Aging: Perspectives from the Behavioral Sciences*, 1–34. Cambridge, England: Cambridge University Press, 1990.

Baltes, P. B., Lindenberger, U., and Staudinger, U. M. "Life Span Theory in Developmental Psychology." In W. Damon and R. M. Lerner (eds.), *Handbook of Child Psychology*, Vol. 1: *Theoretical Models of Human Development* (6th ed.), 569–664. New York: Wiley, 2006.

Baltes, P. B., and Mayer, K. U. (eds.). *The Berlin Aging Study: Aging from 70 to 100*. New York: Cambridge University Press, 1999.

Baltes, P. B., and Smith, J. "New Frontiers in the Future of Aging: From Successful Aging of the Young Old to Dilemmas of the Fourth Age." *Gerontology*, 2003, *49*, 123–135.

Fillit, H. M., and others. "Achieving and Maintaining Cognitive Vitality with Aging." *Mayo Clinical Proceedings*, 2002, *77*, 681–696.

Freund, A. M., and Baltes, P. B. "Life-Management Strategies of Selection, Optimization, and Compensation: Measurement by Self-Report and Construct Validity." *Journal of Personality and Social Psychology*, 2002, *82*, 642–662.

Jopp, D., and Smith, J. "Resources and Life-Management Strategies as Determinants of Subjective Well-being in Very Old Age: The Protective Effect of Selection, Optimization, and Compensation." *Psychology and Aging*, 2006, *21*, 253–265.

Kunzmann, U., Little, T., and Smith, J. "Is Age-Related Stability of Well-Being a Paradox? Cross-Sectional and Longitudinal Evidence from the Berlin Aging Study." *Psychology and Aging*, 2000, *15*, 511–526.

Maas, I., Borchelt, M., and Mayer, K. U. "Generational Experiences of Old People in Berlin." In P. B. Baltes and K. U. Mayer (eds.), *The Berlin Aging Study: Aging from 70 to 100*, 83–110. New York: Cambridge University Press, 1999.

Smith, J., and Baltes, M. M. "The Role of Gender in Very Old Age: Profiles of Functioning and Everyday Life Patterns." *Psychology and Aging*, 1998, *13*, 676–695.

Smith, J., and Baltes, P. B. "Profiles of Psychological Functioning in the Old and Oldest-Old." *Psychology and Aging*, 1997, *12*, 458–472.

Smith, J., Borchelt, M., Maier, H., and Jopp, D. "Health and Wellbeing in Old Age." *Journal of Social Issues*, 2002, *58*, 715–732.

Steinhagen-Thiessen, E., and Borchelt, M. "Morbidity, Medication, and Functional Limitations in Very Old Age." In P. B. Baltes and K. U. Mayer (eds.), *The Berlin Aging Study: Aging from 70 to 100*, 131–166. New York: Cambridge University Press, 1999.

Suzman, R.M., Willis, D. P., and Manton, K. G. (eds.) *The Oldest Old*. New York: Oxford University Press, 1992.

Vaupel, J. W., and others. (1998). "Biodemographic Trajectories of Longevity." *Science*, 280, 855–860.

Verhaeghen, P., Borchelt, M., and Smith, J. "The Relation Between Cardiovascular and Metabolic Disease and Cognition in Very Old Age: Cross-Sectional and Longitudinal Findings from the Berlin Aging Study." *Health Psychology*, 2003, *22*, 559–569.

Yang, L., Krampe, R., and Baltes, P. B. "Basic Forms of Cognitive Plasticity Extended into the Oldest-Old: Retest Learning, Age, and Cognitive Functioning." *Psychology and Aging*, 2006, *21*, 372–378.

CHAPTER

11

CHALLENGES OF PRODUCTIVE AGING IN JAPAN

SHIGEO MORIOKA

There is no question that longevity is a universal wish of mankind. How best to achieve a long-living society benefiting both the elderly and society as a whole, however, is still unclear. How can society help older persons to remain healthy? How can generations work harmoniously to attain a productive society?

This chapter discusses Japan's public programs designed to facilitate older persons' efforts to lead productive lives. It outlines the universal pension, health care, and long-term care programs in Japan as well as challenges faced by these programs. The author believes that public programs by themselves are not sufficient for a society to realize productive aging. It is imperative that the elderly themselves are diligent and self-reliant in preparing themselves for productive old age.

Japan has experienced a dramatic demographic change in the last several decades. In 1947, as Japan entered on the path of recovery following the end of World War II, the average life expectancy in Japan was 50.06 years for men and 53.96 years for women. Today, the figures have risen to 78.64 years for men and 85.59 years for women. This represents a dramatic increase of approximately twenty-nine years for men and thirty-two for women. Over the past six decades or so, improvements in public health led to a lower infant mortality rate, and this in turn resulted in a gradual decline in the fertility rate (the number of births in the year divided by the population of the previous year) and a progressively lower dependency ratio. As education became more widely available and technical innovations took place, Japan's economy grew rapidly, backed by the phenomenon of "population dividends," as described by Bloom and Canning (2000). It is also significant that with its pacifist constitution and under the protection it has been receiving through the Japan-U.S. Security Treaties, Japan has not taken part in any wars for over sixty years. As a result, Japan has maintained an extremely low level of military spending, only about 1.0 percent as a percentage of GDP, over this period. This has had the effect of both promoting economic and industrial development and establishing social security systems.

Population aging is forecast to continue in Japan. The National Institute of Population and Social Security Research estimates that the percentage of elderly age sixty-five or over will continue to rise sharply in coming years (The National Institute of Population and Social Security Research, 2006). The 2005 figure of 21.0 percent is predicted to climb to 27.8 percent in 2025 and to reach 35.7 percent by 2050. A particularly large percentage of the population is composed of the older elderly, aged seventy-five and over. The 2005 level of 9.5 percent is expected to increase to 16.7 percent in 2025, reaching 21.5 percent in 2050. In response to these changes in the population structure, systematic reforms are being swiftly implemented to ensure the sustainability of the public pension schemes and health and long-term care insurance systems that support the well-being and standard of living of the elderly.

JAPAN'S SOCIAL SECURITY SYSTEM: ITS ROLE AND RELATED ISSUES

The concept of the social security system in Japan includes the systems of pension security, health care and long-term care, and public aid. The national pension and health and long-term care insurance systems universally cover the population in Japan. The following discussion outlines these programs, focusing on the challenges they experience in their effort to maintain sustainability.

Pension Schemes

The part of Japan's social security system that provides livelihood support for the elderly is a two-tiered universal coverage system that consists of the national pension and the employee's pension, which was launched in 1961. The 2004 reforms of the pension system provided the following: (1) to avoid limitless future increases in insurance premiums, the premiums will be increased gradually until 2017 (employees' pension premium rate based on standard monthly wage will rise from the prereform rate of 13.58 percent to 18.3 percent from 2017 onward, and national pension premiums from the prereform level of 13,300 yen to 16,900 yen); after that, an insurance premium standard will be fixed; (2) the amount of pension benefits that people receive will be decided based on their wages and the cost of living. The pension benefit level of standard pensioner households will be set at over 50 percent of the average income of working households (prior to the reforms this was 60 percent). The policy is intended to limit growth in the amount of pensions paid by gradually increasing insurance premiums to a level where they will be fixed in the future. The Ministry of Health, Labor and Welfare (MHLW) expects that these reforms could reduce the total benefit costs, projected to reach 73 trillion yen in 2025, to around 62 trillion yen—and ultimately make it possible to maintain the pension system.

It is significant that these reforms treat the pension system not as a form of livelihood insurance, like the Public Assistance System, but rather as a system that ensures protection against the financial risks of old age. The reforms also establish a balance between burden and payment to make the system sustainable. When universal public pension coverage was instituted under the national pension system in 1961, the average life expectancy in Japan was 66.03 years for men and 70.19 years for women. Since then, both figures have increased by about ten years. Therefore, it would be natural for the retirement age to be over sixty-five, and thus it is possible that the age at which pension payments begin will be raised above the current age of sixty-five.

Health Care and Long-Term Care

Japan's health insurance system was established as a system of universal health care in 1961. This was shortly after the years of high economic growth began, and it is an event of great significance in the growth of Japan's average life expectancy. Japan's health care system is operated through a combination of tax and insurance systems and ensures free access to medical institutions.

According to the World Health Organization (WHO), Japan's life expectancy of 74.5 years is the highest in the world. WHO's World Health Report 2000 also placed Japan first in its survey of health care system attainment and performance among all member states. According to the OECD's Health Data 2005, Japan's expenditure on health as a percentage of GDP (7.8 percent) is lower than that of the United States (13.9 percent), Germany (10.8 percent), and France (9.4 percent). This makes Japan one of the lowest spenders on health care among the advanced nations. Japan's health care system has made an efficient and significant contribution toward the improvement of its citizens' quality of life.

But even in Japan, national medical care expenditure is increasing much more rapidly than national income. It rose from 6.1 percent (16 trillion yen) in 1985 to 8.6 percent (31.5 trillion yen) in 2003, and is expected to rise to 12.2 percent in 2025. Medical expenditure for the elderly as a percentage of the total amount of national medical care expenditure has also been growing steadily, from 25.4 percent in 1985 to 36.9 percent in 2003. Thus there is mounting concern that the burden on the public will increase.

The Partial Amendments to the Health Insurance Act, passed by the Diet on June 14, 2006, indicate the direction of subsequent health care system reforms in Japan. The amendments, made in a context of steeply rising medical expenditure for the elderly, consisted mainly of measures to increase the size of copayments by the elderly and to curb medical costs by reducing the incidence of lifestyle-related diseases.

The main measures that were adopted include the following:

- Promoting medical checkups and health guidance, setting numerical targets for reducing the incidence of lifestyle-related diseases, reducing the time needed for treatment, and enhancing the quality of regional healthcare to improve patients' quality of life

- Increasing the amount of copayments by elderly patients—for example, by raising the copayment rate of patients aged seventy to seventy-four from 10 percent to 20 percent, reducing the coverage of public insurance benefits, and, as a countermeasure to the declining fertility rate, increasing support for those giving birth to and raising children

- Establishing a medical system exclusively for the older elderly, aged seventy-five and over, and collecting new insurance premiums

MHLW expects these reforms to lead to an eight trillion yen savings in medical payments in the year 2025.

The Long-term Care Insurance System for the elderly (people aged sixty-five and over) was initiated in 2000 and substantially revised in 2005. The revisions included the following:

- Preparing long-term care services focused on prevention and consisting of improvements in physical exercise, nutrition, and oral functions, for elderly people who are expected to require long-term care or whose condition is likely to be sustained or improved even if they do require long-term care

- Adopting a system of fees for facility users (who until then had been covered by Long-term Care Insurance benefits) to pay for their accommodation and meal expenses

- Creating in communities a flexible, small-scale system of home and institutional care

MHLW expects these reforms to help reduce the total cost of Long-term Care Insurance in 2025 from nineteen trillion yen to approximately sixteen trillion yen.

Although the debate about health care costs for the elderly tends to focus on the perceived burden on elderly people, Suzuki and others (2001) point out that if end-of-life health care expenditure is eliminated from the equation, health care expenditure does not rise with increasing age. In other words, the greater expenditure on health care for the elderly can be explained by the fact that elderly people are more susceptible to terminal illness. Thus the rise in health care expenditure occurs because most people grow old before dying. Since this is a demographic phenomenon, it is reasonable to expect that the society willingly share the burden collectively.

One real issue in elderly health care in Japan is *social hospitalization*, which occurs when elderly people undergo extended hospitalization because a long-term care environment cannot be provided by long-term care facilities or family caregiving. According to the OECD's Health Data 2005, the average length of hospital stays in Japan is 36.4 days, compared with 13.4 days in France, 7.6 days in the UK, and 6.6 days in the United States. Reduction of social hospitalization will require a reassessment of the different roles of health care and long-term care. A system must be created to accommodate those who need care services to support their daily activities but not extensive medical care, so that they can lead a dignified life either in a long-term care facility or at home under the long-term care system. There has also been discussion of respecting the wishes of the individual and family in decisions about terminal care and dying with dignity.

Health Promotion

The philosophy of health promotion is essential for the realization of healthy longevity. Japan has kept in step with the international New Public Health Movement through its "21st Century Measures for National Health Promotion: Healthy Japan 21," a nationwide health improvement program led mainly by MHLW. The program addresses the issue of lifestyle-related diseases and their possible causes, based on the following nine categories: nutrition and lifestyle, physical activity and exercise, relaxation and mental health care, smoking, alcohol, dental care, diabetes, circulatory diseases, and cancer. Local and municipal units have formulated basic policies, examined current conditions, set targets, and defined countermeasures to be implemented by around 2010 to make the nation healthier. The Health Promotion Law, enacted in 2002, made the content of Healthy Japan 21 statutory. The law provides for standardization of medical health examinations on a nationwide basis and promotes research and comprehensive counseling and consultation programs not only on nutrition (which has been traditionally emphasized) but also on lifestyle habits including second-hand smoke.

Since 2005, the government has also been promoting its Health Frontier Strategy, which supports scientific progress in methods for prolonging healthy longevity. The program aims to extend healthy life expectancy by about two years by 2014, by setting numerical targets for the following measures dealing with lifestyle-related diseases and reducing the need for long-term care.

1. Promotion of measures against lifestyle-related diseases to reduce disease and mortality rates:

    ■ Measures against cancer: Improve five-year survival rate by 20 percent

    ■ Measures against heart disease: Reduce mortality by 25 percent

    ■ Measures against strokes: Reduce mortality by 25 percent

    ■ Measures against diabetes: Reduce incidence by 20 percent

2. Reduction of persons requiring long-term care services by preventing health conditions that necessitate long-term care, thereby reducing the proportion of people who are disabled enough to receive care services from one in seven to one in ten

This kind of health promotion will encourage elderly people to do their utmost to be self-reliant.

The employment rate of the elderly in Nagano Prefecture is the highest in Japan, and Nagano's expenditure on health care for the elderly is the lowest. This suggests that elderly people who are still actively participating in society are highly self-reliant. It also suggests that remaining self-reliant for as long as possible is good for elderly people's quality of life, which is significant for all of society. This tells us that the most important issue for the future of social security is how to reduce the elderly's need for services by promoting good health.

ECONOMIC GROWTH AND THE PARTICIPATION OF THE ELDERLY IN THE LABOR MARKET

The interaction between economic growth and labor-force participation by the elderly is complex. During Japan's economic bubble, which lasted up to the early 1990s, many businesses enthusiastically engaged in property investments that were revealed by the collapse of the bubble to be bad assets. These were a drain on Japan's banks, which in turn exerted pressure on other corporations. Japan suffered from an economic recession for more than ten years, and economic growth even fell into the negative range in 1998. Deflation persisted during this period, and the labor market showed a significant decline in hiring of both young and elderly people due to ongoing corporate efforts to restructure business. A sense of crisis pervaded Japanese society, and people questioned the future sustainability of the social security system. The result was the various reforms discussed thus far.

Capital investment finally started to pick up in 2002, mainly in the export sector. According to Cabinet Office statistics, the GDP rose by 1.7 percent in 2004 and by 3.2 percent in 2005, with all industry sales showing a 6.2 percent year-on-year rise in 2005. The trend continued in 2006, with capital investment during the first quarter climbing 16.6 percent higher than the first quarter of 2005. The employment situation is also improving. The overall unemployment rate fell from 4.6 percent in 2004 to 4.3 percent in 2005, and to 4.1 percent during the first half of 2006. There has been much speculation about the negative effect of Japan's aging population on the economy. However, the present partial recovery of the economy has brought Japan to a point where we should be able once again to find a clear direction for the future.

The most serious challenge that must be addressed in the discussion of population aging and economic growth is the diminishing number of workers in the labor force because of the continuously declining total fertility rate. This demographic situation suggests a real possibility of labor shortages. Naoki Mitani and others (2006) created estimates of the working population based on two scenarios. In one, no progress is made in participation in the labor market by elderly people, women, and young people.

In the other, their participation is increased as a result of various policies. In the no-progress scenario, a working population of 67.28 million in 2004 diminishes by 4.91 million by 2015 and by 11.31 million in 2030. The other scenario, in which these groups participate in the labor force, shows the working population declining by 1.92 million in 2015 and by 6.16 million in 2030. The latter scenario presupposes that the proportion of businesses providing work for people until they are at least age sixty-five will have risen by 2030 to equal the number of businesses that currently provide a workplace to people until they are age sixty. This means, in effect, that the current retirement age of sixty, which is observed by most businesses, must be raised.

The labor force participation rate for elderly people in Japan is extremely high. In 2004, the workforce participation rate of the elderly aged sixty to sixty-four was 70.7 percent for men and 39.7 percent for women in Japan. According to the International Labour Organisation (ILO) LABORSTA, in America the participation rate was 57.0 percent for men and 23.3 percent for women; in Germany, 37.7 percent for men and 19.7 percent for women; and in France, 19.0 percent for men and 2.5 percent for women. Also, over half of Japanese older people without jobs expressed a desire to work.

Raising the employment rate of elderly people and women would clearly help to alleviate a problem caused by a drastic decline in the labor supply. This would call for a movement throughout the whole of society to secure employment of the elderly. The effort to increase workforce participation must become a matter of strategy for business, a policymaking target for government, and a motivational goal for the elderly themselves.

During the prolonged recession of the 1990s, businesses tended to remain in the black by cutting labor costs, which encouraged employees to retire early. Hiroshi Yoshikawa (2004) analyzed these restructuring trends by sector and size of business and found that it was not necessarily the small-to-medium, nonmanufacturing businesses that carried out restructuring. Instead, the major manufacturing industries, which had been considered the "model pupils" of the Japanese economy, were at the forefront of the restructuring trend. Now, however, the level of investment in technological innovation is already rising. Going forward, corporations will compete for high-quality services. According to Cabinet Office research, 46 percent of businesses expect the retirement of the Japanese "baby boom generation" (defined in Japan as people born soon after the end of World War II; that is, between 1947 and 1949) to seriously impact the process of transmitting skills and techniques to the next generation. This means businesses must reform the old-fashioned, rigid promotion practices of seniority-based personnel systems and start to employ elderly people. For example, they will need to consider adopting both more flexible ways of working and new methods for taking skills and the desire to work into account.

On the policymaking front, only meager results can be expected if efforts are limited to merely preparing legal mechanisms for raising the retirement age and to intervening in corporate retirement practices. Progress must be made in ensuring more flexibility in the tax system and modes of employment and in creating business incentives to employ elderly people (Osako, 2006).

The aging of the population could also lead to changes in the elderly's attitudes toward saving that would affect the formation of capital stock. In 2004 the average annual income of elderly households was 2.9 million yen, whereas the average figure for total households was 5.79 million yen. However, elderly households tend to be composed of fewer members, so that the per-person figure was 1.84 million in elderly households and 2.03 million in total households. The average savings for total households came to 16.92 million yen in 2004, whereas the average figure for households with a household head aged sixty-five or over was 25.04 million yen, according to the MHLW's Comprehensive Survey of Living Conditions of the People (2004). More than half of the private financial assets in Japan are thought to be owned by people over the age of sixty. All this illustrates the fact that there is very little real disparity in income, and elderly people actually have more savings than other households.

Another point was raised in a recent attitude survey: 35.8 percent of elderly people said they would compensate for shortfalls in living expenses by economizing and 27.1 percent said they would do so by using up their savings. Only 26.4 percent said that they would live with or seek assistance from their children. This suggests that the idea of self-reliance is taking root among the elderly. MHLW's Nationwide Survey of Recipients showed that 37.9 percent of the 1.29 million public assistance recipients are age sixty-five or over.

These facts are noteworthy when examined in terms of the national economy, because they suggest that household savings, which fell from 43 trillion yen to 22 trillion yen between 1991 and 2003, could decline still further—potentially threatening the formation of the nation's capital stock. It is absolutely crucial that employment rates be increased to ensure a stable lifestyle for the elderly.

SOCIAL PARTICIPATION OF THE ELDERLY

The preceding discussion touched on matters of health and care and income and financial future. The issue of family and loneliness—that is, the question of ties with society and communication—is as important as the labor issue. Elderly people who maintain their social ties and contribute to society tend to better retain their mental and physical functions—and thus are better able to fulfill their responsibility to pass on their abilities to that society.

Fewer elderly people live with their children than in the past, and there has been a considerable increase in the number of elderly households consisting of just one person or a couple. According to MHLW's Comprehensive Survey of Living Conditions of People on Health and Welfare 2005, 59.7 percent of elderly people aged sixty-five and over lived with their children in 1990, but this figure had fallen to 45.5 percent by 2004. During that period, the number of households consisting of elderly couples increased from 25.7 percent to 36.0 percent, and single-person households from

11.2 percent to 14.7 percent. The Cabinet Office's 2006 International Study on Living and Consciousness of Senior Citizens found that whereas 53.6 percent of elderly people in 1990 said that they always wanted to live with their grandchildren, the figure had fallen to 34.8 percent by 2005.

Conversely, we find increasing participation in volunteer activities by elderly persons. According to the Cabinet Office's Attitude Survey on Participation in Local Communities by the Elderly (2003), the number of people saying that they had participated in some form of volunteer activity by themselves, with friends, or in some group over the past year rose from 36.4 percent in 1988 to 54.8 percent in 2003. This was a significant increase. Elderly people participate in a varied range of activities, including public health, health care and welfare, child rearing, community safety programs, and social education. This finding further confirms that elderly people are becoming more self-reliant.

The baby boom generation has a significant role to play. It will exert a fundamental influence on the future direction of elderly people's participation in the labor market and society. During the period when this generation was born, the fertility rate reached the phenomenal level of 3.3 to 3.5 percent, and 6.8 million people—about 5 percent of the current population—were born. They will retire en masse from their work when they reach sixty, the age at which most companies let their employees retire. This event is expected to have an impact so great that the issue has come to be known as "the year 2007 problem."

One major concern is that baby boomer retirement may affect the transfer of skills within industry. On the consumption front, there are also hopes that this mass retirement will lead to the creation of a large new market over the next few years. Even more significant, this generation will go on to set lifestyle standards for elderly people in later years. It is hoped that they will serve to establish in Japan a lifestyle in which elderly people participate not just in work, but also across the whole spectrum of social activity. As Yukiko Kudo (2006) points out, there will be demand in the future for ways of work in which, "Instead of the linear life pattern where, at one stage people study, then work, then reach retirement and then go on to volunteering, people will study, work and volunteer at various stages of their life, choose what activities they are involved in, and create a personalized way of living" (p. 166).

OTHER ISSUES AND PROSPECTS CONCERNING THE LONGEVITY SOCIETY

I would like to raise a few more points about the increasing longevity of the population. The decline in the number of children will have a major medium- to long-term impact on Japan. The fertility rate has diminished alarmingly in recent years, with the total fertility rate plummeting to 1.25 percent in 2005. Births started to increase in 2006 because of the improving employment situation, with 11,618 more births in the first half of the year than in the first half of 2005. The Law for Measures to Support the Development of the Next Generation, enacted in 2003, mandates the formulation of action plans for easy-to-use child-care leave systems and shorter working hours. Not only national and local government entities, but also businesses enterprises with 301 or more employees are subject to this requirement. We need to further promote such measures to assist child-rearing. There must also be a strengthening of mechanisms that enable those outside the child-rearing generation to assist in bringing up children.

Supportive and cohesive communities are important for the well-being of the elderly, and efforts are needed in Japan to develop and nurture such communities. Japan used to consist of various self-sufficient regions with their own distinctive economies and cultures. In recent years the foundation of regional economic strength has undergone continuous weakening, along with a growing emphasis on the need to reconstruct both urban and rural communities. Regional power must be reestablished and enhanced. This includes promotion of small and self-sufficient regional units, sometimes referred to as "compact cities," where elderly people can lead their lives without having to go beyond walking distance from their homes. This is beneficial from the point of view of (1) regional economic independence, (2) developing better systems for the support of elderly people who require care in the various different regions of Japan, (3) strengthening networks through which the elderly can participate in society, and (4) developing housing where people can live with a sense of security.

Longevity is increasing everywhere throughout the developed world. In some countries it is increasing at an even faster rate because of rapid economic growth. There are regions where population explosions coexist with extremely high infant mortality rates. As Robert N. Butler has pointed out:

> So long as there is "shortgevity" and nations have huge populations with 35–40 percent of the population under 15 years of age, there will be too few healthy, productive citizens to buy, sell and exchange the goods and services with the developed world. The latter must do more about the inequalities of wealth, longevity and health for their own interest [2005, p. 6].

Countries that enjoy high rates of longevity have a responsibility to share with other countries information about their policies on aging as well as their successes and failures in dealing with longevity issues.

IN CONCLUSION

I have discussed some of the vast array of issues that Japan currently faces and have taken a look at directions for the future. Much can be expected from elderly people in the areas I mentioned, including health promotion, participation in the labor force and other sectors, support for child rearing, regional revitalization, and fulfillment of Japan's role in international society. In 2006, Hiroshi Shibata drew an analogy between the human body and the elderly person. He pointed out that just as every single part of the human body has a crucial function in biology, "surely every elderly person plays a vital role in society. From now on the elderly should feel that they are leading society, and realize productive aging" (p. 5).

There is a tendency among some to perceive the elderly as weak. However, Tsutomu Hotta (2006) has said that

We should reconsider the notion that people over sixty-five are "elderly." Social security has gone beyond the realms of Article 25 of the Constitution [which states "1) All people shall have the right to maintain the minimum standards of wholesome and cultured living. 2) In all spheres of life, the State shall use its endeavors for the promotion and extension of social welfare and security, and of public health."] and entered those of Article 13 [which states: "All of the people shall be respected as individuals. Their right to life, liberty, and the pursuit of happiness shall, to the extent that it does not interfere with the public welfare, be the supreme consideration in legislation and in other governmental affairs."]; we need to create a strong society based on self-reliance and mutual assistance [p. 5].

By achieving productive aging, elderly people in Japan will demonstrate that the long-lived society can be rich in possibilities.

SELECTIVE LEGISLATION IMPACTING THE LIVES OF THE ELDERLY IN JAPAN

1922   Enactment of the Health Insurance Law (health insurance system primarily for skilled workers)

1923   Enactment of the Pension Law (national pension system for public servants and veterans)

1938   Enactment of the National Health Insurance Law (voluntary health insurance system for residents organized by municipalities)

1941   Enactment of the Worker's Pension Law (universal pension scheme for male workers employed by enterprises with ten or more employees)

1950   Enactment of the New Public Assistance Law (public assistance for all persons whose income does not meet a set minimum)

1961   Implementation of the Revised National Health Insurance Law (the first universal health insurance plan)

1961   Implementation of the National Pension Law (the first universal pension scheme covering the employed, the self-employed, and homemakers)

1963   Enactment of the Welfare Law for the Elderly (law mandating medical and social services for the elderly, emphasizing long-term care programs)

1973   Revision of the Welfare Law for the Elderly (medical services made available at no cost for all senior citizens aged seventy and over)

1982   Enactment of the Health and Medical Service Law for the Elderly (expansion of funding for health care costs to include nearly all employees regardless of age)

1995   Enactment of the Basic Law on Measures for the Aging Society (comprehensive national framework of services for the elderly, including long-term, intermediate, and home-based care)

2000   Implementation of the Long-term Care Insurance Law (universal long-term care insurance coverage for those aged sixty-five years and over, enacted in 1997)

2004   Amendment of the National Pension Law and Related Legislation (emphasis on attaining program sustainability through stabilization of premiums and containment of benefit escalation)

2005   Revision of the Long-term Care Insurance Law (emphasis on preventive care and cost containment)

2006   Implementation of the Revised Law Concerning the Stabilization of Employment of Older Persons (expansion of employment opportunities for older workers through a raising of the mandatory retirement age and other measures)

2006   Comprehensive Revision of Health Care System, involving several existing acts of legislation (emphasis on preventive care for lifestyle-related diseases and cost containment)

REFERENCES

Bloom, D. E., and Canning, D. "The Health and Wealth of Nations." *Science*, Feb. 18, 2000, *287*.

Butler, R. N. "The Health and Wealth of Nations: Do Health and Longevity Create Wealth?" Unpublished paper presented at the Symposium of Joint Committee, ILC Partnership, Rio de Janeiro, Brazil, June 2005.

Economic Planning Agency, Government of Japan. *Japan in the Year 2000: Preparing Japan for an Age of Internationalization, the Aging Society and Maturity*. Tokyo: The Japan Times, 1983.

Hotta, T. "Elderly People in the 21st Century: Thoughts on Living a Dignified Life" (in Japanese). ILC-Japan's *Long-lived Society Global Information Journal*, 2006, *2*, 5.

Kudo, Y. *Gerontology: Opening up a New Society for the Elderly* (in Japanese). Tokyo: Kadokawa Shoten, 2006.

Mitani, N., and others. *Labor Market Supply and Demand Estimates* 2005 (in Japanese). Tokyo: The Japan Institute for Labor Policy and Training, 2006.

National Institute of Population and Social Security Research (Japan). *Japan Population Estimate* (in Japanese). Tokyo: National Institute of Population and Social Security Research, 2006.

Osako, M. "Toyota, Sanyo Electric and Others Design Measures to Comply with the Revised Senior Employment Opportunity Expansion Law" (in English). *ILC-Japan Web Journal*, 2006. [http://longevity.ilcjapan.org]. Accessed Nov. 1, 2006.

Shibata, H. "International Information and the Lifestyles of Elderly People Today" (in Japanese). ILC-Japan's *Long-lived Society Global Information Journal*, 2006, *1*.

Suzuki, W. and others. "Is Longevity a Major Cause for Elderly Health Cost Expansion?" (in Japanese). Japan Center for Economic Research Discussion Paper No. 70, 2001.

Yoshikawa, H. "The Decade of Loss: Finance and the Real Economy" (in Japanese). *Ministry of Finance, Policy Research Institute Financial Review*, Sept. 2004, 35.

CHAPTER

12

HEALTHY AGING IN THE NETHERLANDS

C.I.J.M. ROSS-VAN DORP

Many countries are confronted with the challenge of an aging population, and the Netherlands is no exception. There are currently more than 2.3 million people aged sixty-five and older in the Netherlands—approximately 14 percent of the total population. In France that figure is 16.2 percent, in Germany 16.9 percent, and in Sweden 17.2 percent. Studies and demographic scenarios show that by 2030 there will be approximately four million people over sixty-five in the Netherlands. That is approximately 25 percent of the total population, twice as many as now. There will be six retirees for every ten workers; the ratio now is three retirees for every ten workers.

The challenge is for a population whose average age is rising to provide care for more and more old people. The trend will gain momentum after 2010, when the baby boom generation, born shortly after the Second World War, starts to retire.

This chapter examines the main characteristics of the population of the Netherlands and the future challenges and trends. I shall then touch on elements of the policy that the Dutch government established in 2005. The main thrust was that investing now in human and other resources—including health, training, entrepreneurship, housing, transportation infrastructure, intergenerational solidarity, and social cohesion—is the best way of meeting the challenges society faces.

140

HEALTH IN THE NETHERLANDS

The Dutch government is regularly informed about public health, the position occupied by elderly people in society, and the development of the care system.

Public Health

In 2006, the National Institute of Public Health and the Environment (RIVM) produced a publication on trends in public health in the Netherlands. Its conclusions can be summed up as follows:

- Dutch people live longer and enjoy good health longer than ever before. Since 1950, average life expectancy has risen for men from 70.4 to 76.7, and for women from 72.6 to 80.9. Because this has been rising more slowly in recent years, it is now about average for the EU.

- There is still plenty of room to improve public health. There are considerable regional differences in health status. People living in socioeconomically deprived areas tend to have more health problems.

- Poor diet and obesity raise concern about the future health status of certain population groups. Twenty-five years ago, one-third of the population was overweight. That proportion has now risen to one-half. There also has been no reduction in smoking among young people, and alcohol consumption has increased. All these factors will seriously affect future health care needs. For example, obesity is the main cause of diabetes and cardiovascular disease.

- Cardiovascular disease is still the main cause of death in the Netherlands, but it is claiming relatively fewer victims. However, the incidence of diabetes and asthma is rising. The number of victims claimed by smoking-related diseases (COPD and lung cancer) is now stable. The rate among men has dropped sharply, but the rate among women has risen sharply.

- Although illnesses are increasing, they are placing fewer constraints on people, thanks to medical aids and technology. However, this trend is not as strong in the Netherlands as in the United States, among others.

Position of the Elderly in Society

The Dutch government regularly asks the Social and Cultural Planning Office (SCP) to produce reports on social issues. In 2006, it produced a *Report on the Elderly* (2006b), identifying the following trends.

- Educational levels among those over fifty-five are still rising.

- Those aged fifty-five to sixty-four are working longer.

- Many elderly people are active in the community.

- Elderly people's incomes have risen in recent years.

- From the age of seventy-five, people do less volunteer work and engage in fewer leisure pursuits.

- Those over seventy-five have relatively more health problems: in 2003, two-thirds were suffering from a chronic illness.

Development of the Health Care System

The main indicators for the health care system are regularly reviewed by the Dutch government. The RIVM's Dutch Healthcare Performance Report, which was published in 2006, indicated that attention should be focused on the following:

- *The growing demand for care.* Both the volume and price of care rose sharply in the 2001–2004 period. In the same period, costs rose from €47 billion to €60 billion; that is, from 8.1 percent to 9.2 percent of GDP. Costs per capita are therefore higher than the average in both the OECD and the EU.

- *Trends among care workers.* Despite the fact that there were fewer hard-to-fill vacancies in the 2001 to 2004 period, staff shortages are expected to increase between 2006 and 2008.

- *Choice.* Clients want more freedom to choose. With the "personal budget" arrangement for long-term care, clients can make their own arrangements without interference from the insurer. The number of people with a personal budget rose from ten thousand in 1998 to eighty thousand in 2005 (an increase from 2 percent to more than 10 percent of total long-term care beneficiaries).

- *Satisfaction.* Clients are highly satisfied at the standard of Dutch health care, but 36 percent are less confident about the future.

- *Nursing and care homes.* In these institutions the burden of care is extremely heavy, affecting the quality of the services provided. Standards need to be improved. New technologies could be introduced to provide support.

CENTRAL GOVERNMENT'S POLICY PLANS

As indicated in the introduction, many countries are confronted with the consequences of an aging population. But the issue can be viewed from various angles. Some experts say that it is a demographic time bomb that will have disastrous social consequences. They point, for example, to the growing number of elderly people suffering from dementia. In the Netherlands, that number is projected to increase from 175,000 to 320,000 by 2030.

Though not wishing to make light of these experts' views, the Dutch government feels that they are being overly pessimistic. We need not view the increase in the number of elderly people as a threat. Living a longer, healthy life enriches both the individual and society. But society needs to be prepared for this new situation.

The Dutch government has therefore made a number of long-term policy plans that aim to maintain high levels of care for the elderly in the years to come while ensuring that they continue to play an active and independent role in society. The government has put together a comprehensive package of measures, grouped into seven main tasks:

- Ensuring that people stay fit and healthy

- Enabling people to play an active role in society in later life

- Maintaining income levels

- Ensuring adequate housing

- Enabling the elderly to move around in freedom and safety

- Ensuring care

- Safeguarding the right to die with dignity

The State Secretary at the Ministry of Health, Welfare, and Sport is specifically responsible for ensuring that policy for the elderly is cohesive, with attention paid to all elements.

I will now examine each of the seven tasks in more detail, setting out the main outlines of policy and describing a number of measures.

Ensuring That People Stay Fit and Healthy

It has been established that lifestyle has a very great influence on later demand for care. The aim is therefore to influence people's lifestyles at an early stage so that they have less need of care services in the future.

An important issue is exercise. In the Netherlands, 57 percent of those aged sixty-five and over take less than thirty minutes of exercise a day. A campaign launched in 2005 aimed to increase this percentage by promoting walking, cycling, sports, and doing chores around the home. A program was also set up to provide various forms of exercise for elderly people with a disability. Contact was also sought with sports associations. A task force will launch activities to get people over-fifty to join sports clubs. Staff members are also being trained to help them exercise properly.

Another important issue is nutrition. The ministry stimulates activities that encourage elderly people to eat healthily, through organizations such as the Municipal Health Services (GGD), the Netherlands Heart Foundation, and the Netherlands Nutrition Center.

Older women from the ethnic minorities are a group of particular concern. A study conducted by the Social and Cultural Planning Office in 2004 shows that this group lags behind when it comes to both exercise and diet (2004). Central government is now considering activities specifically targeting this group.

A third area the government is focusing on is fall prevention. Every year in the Netherlands, fifteen thousand people are admitted to hospital with a hip fracture. The government has launched a campaign to address this issue.

Enabling People to Play an Active Role

According to the Social and Cultural Planning Office's 2006 *Report on the Elderly* (2006b), 40 percent of those aged fifty-five to sixty-five are in paid employment. However, among those aged sixty to sixty-five, this figure is only 19 percent. The government wants to see this percentage increase. Between 1992 and 2004, the employment rate among those aged fifty-five to sixty-five rose from 25 percent to 40 percent, mainly because more women were working outside the home. But this percentage is still much lower than in the United Kingdom or the United States, for example, where 60 percent of people in this age group work.

Measures have been introduced to address this, such as less generous early retirement schemes, life-course savings schemes, and tighter procedures for making older employees redundant. Special facilities have also been created for older entrepreneurs.

Apart from encouraging older people to stay in work, the government is also supporting organizations that develop new methods to make volunteer work more attractive.

Computer technology enables older people to remain socially active for a longer period, and the government has asked housing associations to invest in small-scale housing projects using domotics (automated technology services that make a home "smart" and easier to live in, particularly for the elderly). However, reliance on the computers also has its downside. Elderly people who are unable to use computers may become more isolated. Older people using computer-driven aids also run the risk of becoming dependent on them, so that they are no longer able to perform certain functions independently.

As part of its efforts to make life a little easier for older people, the government will be introducing a citizen service number in 2007. This unique identification number will be used by all agencies, so that applying for facilities and services will be much simpler.

Maintaining Income Levels

An assured income is an important basis for playing an active role in society. In the Netherlands, it is considered to be the government's task to guarantee a minimum income for old people. Everyone who has reached the age of sixty-five is entitled to an old-age pension under the General Old Age Pensions Act. Expenditure on old-age pensions now amounts to 5 percent of GDP; the projected population aging will cause this to rise to 9 percent by 2030. The main steps the government is now taking to compensate for this increase include encouraging more older people to continue working, adapting other collective schemes, and reducing the government deficit so that less of its revenue goes to servicing debts. A discussion is currently under way in the

Netherlands about raising the retirement age and requiring retirees themselves to contribute to their own pensions. The two measures have led to considerable controversy.

Apart from the basic old-age pension, the government also provides for health insurance compensation schemes for people with a minimum income (health care benefit and tax relief for exceptional medical expenses) and supplementary assistance for people who are not entitled to a full old-age pension. Actual disposable income per household of those aged sixty-five to seventy-four rose by 2 percent in the 2001–2003 period. For people over seventy-five, the increase was 6 percent in the same period (Social and Cultural Planning Office, 2006b). Because the old-age pension is indexed to the cost of living, retirees will maintain the same level of prosperity.

Ensuring Adequate Housing

Older people increasingly wish to live in their homes for longer than they did in the 1980s and 1990s. However, given the fact that people need more care as they get older, both homes and care services will have to be tuned to their individual needs. In the future, this responsibility will fall more to individuals and civil society organizations, particularly housing associations. Local factors often play a role on the housing market. Housing associations, project developers, and the local authorities are better equipped than central government to respond to these factors. In the long term, therefore, central government is more likely to play a supporting role than to act as initiator. But because it is responsible for coordination, it will have to continue monitoring the efforts of the parties involved. This could lead to the introduction of incentive schemes that encourage them to respond to changing trends.

The Netherlands faces a considerable challenge in devising housing and care programs. On September 15, 2003, I informed parliament of quantitative housing, care, and welfare needs up to 2015. On July 5, 2004, I sent parliament the "investing in the future" action plan. A total of 255,000 extra homes will be needed, with stair-free internal and external access. This figure can be reached through new developments (104,000 homes), renovation (29,000 homes), creating community-care support centers (35,000 homes), and by ensuring a faster throughput of young people from appropriate homes (87,000 homes). Central government supports this process with grants and incentives for private investors. In future, elderly people will be responsible for paying their own living costs when they receive care in their own homes. In many cases, these costs are now reimbursed under the Exceptional Medical Expenses Act. The thinking is that elderly people will have more freedom of choice and there will be more opportunity for those in the home construction industry to build alternative types of accommodation (for example, complexes combining housing with care services). As indicated previously, combining housing with care and welfare services will be the task of the local authorities. The Social Support Act, which takes effect in 2007, will give them greater opportunity to do so. This act presents the local authorities with the tools and resources needed to provide better welfare services, such as help in the home and local transportation. The act targets the more vulnerable social groups that need extra support.

Enabling the Elderly to Move Around in Freedom and Safety

If individuals are to develop, they need to be mobile. If elderly people are to travel beyond their own homes and immediate environment, they need access to public transportation. Initiatives to accomplish this include adapting buses and trains to improve access. In 2004, 25 percent of buses were wheelchair-accessible, and this is now required of all new buses. Bus stops are also being adapted. There are plans to adapt trains, but that takes more time, as buildings and rolling stock in this sector have a longer life. Because more than 25 percent of those over sixty-five have physical limitations (Social and Cultural Planning Office, 2006a), local authorities also provide facilities enabling people to use their own cars or special local services. By 2005, transportation-on-demand in one form or another had been introduced in 80 percent of all municipalities.

In addition to mobility, elderly people need the right immediate environment. This should be age-proof. Residential planning must take into account the future care needs of elderly residents and their need for safety. In new developments, these requirements can be considered at the design stage. In existing residential areas in major cities, land-use planning falls under central government's urban policy. Within this framework, extra attention is devoted to neighborhood safety through community schemes and the reintroduction of community police officers.

As people age they become more vulnerable to abuse, and it is important that they be given assistance and attention. In the Netherlands, approximately 5 percent of those over sixty-five who live independently are confronted with abuse. There is a network of organizations responsible for identifying and dealing with such cases.

Ensuring Care

In the years to come, the growing elderly population will need considerably more care services—and these must be of a high quality. The growing number of elderly people suffering from psychogeriatric conditions form a particularly vulnerable group in our society. The Dutch government has given high priority to the care of people suffering from psychogeriatric conditions and has developed a national plan specifically for them. Care provision will need improvement, with closer coordination among the various geriatric disciplines. There will also be a need for more places to cater to this group, either institutions or independent units.

Growing demand for care will lead to a growing need for care workers. Since the job market is on the upturn, this could create problems. To meet future care needs adequately, care providers will need to be more innovative and increase their productivity. A first step has been taken for the short term with the conclusion of a covenant with care providers' sector organizations. For the same budget, they have agreed to provide care for 1.25 percent more people each year between 2005 and 2007. They achieved this objective in 2005. The covenant also included agreements on extra resources for innovation, information and communication technology (ICT), and reducing the administrative burden. In the long term, the government expects more competition to be an incentive for higher productivity and innovation.

The government is also engaged in activities to organize the care process more efficiently. It has launched initiatives to restructure long-term care tasks. In nursing homes, some tasks and responsibilities are being transferred from doctors to nurses, and courses have been set up for nurse practitioners.

Care of the elderly amounts to more than simply long-term care. The part played in the process by the family doctor and the influence of medicines are both vital factors. The government is looking at ways of producing a cohesive package of geriatric care services.

Another factor determining the pressure on the care sector is informal care. The government is investing in supporting informal caregivers. The Social Support Act, in combination with opportunities for respite care, should enable informal caregivers to continue playing a major role in the care of the elderly.

As I have already pointed out, it is not only the availability of care services that matters, but also their quality, and many activities have been launched to improve it. For example, efforts are being made to promote small-scale housing for elderly people. At the same time, multiple-bed wards in nursing homes, where ten thousand patients are now accommodated, will become a thing of the past. By 2010, they will all have been scaled down.

Another action program aims to improve quality by ensuring more transparency from institutions, stepping up supervision, and setting up projects to implement good practices. A set of indicators has been developed to test organizations' performance. They are required to publish an annual report, which will give an accounting of their scores.

The Right to Die with Dignity

Each year, approximately 140,000 people die in the Netherlands. Nonacute, incurable illnesses—to which elderly people in particular are prone—account for about one-third of these deaths. Because the population is aging, the incidence of these illnesses will increase, and demand for palliative care will increase. Palliative care encompasses not only pain control—that is, alleviating the physical symptoms of illness—but also the psychosocial, emotional, and spiritual implications of approaching death.

Most terminally ill people want to die in familiar surroundings. Thanks to the efforts of volunteers, incurably ill people can stay in their own homes for longer. The government has earmarked an extra €2.25 million a year for the coordination of volunteer home care and informal care. Extra money (€4.8 million) has also been allocated to equip palliative units in nursing homes, and the government is encouraging the formation of networks to improve the quality of palliative care.

MONITORING POLICY

The Dutch government believes that the effects of policy should be measurable. Thirteen indicators have been defined for this. There are indicators for exercise (number of elderly people taking regular exercise), fall prevention (number of fractures as a result of falls), the employment rate among people aged fifty-five to sixty-four, and targets for the number of homes to be adapted. The initial value in 2005 is presented as a starting point. The government has set itself target values for the period up to 2010. Major progress is expected under the headings "moving around in freedom and safety" and "ensuring care." As far as volunteer work is concerned, the main aim is to maintain current levels.

CONCLUSION

I much appreciate having had the opportunity to contribute to the debate on aging. The policy initiatives launched in the Netherlands and the reasons underpinning them may possibly serve as inspiration to other countries confronted with the same issues. The Netherlands, too, regularly looks at what other countries are doing in order to learn new ideas. In this context, it is very important for countries to continue exchanging information, both within the EU and globally. Good examples include the seminar on long-term care held in Brussels on September 13, 2006, which was organized by AARP in collaboration with the EU, and the EU project on healthy aging, to which the Netherlands will be making an active contribution in the next few years.

REFERENCES

Social and Cultural Planning Office. *Gezondheid en welzijn van allochtone ouderen* (Elderly from the ethnic minorities: Health and welfare). The Hague: Social and Cultural Planning Office, 2004.

Social and Cultural Planning Office. *Ondersteuning Gewenst* (Support Needed). The Hague: Social and Cultural Planning Office, 2006a.

Social and Cultural Planning Office. *Report on the Elderly*. The Hague: Social and Cultural Planning Office, 2006b.

CHAPTER

13

AGING IN SPAIN: WORKING TOWARD CREATING NEW RIGHTS IN THE WELFARE STATE

JOSÉ LUIS RODRÍGUEZ ZAPATERO

In Spain today, more than 7.3 million people are aged sixty-five and over—some 16.6 percent of the total population. The dependency rate—that is, the number of people over sixty-five divided by the number of nondependent people—is 24.4 percent.

In regard to aging in Spain, we also have to consider the phenomenon known as "the aging of aging"—the fact that the number of people over eighty has doubled in just twenty years. Currently, more than 815,000 people in our country are over eighty-five.

Because in Spain an estimated 32 percent of people over sixty-five have some kind of disability, a progressively aging population produces dependency situations that need appropriate attention.

Population pyramids for Spanish citizens and foreigners for 2000 and 2005 widen in the middle sector because of the arrival of young foreigners (attributed to immigration). This trend slows down the aging of the Spanish population and also has significant effects on the norms governing the growth and aging of the Spanish population pyramid. Consequently, the demographic growth in Spain has reached its highest point in the last five years, with 76.4 percent of this effect attributable to the increase of foreigners in the population.

As is the case with other countries in Europe, the Spanish population is experiencing a significant phenomenon of aging. Because of lower birth rates and decreased mortality, the aging support structure for the Spanish population will need to be strengthened over the next few decades.

In Spain, life expectancy at birth is 77.2 years for men and 83.8 years for women, above average for European Union (EU) countries. Eurostat calculates healthy life expectancy, or healthy life year (HLY), for men and women in the fifteen EU member states (except Luxembourg). With regard to men (in 2003, the last year for which figures are available), Italy has the highest HLY at 70.9 years, followed by Belgium at 67.4, and Spain at 66.8 (see Table 13.1). For women, Italy at 74.4, Spain at 70.2, and Austria at 69.6 had the highest HLY (see Table 13.2).

HEALTH-DETERMINING FACTORS FOR THE ELDERLY

The health of older people is influenced by the same biological, environmental, and social factors that affect the population as a whole. In addition, older people experience a sustained increase of chronic disease and also functional and sensory deterioration that often leads to dependency-generating disabilities that correlate with declining health.

Although deterioration is a generalized biological process, we know too little about the mechanisms of aging to radically alter them with biological intervention. However, countries with higher per-capita incomes have enjoyed some success in slowing both the decrease in the quality of life associated with aging and the rate of declining health because of dependency. In wealthier countries, significant physical deterioration generally occurs at an age ten to fifteen years older than was the case fifty years ago; for many it now begins around age eighty.

The important social changes taking place in developed societies also influence the experience of illness, disability, and the loss of autonomy. Decisive factors include the decreasing importance of traditional families, the advent of new kinds of family units, the gradual inclusion of women in the workplace, and the social relevance of the role played by people according to their age. For people in these countries, providing social and health care services that maintain quality of life becomes much more critical.

But many social and health care services fail to adequately focus on the aging population.

Conversely, housing conditions and, in general, the urban environment, levels of education, and purchasing power all play key roles in the state of our citizens' health. These same factors—especially educational levels—significantly influence health-related behavior regarding food and nutrition, adequate use of health care and social services, and physical activity.

TABLE 13.1. **Healthy Life Expectancy at Birth for Men in European Union Countries (fifteen members).**

	1995	1996	1997	1998	1999	2000	2001	2002	2003
European Union (15M)	–	–	–	–	63.2[a]	63.5[a]	63.6[a]	64.3[a]	64.5[a]
Austria	60.0	62.3	62.2	63.4	63.6	64.6	64.2	65.6[a]	66.2[a]
Belgium	63.3	64.1	66.5	63.3	66.0	65.7	65.6	65.9[a]	67.4[a]
Denmark	61.6	61.7	61.6	62.4	62.5	62.9	62.2	62.8[a]	63.0[a]
Finland	–	54.6	55.5	55.9	55.6	56.3	56.7	57.0[a]	57.3[a]
France	60.0	59.6	60.2	59.2	60.1	60.1	60.6	60.4[a]	60.6[a]
Germany	60.0	60.8	61.9[a]	62.1[a]	62.3[a]	63.2[a]	64.1[a]	64.4[a]	65.0[a]
Greece	65.6	66.9	66.4	66.5	66.7	66.3	66.7	66.7[a]	66.7[a]
Ireland	63.2	64.0	63.2	64.0	63.9	63.3	63.3	63.5[a]	63.4[a]
Italy	66.7	67.4	66.0	67.9	63.7	69.7	69.8	70.4[a]	70.9[a]
Luxembourg	–	–	–	–	–	–	–	–	–
Netherlands	61.1	62.1	62.5	61.9	61.6	61.4	61.9	61.7[a]	61.7[a]
Portugal	59.6	56.2	59.3	59.1	58.8	60.2	59.5	59.7[a]	59.8[a]
Spain	64.2	65.1	65.5	65.2	65.6	66.5	66.0	66.6[a]	66.8[a]
Sweden	–	–	62.1	61.7	62.0	63.1	61.9	62.4[a]	62.5[a]
United Kingdom	60.6	60.8	60.9[a]	60.8[a]	61.2[a]	61.3[a]	61.1[a]	61.4[a]	61.5[a]

Note: – = data not available.

[a] Estimated figure.

TABLE 13.2. **Healthy Life Expectancy at Birth for Women in European Union Countries (fifteen members).**

	1995	1996	1997	1998	1999	2000	2001	2002	2003
European Union (15M)	–	–	–	–	63.9[a]	64.4[a]	65.0[a]	65.8[a]	66.0[a]
Austria	–	–	–	–	–	68.0	69.5	69.0[a]	69.6[a]
Belgium	65.4	68.5[a]	68.3[a]	65.4[a]	68.4	69.1	68.8	69.0[a]	69.2[a]
Denmark	60.7	61.1	60.7[a]	61.3[a]	60.8	61.9	60.4	61.0[a]	60.9[a]
Finland	–	57.7	57.6	58.3	57.4	56.6[a]	59.9	56.8[a]	56.5[a]
France	62.4	62.5	63.1	62.8	63.3	63.2[a]	63.3	63.7[a]	63.9[a]
Germany	64.3	64.5	64.3	64.3[a]	64.3[a]	64.6[a]	64.5[a]	64.5[a]	64.7[a]
Greece	69.2[a]	69.6	68.7	68.3	69.4	68.2	68.6	68.5[a]	68.4[a]
Ireland	–	–	–	–	67.6	66.9	66.5	65.9[a]	65.4[a]
Italy	70.0	70.5[a]	71.3	71.3	72.1	72.9	73.0[a]	73.9[a]	74.4[a]
Luxemburg	–	–	–	–	–	–	–	–	–
Netherlands	62.1[a]	61.5	61.4	61.1[a]	61.4	60.2	59.4	59.3[a]	58.8[a]
Portugal	63.1	60.5	60.4	51.1	60.7	62.2	62.7	61.8[a]	61.8[a]
Spain	67.7	68.4	68.2	68.2	69.5	69.3	69.2[a]	69.9[a]	70.2[a]
Sweden	–	–	60.0	61.3	61.8	61.9	61.0	61.9[a]	62.2[a]
United Kingdom	61.2[a]	61.8[a]	61.2[a]	62.2[a]	61.3[a]	61.2[a]	60.8[a]	60.9[a]	60.9[a]

Note: – = data not available.

[a] Estimated figure.

CHALLENGES FOR SOCIETY

Public officials must promote the social integration of older people by recognizing their abilities and permitting them to actively contribute to society for as long as possible.

We should view aging as simply another stage in life, one that an ever-growing number of people should be able to face under the best social, economic, and personal conditions. But we must also be realistic about the inevitability of old age and avoid promoting irrational and unrealistic expectations.

We should strive to adapt social and health care services more efficiently to human needs, especially the needs of older people. Public services should pay special attention to the inequalities of gender, social class, educational level, and ethnicity that exist in the aging population.

CREATING A NATIONAL DEPENDENCY SYSTEM IN SPAIN

On December 11, 2006, the Spanish Parliament approved the Bill to Promote Personal Autonomy and Care for Dependent Persons. This bill creates new rights for people who are dependent (the elderly and seriously disabled) and need assistance with the activities of everyday life. Today, 22 percent of Spanish senior citizens live alone. Our government believes it should guarantee that older people are never neglected or left alone at the end of their lives. A society committed to ethical principles and values cannot allow this to occur.

In reality, family members care for a large percentage of dependent persons. Specifically, women represent about 83 percent of family caregivers. The Bill to Promote Personal Autonomy and Care for Dependent Persons responds to the belief that the decency of a society is measured by the way it treats its elderly. The actual text of the Spanish Constitution (in Articles 49 and 50) addresses care for the disabled and the elderly, and also the need for a government system of social services to ensure the well-being of our citizens.

In 1978, the fundamental elements of the welfare state focused on health care, education, and Social Security for all citizens. Since then, social development in Spain has increasingly focused on social services that meet the needs of all citizens and has created new social demands that must be incorporated in our model for the welfare state.

Spain addresses care for dependent people from a dual perspective. We will combine protections for people who lack personal autonomy and those who take care of them with measures aimed at promoting autonomous living for the disabled and the elderly. Our territorial model, wherein health care and social services are managed at the autonomous community level (there are seventeen such regions in Spain), gives us a firsthand perspective of the needs and problems of our people—a perspective that in turn ensures more efficient management and guarantees the principles of equality and solidarity throughout Spain. All of this promotes social unity.

Once the Spanish Parliament passed the Bill to Promote Personal Autonomy and Care for Dependent Persons, in December 2006 the Spanish government and the governments of the Autonomous Communities reached agreement on immediate implementation, to ensure that any citizens who lack personal autonomy will have the right to access the set of services they need to accomplish normal, everyday activities. This will significantly increase the well-being of those people and their families while giving the government the tools it needs to achieve important and decisive social progress in Spain. The bill establishes universal, public, and equal access to those services.

The creation of a National Dependency System will guarantee the rights established by the law. The project is a broad social program that will affect a wide range of political arenas—the economy, social services, health care, the job market, vocational training, and social welfare—and require the utmost administrative cooperation and coordination. Implementation of the National Dependency System will have a huge, direct impact on the well-being of more than 1.1 million dependent people and their families. It will also have a positive economic impact and generate new jobs. Specifically, it will add many women—who were previously caregivers—to the job market.

Allocation of public resources will be vitally important between 2007 and 2015, as the National Dependency System is gradually implemented. During that period, the General Government Administration will contribute nearly €13 billion and the autonomous communities will contribute a similar amount. It is this legislature's most aggressive government investment initiative, representing approximately 2.6 percent of GNP.

Developing this fourth pillar of the welfare state over the next few years is the Spanish government's primary social policy goal. Creating this wide-ranging social services network will be one of our society's major challenges. This government's main political objectives are to oppose social exclusion, protect the vulnerable and ensure equal opportunity, battle against discrimination, encourage social cooperation and volunteerism, and absolutely improve quality of life for its citizens—all the while meeting criteria for and commitments to budgetary stability.

ANALYSIS OF MACROECONOMIC DATA AND SOCIAL SPENDING IN SPAIN

Spain has recently enjoyed high and sustained economic growth. During the first quarter of 2007, GNP grew by 4.0 percent—one-tenth more than in 2006 and much higher than the 2.1 percent EU average.

Industry is also showing very positive numbers, with growth of industrial production at 4.4 percent and extraordinarily favorable investment in capital goods. All this reflects confidence in our economy's present and future.

More than seven hundred thousand jobs will be created in 2006, many which will be permanent. The unemployment rate is 8.5 percent, which means a reduction of three points in the three years of this legislative session.

Social Security is also markedly improved. Our pension system (an allotment system) is in the best shape ever, with more than 19.1 million Social Security members—an additional 2.1 million in the last three years—at a ratio of 2.6 workers for each retired person. The Social Security system is critical because it provides security for retirees as well as social and financial protection in the event of various contingencies. Social Security is the main component of the Spanish welfare state. The good financial health of this system has led over the last three years between 20 and 25 percent increase in the minimum pensions paid to some three million retirees, and we are committed to increasing minimum pensions to 26 percent by the end of this legislative session (2004–2008). The Social Security Reserve Fund has almost tripled over the last three years. The amount contributed to the fund in 2006 was €7.8 billion, which means that the balance of the Social Security Reserve Fund will surpass €40 billion—4 percent of GDP.

Thus we see both how the Spanish economy is expanding and creating jobs, and the robust financial health of the Social Security system.

The creation of a National Dependency System will engender reforms that look to the future. It is an exercise in responsibility and commitment that we must never lose sight of, because our population, like all other European societies, is aging. By 2020, our elderly will represent 20 percent of the overall population. Our life expectancy, which has increased by eight years since 1970 and now exceeds the Organization for Economic Cooperation and Development (OECD) average, should continue to grow by one year of life expectancy every ten years. The statistics on economic and budgetary perspectives are positive. In 2007 it is expected that the economy will continue to grow at a high rate, employment will continue to increase by more than six hundred thousand jobs, and unemployment should drop to under 8 percent. As a result of our priorities, the social spending budgeted for 2007 grows significantly. The line item for caring for dependent persons doubles the figure for 2006.

Based on the preceding analysis of macroeconomic data, I can state that the growth of our economy and the outlook for its future will permit us to make the necessary budgetary commitment to the creation and strengthening of the National Dependency System.

KEY ELEMENTS OF THE SOCIAL WELL-BEING POLICIES

One major concern for any responsible politician is the growth of health care spending in relation to national wealth and efficient planning of social services. In Spain, citizens are reasonably satisfied with the functioning of the National Health Care System, which provides universal coverage and entails a large monetary contribution from the public sector. Health care expense per capita in 2003 was $1,835 (adjusted by buying power parity), one-third the cost of health care in the United States. The system's efficiency has been widely recognized by international organizations such as the World Health Organization (WHO), as well as by the Spanish citizenry and others residents of Spain who benefit from its services.

Implementing the fourth pillar of the welfare state will affect the planning of health care services by reducing the splintered and fragmentary nature of its components: community care and public health (collective services provided to the population), primary care, and specialized care (hospitalization). The greatest challenges to health care planning will be to avoid the duplication of activities after health care services are combined with the new social services and to take advantage of the synergies between them. Effective coordination of health care services and social services will be the key to avoiding duplication and to using resources more efficiently.

As things stand today, hospital medical and urgent-care services handle much of the elderly's needs. Creation of the National Dependency System will change this and, as a result, make the National Health Care Service more cost-effective.

In the near future, the National Health Care System will confront the challenge of developing programs and services aimed specifically at the aging population, strictly and clearly evaluating their impact in terms of efficacy, efficiency, and fairness.

Increased emphasis will be also be placed on preventive care that fosters greater personal autonomy. In Spain, the Ministry of Health and Consumer Affairs is conducting advertising campaigns, aimed at people over age sixty-five, that inform about and explain specific practices geared toward preventing the loss of personal autonomy.

Other political actions by the Spanish government to improve the health of our citizenry, specifically the elderly, include promoting rational use of medications and health care products to reduce inappropriate consumption. Sections of the recently approved and published Law on Guarantees and Rational Use of Medications and Health Care Products address this.

For the creation of the fourth pillar of the welfare state and the concomitant increase in the social rights of citizens to succeed, all sectors of society, especially the elderly, must actively participate. To adequately meet their needs, we must strengthen channels of communication with this segment of the population.

The National Dependency System is my government's commitment to social policies that reflect the principles and ethical values of the citizenry. To meet this challenge, everyone involved must participate, to which end the government will work in coordination and cooperation with regional and local governments as well as with social and economic agents. Only through a concerted effort by everyone involved will we continue increasing the social rights of our citizens.

CHAPTER

14

HEALTH AND AGING IN SWEDEN

BARBRO WESTERHOLM

The twentieth century brought a victory for Sweden: the average life expectancy was increased by a quarter of a century. A hundred years ago in Sweden, a newborn girl could expect to live until she was fifty-eight years old and a newborn boy until the age of fifty-five. In contrast, the average expected life span for a girl born today is eighty-three years and for a boy, seventy-eight years.

Behind this success are many factors. Improved housing, clean water, efficient sanitation, better working conditions, and better food have all contributed to the increased life span. The development of the health care sector and the introduction of modern medicines and vaccines and other treatment methods have also played an important part. Smallpox, polio, measles, and diphtheria are no longer seen in Sweden. Tuberculosis is rare. Pneumonia is no longer a killer, thanks to the availability of antibiotics. Cancer and cardiovascular diseases are not the threat today that they once were, thanks to the availability of effective treatments.

Most of the years gained are healthy years. In the younger group—those in their sixties and seventies—hips, knees, eye lenses, and coronary vessels may have to be changed, but when this is done, health is regained. In their eighties, people begin to experience more troublesome health problems. Many of the elderly develop multiple health problems (multimorbidity), which limit their everyday lives.

DEMOGRAPHIC DEVELOPMENTS

As of 2006, about 17 percent of the Swedish population (9.1 million inhabitants) are aged sixty-five or over. The number will increase during the next thirty years. The increase will first be seen in those aged sixty-five to seventy-nine years. Thereafter the number of those aged eighty and over will increase in size. In 2005, 487,000 people were eighty and over; in 2050 there are expected to be 912,000. Unless there is a remarkable improvement of the health situation among those eighty and over, this will be a challenge to society. Women will still be in the majority among the elderly, but their percentage is projected to decrease from 64 percent in 2005 to 56 percent in 2050.

NATIONAL OBJECTIVES ON POLICY FOR THE ELDERLY

The Swedish policy for the elderly (Ministry of Health and Social Affairs, 2005) aims at enabling older people to live independently with a high quality of life. Those who are in need of care and social services are entitled to high-quality help.

RESPONSIBILITIES FOR CARE

Responsibility for the care of the elderly rests on three levels: (1) the national level, parliament and government, where policy goals through legislation and financial control measures are determined; (2) the county level, where the eighteen county councils are responsible for the provision of health and medical care; and (3) the 290 municipalities, which have a statutory duty to meet the social service and housing needs of the elderly and also provide some health care.

In Sweden, municipalities and county councils have a high level of autonomy by international standards. The National Board of Health and Welfare and the twenty-one county administrative boards are responsible for supervision, follow-up, and evaluation of municipal and county council care services.

FUNDING AND EXPENDITURE

Care and services for the elderly are to a great extent (more than 80 percent) financed by taxes levied by the municipality from its residents. State grants amount to about 10 percent of the budget. Fees or rates finance about 4 percent of the costs. The cost in 2005 amounted to SEK 158 billion ($145), equal to 6.5 percent of the GNP.

LEGISLATION

There are two main laws that form the basis of the support and care of the elderly:

The Health and Medical Services Act
According to this act, health care should be available to all members of society. It ensures a high standard of general health and care for every citizen on equal terms.

The county councils are responsible for medical services provided by doctors in health care services, while the municipalities must offer good health care and medical services, including rehabilitation and assistive technology in special forms of housing accommodation and daytime activities. Municipalities are responsible for home nursing by agreement with the county councils. The municipalities have the duty to employ personnel with suitable training and experience.

The Social Services Act

This act sets out the duty of municipalities to provide social services and care for older people. Any person who is unable to provide for his or her needs or to obtain provision for them in any other way is entitled to assistance toward livelihood and living in general.

According to the act, municipalities should endeavor to ensure that older people are enabled to live independently, in secure conditions, and with respect shown for their self-determination and privacy. The municipalities should facilitate what is needed for the individual to continue living at home by means of help services and daytime activities. The municipalities should also facilitate the situation for family members caring for older people and establish special forms of housing accommodation with service and care for older people in need of special support.

SERVICES FOR THE ELDERLY

The municipalities provide home help service and personal care under the Social Services Act. The tasks include, for example, cleaning and doing laundry and helping with shopping and preparation of meals. Personal care can include assistance with eating and drinking, getting dressed, personal hygiene, and moving about. Daytime activities and short-term care should, according the Social Services Act and the Health and Medical Services Act, be given to those in need. Daytime activities are provided in the form of treatment and rehabilitation; short-term care in the form of temporary housing combined with treatment, rehabilitation, and care, partly for purposes of relief and alternate care.

There are special housing accommodations for older people with need of extensive care and attention. It includes housing that in earlier legislation was classed as service blocks, old people's homes, group housing, and nursing homes.

MAJOR HEALTH PROBLEMS AMONG THE ELDERLY IN SWEDEN

Cardiovascular Disease. The most common long-term disease in elderly people is cardiovascular diseases. In Sweden nearly half of the people over age sixty-five have some form of cardiovascular problem. Mortality in this disease group has fallen by nearly one-third over the last twenty years. Important interventions are the reduction of smoking, treatment of hypertension, initiation of physical activity, and weight reduction.

Cancer. The risk of contracting cancer is closely related to age. One out of three Swedish people will contract cancer at some time in life. The disease causes one in five deaths. The most common form of the disease among women is breast cancer and among men, cancer of the prostate. Other common forms are cancer of the lung and of the gastrointestinal tract.

Diabetes. Type 2 diabetes is currently one of the most rapidly increasing diseases in Sweden, for two reasons: the increasing number of overweight people and particularly overweight men.

Mental Illness. Mental illness is a major problem among older people in Sweden. It is estimated that about 150,000 older people suffer from depression and 100,000 from anxiety. Some 100,000 have some kind of psychotic condition. Women form the majority of this group. The risk of suicide, however, is higher in elderly men than in women of the same age.

Dementia increases markedly with age. About 1 percent of people age sixty-five to sixty-nine suffer from some form of dementia. This figure rises to 3 percent among people aged seventy to seventy-four. Prevalence then doubles every five years. Among those over ninety, it is estimated at 21 percent.

Osteoarthritis and Osteoporosis. Osteoporosis and osteoarthritis (or osteoarthrosis, as it is more commonly known in Europe) are common in older people and especially among women. About 22 percent of Swedish women between sixty and sixty-nine, 31 percent of those aged seventy to seventy-nine, and 36 percent of those aged eighty to eighty-nine have osteoporosis in the neck of the femur. An estimated seventy thousand fractures occur each year as a result of osteoporosis.

Hearing Impairment. Hearing impairment is one of the most common disabilities of age. One in ten of those over sixty is expected to suffer from it. More than two-thirds of the ninety-year-olds who otherwise enjoy good health have a hearing problem.

Sight Impairments. Nearly 15 percent of people over sixty-five are estimated to have impaired sight. Half of these are unable to read a newspaper even with the aid of spectacles because of cataracts, glaucoma, and macular degeneration. The consequences include a greater risk of fall accidents and fractures.

Incontinence. Urinary incontinence is widespread and is still a taboo subject for many older people. Many feel ashamed and guilty about their problem. It is estimated that about half a million Swedish people experience incontinence, but only 25 to 50 percent of them actually consult a doctor. It can be classified as a hidden public health problem.

Dental Health. Dental health is an area that is attracting increased attention. In the 1970s, less than half of those aged seventy and over had their own teeth; today, the figure is more then 90 percent. However, despite the importance of dental health, many older people encounter long waiting lists for subsidized dental care. And there are major disparities, both regionally and according to class. Former blue-collar workers have a much worse tooth status than white-collar workers. Toothlessness is more common among immigrants than among native Swedish people.

Accidents and Injuries. Fall injuries among older people are a widespread public health problem in Sweden. The number of older people with hip fractures has doubled over the last decade. One out of three eighty-year-old women is expected either to have already suffered a hip fracture or to suffer one in the future. Fall accidents are more common among women than men, and they also increase with age.

Musculoskeletal Pain. Aches and pains are common among elderly people. The main reasons are rheumatoid arthritis, osteoarthritis, and cancer.

Multimorbidity. Elderly people treated in patient facilities or living in special housing accommodations often suffer from several concurrent diseases and conditions after injuries (stroke, fractures, and so on) and multiple concurrent treatments. This group of elderly patients often needs significant care and presents a challenge when it comes to diagnosis, treatment, care, and rehabilitation.

Elder Abuse. This is a hidden, neglected problem in Sweden. According to an investigation made in Northern Sweden, among those aged sixty and over, 16 percent of women and 13 percent of men have been exposed to some kind of abuse (neglect, threats, physical abuse, sexual abuse, and financial abuse).

Causes of Death in Older People. Cardiovascular disease is the dominant cause of death among both women and men in Sweden. Tumors are a common cause of death among women ages sixty-five to seventy-four. The number of women dying from a tumor decreases after the age of seventy-five. Mental illness—especially Alzheimer's disease—is the third biggest cause of death among women over seventy-five.

Socioeconomic Disparities. Life expectancy is longer in socioeconomically strong counties. The socioeconomic disparities become even clearer on the municipality and parish level. The variation in average life expectancy on the municipality level is greater for men than for women. This is also true on the county level. There are strong links with socioeconomic variables such as education level, working life, income, and housing.

The Health of Elderly Immigrants. In Sweden, foreign-born nationals make up to ten percent of those over sixty-five. This percentage is projected to increase quickly over the next few years. It is a heterogeneous group, and we have to confess that we lack data on their health and their life situation. We know that they generally have a good level of education but they have faced unemployment more so than native-born Swedes. Twice as many immigrants as native Swedish people—9 percent—feel that they are in a poor state of health. More of them are also afflicted with some kind of long-term illness or significant disability.

NATIONAL DEVELOPMENT PLAN FOR CARE AND SOCIAL SERVICES FOR THE ELDERLY

In March 2005, the government of Sweden presented a bill containing its plan for development of care and social services for the elderly during the next ten years. New initiatives and economic investments in care and services for the elderly were necessary so that the municipalities and other sectors in society would be able to meet the local need.

Resources were allocated to improve care and social services for the seriously ill. It was obvious that the quality of care had to be improved and more resources allocated for measures concerning rehabilitation, nutrition, medical drug reviews, and greater physician involvement, including the following:

- Extending and strengthening home nursing

- Improving physician involvement in home nursing, both in ordinary dwellings and in special housing accommodations

- Introducing medical drug reviews to ensure follow-up after prescribing medicines for the elderly

- Ensuring early diagnosis and adequate care of people with dementia, through teamwork, collaboration, and competence

Another development area in this bill concerned safe living arrangements. Couples who are both in need of special living arrangements should be reassured that they can continue to live together if they wish. Other parts of the bill dealt with services for the elderly with different language and cultural backgrounds, quality control of care and services for the elderly, and strengthened legal security for people who have been approved for support.

The bill stresses the necessity of continued investments in research and development in the care of the elderly. It will promote cooperation among industry, research, authorities, and personnel to develop new techniques and introduce new technical solutions in care and services for the elderly, including the development of personnel skills. The bill also recognizes that prevention and health promotion should be stimulated.

Since October 2006, Sweden has a new government that intends to further strengthen the care and services for elderly women and men.

THE SITUATION TODAY IN THE CARE OF THE ELDERLY

Every year, Swedish municipalities and county councils present an overview of the situation in the care of the elderly. The following conclusions can be drawn from the publication presented in November 2006 (Sveriges Kommuner och Landsting, 2006).

The economy of older people is mainly dependent on what income they have had during their working life and how long they have been working. It also depends on whether they have savings. The greatest difference is usually between those who live as a couple and those who are single. Single women, as a rule, have less money to live on than men. About 20 percent of single people aged sixty-five to sixty-nine will also have a future income below what is needed for a reasonable standard of living. People born abroad and who have come to Sweden as adults will have a smaller pension than those who spent their entire work lives in Sweden.

About half of the elderly people have both a partner and children. Many have children within ten kilometers and see their children at least once a week. It seems that the elderly have a closer network today than in the past. Many help someone outside their own home. There are some who feel lonely and wish for more social contacts, but they are in the minority. The feeling of loneliness is most common among those who have lost their spouses and who lack relationships with other people.

Sweden has five national minorities—Lapps, Swedish Finns, Tornedalingar (Torne Valley Finns), Romanies, and Jews. The number of people aged sixty-five and over who were born abroad now amounts to about 170,800, corresponding to 11 percent of the population in that age group. The number is expected to increase in the years to come. Almost 50 percent were born in another Nordic country, 90 percent in a European country, and only 10 percent born outside of Europe. The efforts to help those born abroad who are in need of care have increased over the years but are still not sufficient. One challenge is to get personnel who speak the language of older immigrants. In the area of Stockholm alone, nearly two hundred different languages are spoken!

There are 483,000 people over age eighty and 73,000 over age ninety. Of these, about 104,800 live in special housing accommodations. Services are received by 132,300 in their own homes; 32,300 have both services and care in their own home. Approximately 10.6 percent of the services and care come from private entrepreneurs. About 240,000 people work in this sector.

Housing

Most of the elderly—94 percent of those aged sixty-five and over—live in ordinary homes and flats. The goal has been that older people should be able to stay in their own homes until they die. This vision has been questioned recently. When old people become widowed and afflicted with multiple health problems, many of them want to move to a more sheltered living situation with access to care. Some of them feel imprisoned in their own homes. At present, about 16 percent of those eighty and over live permanently in special housing accommodations. An increasing number of older people want to move to flats or houses for seniors built to suit older people with various disabilities. They want to live with access to home and health care and to facilities where the elderly can meet. There is some interest in the municipalities to build such houses.

Meals

Almost all municipalities offer to send home ready-made food to elderly and disabled people who live in their own homes. Nearly half of the municipalities distribute warm food; others send food that has to be heated. More than half distribute the food daily; others more than once a week. In about half of the municipalities, meals are available in day care centers.

Transportation

For the elderly who cannot use public transportation, it is possible to get mobility service. The most common transportation is a taxi, but there are also special cars built for disabled people that can be used. More than half of those who get this service are eighty and over.

Emergency Medical Alarm

The elderly and people with disabilities can apply for emergency medical alarms. Nearly 160,000 people received such alarms in 2006.

Home Service

Those who cannot cope with daily life at home—tasks such as cleaning, cooking, and so on—can receive home service after an aid worker's assessment. In 2005, 132,300 received such services. The trend is that fewer and fewer people receive home service, and those who get it are suffering from either dementia or multiple health problems. At the same time, the number of available hours has risen. Thus, there are fewer people getting more help today than five years ago.

Short-Term Living

Short-term living is a complement to home service. It is an in-between form of living, an alternative to living in one's own home, special service accommodations, or hospital care. It is used for rehabilitation, care, and respite for a caregiving family member or friend. There were 8,700 people aged sixty-five and over in short-term living as of October 1, 2005—four hundred fewer than in 2004.

Day Care

Another complement to home service is day care, which facilitates living in one's own home. Mainly older and disabled people with dementia or psychological disabilities use it. On October 1, 2005, about eleven thousand people took part in these activities.

Special Housing Accommodations

The service provided is reserved for older people who need extensive service and care. The municipalities assign the flats following a special examination by an aid worker. On October 1, 2005, 100,400 people aged sixty-five and over were living in such housing accommodations.

Support from Relatives and Close Friends

It is estimated that about 70 percent of the care of elderly people is given by relatives and close friends. Since the end of the 1990s, government money has been allotted to support and development of this kind of care.

Health Care

Development in the health care sector has increased the capabilities to treat different diseases and injuries in the very old. This in turn has increased the public's expectations of health care. To cope with these increased demands, the county councils have reorganized the health care in hospitals so that patients stay for a much shorter time than previously. Thus more and more of the care is given outside the hospital. In the oldest patient group, aged eighty-five and over, the average number of days in the hospital has decreased from 10.7 days in 1994 to 7.9 days in 2004.

People aged eighty-five and over constitute 2.5 percent of the population and accounted for 13 percent of days in hospital. Those aged seventy-five to eighty-four constituted 6.4 percent of the population and used 25 percent of treatment days.

Care at End of Life

During the twentieth century, it became common to die in the hospital. This trend is now reversed, and more and more die in special housing accommodations or in their own homes. The possibilities for obtaining advanced medical help in the home have increased in the two decades since the mid-1980s.

Personnel

In November 2005, 254,000 people were employed in the care of the elderly in the municipalities. The majority are assistant nurses, hospital orderlies, and helpers (185,800). The number of nurses was 12,200. Physicians are employed by the county councils and are thus not part of the care team, which sometimes is a disadvantage. Most of the employed are women, and an increasing number are born outside Sweden.

Nongovernmental Organizations

There are five organizations in Sweden for retired people. All together, they include among their members more than half of the inhabitants aged sixty-five and over. Their main task is to form social networks all over the country and to put pressure on decision makers to improve the situation for older people. At the governmental level, they are represented in the Pensioner's Committee, headed by the minister of health and social welfare. An example of success in this effort are the rules that came into force in 2002, which were designed to strengthen safeguards for the individual against excessively high charges. There are similar committees at the county council and municipality levels. Other organizations—such as the Red Cross, the organizations for dementia patients and relatives, and the Council of Relatives—are also important actors in this field.

Goals versus Realities

By international comparison, Sweden is a good country to age in. Despite the facts—the elderly in Sweden are healthier today than before, we have legislation ensuring elderly support and health care when in need, and the economy is stable—there are still problems that must be tackled.

Age Discrimination

Discrimination against older people in the workplace and for access to goods and services is a reality in Sweden. We have the right to retire at the age of sixty-one and the right to work until age sixty-seven, but for those who can and want to stay longer, there are obstacles. There are myths about the capability of older people to work—that they are slow, cannot learn new things, are not flexible, and cannot tolerate stress. But older people are individuals who age individually. An eighty-year-old can seem younger than someone else who is seventy.

There is also discrimination in the care of the elderly. There are examples of older people who have to wait longer for an operation than younger people because they are thought to "have time to wait." Access to rehabilitation has been shown to be better for younger than for older people.

To Decide for Yourself

When the day comes that you can no longer manage everything in your home, you depend on the services provided by the municipality. However, in many older people's experience, decisions about what they are to receive are made over their heads by a social worker. Thus, if you ask for help with cutting the grass in your garden, you may get help with cleaning your floors instead, even though you can manage that yourself.

In Sweden, there has been a vision that older people should be able to live in their own homes until the very last day of life. But as mentioned earlier, for old people who are alone and housebound, home can become a prison. In that situation, many want to move to a house for seniors or special housing accommodations but cannot because there is a lack of this kind of housing.

Quality of Care

The older you are, the more health problems you are likely to develop. To treat this demands competent physicians, nurses, physicists, and other professionals. However, education in geriatrics and gerontology is very weak in Sweden. For instance, a general practitioner does not have to have any training in geriatrics despite the fact that the largest group of patients seen in the doctor's office is the oldest one. The education in pharmacotherapy is also very limited, which is a problem since older patients consume the most medicines.

Inappropriate use of medicines with adverse drug reactions is common in Sweden; overtreatment and undertreatment are the results. It is estimated that about 15 percent of hospitalized patients in medical wards suffer from adverse reactions that could have been prevented. On average, the elderly person in special housing accommodations takes ten different medicines. Four out of five of these residents are known to use psychotropic drugs, and almost one in three to take several such medicines concomitantly.

Elder Abuse

Elder abuse is a public health problem encompassing abuse and burglary by unknown people, abuse within families, and abuse by professional caregivers of the elderly. So far, very little has been done to prevent these crimes and to help the victims. Some local initiatives have succeeded in detecting abuse earlier and helping the victims; these can serve as positive models. Examples of additional actions that must be taken are better statistics gathering; more research, information and education of personnel;

collaboration between professional groups meeting the victims, and establishing contact points to which the victims can turn.

NEEDED RESEARCH

There is a lack of good quality studies on the effect of different treatment methods on various ailments in the elderly and of studies highlighting both the positive and negative effects of concomitant treatments. With so few studies regarding patients aged eighty and over, our base of scientific evidence is weakest for the age groups that most often receive various types of treatments. Thus there is a strong need for clinical treatment research in elderly care.

FINAL WORD

Marit Paulsen, a former member of the European Parliament, has formulated a vision for the care of the elderly:

We should be able to live our whole life. We should be able to become old and frail in the feeling of safety and security that society has the knowledge, will, and resources to take tender care of us during the last part of life, in exactly the same way that our society invests in the first year of life.

REFERENCES

Sveriges Kommuner och Landsting (The Swedish Municipalities and County Councils). Aktuellt om Äldreomsorgen (Facts About the Care of the Elderly). Stockholm: Sveriges Kommuner och Landsting, 2006.

Ministry of Health and Social Affairs. Policy for the Elderly. Fact Sheet No. 14. Stockholm: May 2005.

CHAPTER

15

AGING IN THE UNITED KINGDOM

SALLY GREENGROSS

The improvements in life expectancy now being seen in the UK owe their origins to the last twenty-five years of the nineteenth century, when the first legislation on sanitation, clean water, and hygiene was enacted and housing standards for the poor began to greatly improve. The twentieth century saw enormous improvements in medical development generally, and Britain led the world in the development of geriatric medicine. The introduction of early-years inoculation and vaccination was one factor in the increased survival of new babies, and their survival was to add many years to life expectancy, at a rate never before seen. Across the population as a whole, the National Health Service has since 1948 been the main agent in the hugely improved health enjoyed by most Britons.

We are now adding three months per year to life expectancy at the end of life. Although this is an unprecedented gain, it does not have the same impact as the huge increase in life expectancy at the start of life. Another significant change is that diseases that culled earlier generations are now no longer mass killers. However, we must accept that more of our later years of life are likely to be lived with a range of degenerative conditions that will, at best, limit our capacities and, at worst, remove them. In Britain, as the English Longitudinal Study on Ageing (ELSA) long-term project has shown, there are wide variations in life expectancy, both across socioeconomic groups

168

and across regions of the UK. Addressing these challenges is a priority for policymakers and health professionals alike. The final years of decline are expensive in terms of medical and social care: although dying costs the same at any age, there can be significant economic as well as societal benefits to maximizing productive life and reducing the morbidity period.

The very success of the NHS has led to ever-increasing demands on its capacity and resources. Inevitably it has moved somewhat away from the original promise of care free at the point of delivery—"from cradle to grave"—as its founders envisaged. In post–World War II Britain, health was assumed to be a definable state. Now we recognize that our expectations of health are changing continuously, and access to information on new drugs and treatment drive our expectations to unprecedented new levels. I will return to some of the contemporary debate about that later in the chapter. Britons are intensely proud of the NHS and often have a very strong emotional attachment to it, but they have yet to accept that it needs radical restructuring to meet the needs of an aging population.

For instance, one of the most urgent debates concerns who is responsible for long-term care and how it should be paid for. Provision was never planned into the NHS originally because of the shorter life expectancy when it was established. Most residential care is funded through local authorities in the UK, which means it is considered to be social care paid for according to people's means, and for most not free at the point of delivery, which it would be were it an integral part of NHS services. There are consequences flowing from this for staff standards and quality of care. Argument has been fueled by the decision of the Scottish Parliament to meet personal care costs (though not all accommodation costs) through taxation, but we should be wary of comparisons. It was a much easier decision to make for five million people than it would be for fifty-five million, and Scotland has far fewer variations in socioeconomic determinants of health than have England and Wales.

Overall spending on health care has risen to some £84.5 billion (approximately $160 billion) and has doubled in nine years. Every medical school in the UK has a department of geriatric medicine, as does every general hospital. Individuals dependent on state-funded social care can now receive payments directly to help shape personal decisions, but this is rarely used. A major effort has been made to raise the income level of the poorest older people, and the Sure Start scheme, which originally focused on early childhood by concentrating services on deprived local communities and comprehensive intervention strategies, has now been expanded to older people's schemes, channeling government money into disadvantaged locales. This approach has the dual benefit of not stigmatizing individuals and of spreading outcomes across the entire community.

So there is much to applaud, but the boundaries between health and social care are very difficult to define—particularly, I think, when it comes to the frail oldest. The social needs of older people are not adequately met, and community care is not nearly as comprehensive and integrated as it should be. The fast-escalating trend is to reduce health care in hospitals and provide far more to people in their own homes; budgets are being redirected to meeting this objective, but a coordinated approach between the different services is not easy to achieve, and those who rely on this service really need "one-stop" delivery.

Work, and the relationship between our paid employment and other aspects of our lives, will play an increasingly important and complex role in the new longevity. We all recognize the economic benefits to the individual and society of participation in paid employment, and increased self-worth, achievement, and creativity for the individual are known to contribute to better health and thus life expectancy. The work environment for many in the UK has improved enormously in the thirty years from 1976 to 2006: health and safety issues have due prominence now, technology has cut the toll of physical injury from heavy and manual labor, and there has been a concerted attempt to reinforce basic work rights. We can expect all of these to translate to a longer and healthier working life.

Since the early 1980s, the UK labor market has changed dramatically, away from the "male sole breadwinner" model toward the "full employment" model, with an increase in households in which all adults are working. During the 1980s traditional heavy industries, so long the mainstay of male "jobs for life," all but disappeared, while business deregulation and tax cuts underpinned a much more consumer- and market-oriented view of society and led to an explosion of new service-sector jobs. The expansion of university education has also created new career options for many. But housing costs also rose sharply, which accounts for why, several decades on, Britain has some of the longest working hours in Europe and a high incidence of dual-income households. This is so partly because women are choosing to work more, and partly because home ownership is firmly entrenched in the British psyche.

Employers and employees have had to adapt to this new reality—particularly employees, when balancing competing commitments to work and to their family care responsibilities, which traditionally have been child care but now also involve care of older people. Although there is no formal definition of "work-life balance," we all have an idea of what we mean by it. In the UK, the Work Foundation defines it thus:

> Work-life balance is about people having a measure of control over when, where and how they work. It is achieved when an individual's right to a fulfilled life inside and outside paid work is accepted and respected as the norm, to the mutual benefit of the individual, business, and society.

A government strategy document published in January 2003 set out the following key "drivers of change" behind the need for work-life balance:

- A transformation in the way families organize their work, with a strong trend among couples away from single-earner toward dual-earner families and sustained growth in single-parent employment

- A dramatic increase in the proportion of employees with caring responsibilities

- The combination of a competitive business environment and the current labor market context, bringing new challenges for employers and employees

UK fathers work the longest average hours in Europe—46.9 per week, more than in Portugal, Germany, and Ireland and nearly 12 hours more than in France. Findings from the Health and Safety Executive in 2004–2005 show one in five working people reported that they felt their work was very or extremely stressful. This, again, may be associated with the increasing deregulation of the UK labor market, in which the trend is for short-term contracts, with all their concomitant insecurities, in place of the traditional pattern of relatively secure long-term employment.

Although these figures relate to all age groups, there is no doubt that the opportunities for, and nature of, the work available for older workers will be heavily influenced by our success in achieving a work-life balance.

Various legislative measures have been introduced with the aim of making the labor market more accessible to parents and improving that balance. The key measures currently in place include entitlements to paid maternity and paternity leave, adoption leave, the right to request flexible work hours to accommodate family needs, equalization of employment rights for part-time workers and those on fixed-term contracts and of rules on maximum working hours, and a national minimum wage.

I believe it is fair to say that we owe these rights largely to the influence of the European Union (EU). What has come to be known as "The Social Chapter" was originally the Social Policy Agreement made between all EU states at Maastricht in December 1991, and the phrase is now used as shorthand for all employment directives issued by Brussels. Under the Conservative government the UK originally opted out of the agreement, but that policy changed with the advent of a Labour government in 1997, and the UK has been a signatory with effect since May 1999. The Social Chapter was neither legislation nor did it impose any new laws; rather, it created a mechanism for member states to introduce social legislation.

The directive on working time came into force in the UK on October 1, 1998. It places a general limit of forty-eight hours on the working week, which can be averaged over seventeen weeks, and entitlements to rest periods are also set out. (Individual workers can agree in writing with their employers voluntarily to "opt out" of the forty-eight-hour limit.) But there are problems applying it in the flexible economy Britain has adopted—and it has also caused difficulties within the NHS, in which the long hours worked by junior doctors have long been an established part of the professional structure.

If we are serious about the work-life balance and about recognizing the potential to live more fulfilled lives, a significant challenge remains for all involved to support social and family rights in an adaptable and fast-changing economy.

What role will older workers—a term now applied to anyone over fifty in Britain—play in achieving this aim?

Pressure has built up over the past two decades around the issue of retirement age. The Sex Discrimination Act of 1986 introduced equal retirement ages for men and women in employment. It arose from a test case involving an NHS health authority that was found to have breached the EU's Equal Treatment Directive by requiring a female employee to retire at age sixty-two when men were not required to retire until the age of sixty-five. The government of the day decided to introduce legislation requiring all employers to set equal compulsory retirement ages for men and women.

Twenty years on, there is debate about whether the default retirement age of sixty-five should be abandoned entirely. A formal review is due in 2009, but many campaigners do not want to wait that long. The aim is to allow individuals more choice over timing the end of their working lives and to try and force employers to employ more older people, but this is a politically sensitive move for any government to make. An earlier consultation paper, which raised the possibility of mandatory retirement at seventy or scrapping fixed retirement ages altogether, prompted press headlines of the "work till you drop" variety.

Potentially the biggest change in favor of the rights of older workers has just come into effect. The EU and UK have been lamentably slow, compared to the United States, in introducing anti–age discrimination legislation. To lag forty years behind the United States in this area is amazing, but now we have caught up: the law applies to young as well as old, and the next few years will indicate whether it is going to work. Again, the impetus came from an EU directive, commonly called the "Employment Directive," to prohibit discrimination in employment on the grounds of religion or belief, disability, age, or sexual orientation. The requirement was for the age discrimination strand of the directive to be implemented by December 2006; it in fact came into force in the UK on October 1, 2006. It is hard to predict, at the time of this writing, what the problem areas for enforcement will be, and there remains a potentially far more contentious area to tackle: that of discrimination in the provision of goods and services. Draft legislation on this is expected by the end of this year.

Age discrimination in the labor market can result in significant costs. Individuals see their living standards decline; employers deny themselves the experience and motivation of older workers; society and the economy lose cumulatively. There have been notable success stories in Britain, such as the DIY retailer B&Q, which has gained public approval, and real brand impact, as an employer of those over fifty. They have now abandoned any retirement age and have employees in their eighties. The retail sector generally has a good record in this area; other sectors, such as financial services, much less so—surprising, when you consider the potential market of the "gray pound" (or dollar) and the increasingly imaginative financial products that will be required to meet the evolving needs of older people.

In 2003, the Chartered Institute of Personnel Development (CIPD) carried out a survey titled "Age, Pensions and Retirement: Attitudes and Expectations." The key findings of the survey in relation to age discrimination follow:

- Twenty-one percent of respondents over fifty stated they had been discouraged from applying for a job "because of wording in an advertisement that contained or hinted at an age range."

- Sixty-six percent of all respondents stated that recruitment advertising did not encourage older workers to apply for jobs.

- Seventeen percent of respondents aged fifty and over stated that they had been discriminated against because of their age during an interview.

- Forty-eight percent of respondents stated that the organization that they currently work for does nothing to encourage the employment of older workers.

- Thirty-five percent of all respondents stated that the primary reason for discrimination in the workplace was age.

A recent survey by the CIPD and the Chartered Management Institute (CMI) published in October 2005 analyzed age discrimination in the workplace. The survey of 2,682 managers and personnel professionals produced these findings:

- Fifty-nine percent of respondents reported that they have been personally disadvantaged at work because of their age.

- Twenty-two percent stated that age has an impact on their own recruitment decisions.

- Forty-eight percent of those surveyed had "suffered" age discrimination through job applications.

- Thirty-nine percent stated that their chances of promotion were hindered by age discrimination.

- Sixty-three percent stated that workers between ages thirty and thirty-nine had the best promotion prospects, with only 2 percent citing those aged fifty and over.

- Sixty-one percent reported the perception that career expectations decrease with age.

- Thirty-seven percent stated that there should be more career advice for older workers.

- Seventy-seven percent agreed that career advice and training would be critical in retaining older workers.

The government has under way both skills reviews and assessments of the labor market for those over fifty, and we await legislative proposals. There is plenty of evidence that is cost-effective to retain workers with experience, reliability, and loyalty; these qualities may have become less prized in our fast-changing competitive economies than in the past, but I believe we need to take a more holistic view of what comprises skills if we are not to lose them entirely.

A new Commission for Equalities and Human Rights has been created, bringing together previously separate bodies dealing with discrimination on grounds of gender, race, and disability, including—for the first time—age, sexual orientation, and religious belief. At the time of writing, it is still being set up; it will become active in late 2007. It should provide an ideal mechanism for advancing, and establishing, the idea that we must maximize and protect the potential of every individual. Britain has been much changed in the past twenty-five years by a brand of ideological individualism that has tended to exaggerate differences rather than recognizing and valuing common experience. It is also regrettably true that single-issue activism, originally a positive force for upholding minority rights, has contributed to a societal model of mutually antagonistic special interest groups and often obscures the truer picture of a diverse and aging society.

One result, unsurprisingly, has been a loss of traditional respect for elders and a breakdown of contact and understanding between age groups. This may well be a temporary phenomenon arising from the belief in the value of the nuclear family, one that will reverse. The shape of family life is changing, with many more older mothers, single-parent families, and longer life—creating obligations of care across four, or even five, generations.

Another identifiable theme in the UK since the 1970s has been the move away from persuasion to enforcement: in a range of health and social policy areas, the previous Conservative governments (and their Labor predecessors in the 1970s) invoked the rhetoric of individual choice and, to varying extents, the regulation of the market. Increasingly, and significantly due to the influence of the EU, it is recognized that legislative action is necessary, in contexts as disparate as smoking in shared space to age discrimination in employment.

Attention is now rightly being directed at some of the hidden problems affecting the care of older people, and there is a growing awareness that specific measures are needed to address them. Legislation has been passed to safeguard the rights of vulnerable adults, including those with physical and mental incapacity, and the government has launched a "Dignity in Care" campaign directed at vulnerable elders, but law and policy are still nowhere near achieving the same level of protection as that afforded to vulnerable children. Guidance has been issued on the quality of nutrition in clinical settings and research is being carried out on the same theme within community care.

I referred earlier to the debate around provision of free health care via the NHS, and how improved medical treatments and greater life expectancy have inevitably created many new demands on the system.

Since 1999, the National Institute for Health and Clinical Excellence (NICE) has evaluated new drugs and treatments and issued advice and guidance to health professionals; it is then up to the government to accept their guidance and either allow or restrict provision of that treatment within the NHS. Previously, decisions on availability of treatment had been left to local health authorities, resulting in wide disparities of provision around the country. It can be argued that a health-care system funded from taxation to the extent the NHS is must have some independent arbiter of how taxpayers' money is spent, and prescription drugs represent the second largest cost component in the health service. The independence of NICE and the robustness of their procedures are not in question, and many find it preferable to have such an organization preside over the rationing of treatment, rather than individual clinicians or managers.

But there have been some decisions whereby treatment is not approved at an early stage, on cost-effectiveness grounds, only to be approved once the condition is further advanced. Herceptin for breast cancer and Aricept for Alzheimer's disease are two that have caused significant debate. It strikes many people as perverse that the government should accept such guidance when its own health policy emphasizes early intervention and prevention. In the case of the Aricept decision, in October 2006, prescription through the NHS was denied to early-stage sufferers of Alzheimer's, yet the drug would have cost the NHS £2.50 ($5) per day per patient.

Of course, such decisions carry much greater costs to society—costs that are outside the purview of NICE to calculate. But these are the responsibility of the government, especially if they are serious about coordinating National Service Frameworks and achieving their own public health goals. How are Alzheimer's sufferers to be cared for? Who provides the care, and how it is paid for? What is the cost to the economy when family members who would otherwise be in paid employment provide care? The truth is that they are unlikely to work again if they have significant care duties and will therefore be reliant on public benefits. And, crucially, what are the costs of challenging NICE decisions in court?

I believe that these arguments lead inexorably toward the introduction of a revised form of payments for some health treatments; in particular, we will need to introduce a partnership model between the public funding and individual contribution to meet the costs of long-term care. This is a very challenging decision for any government in Britain to make, but it is, in my view, inevitable in the longer term. It may be easier to achieve this if we move our societal understanding of health care further away from disease control, toward a model that maximizes well-being across the life course.

What other future paths for public action can we identify?

For the government, there must be an overarching strategy on aging across departments, with a coordinator both to monitor implications of an aging society for public services and to ensure delivery of services. The creation of an Older People's Strategy Development Group is a start, but we have not yet sufficiently recognized what the impact of demographic change on public services will be, and much more research needs to be done. It is particularly important to integrate fiscal, economic, and social policy.

This is about not just the increasing numbers of older people, but also the changing expectations of younger people about the nature and extent of their working life and their retirement. Governments need to promote the notion of "productive engagement" in relation to all age groups.

We must do more to address inequalities beyond the purely health sphere, adopting a holistic approach that embraces housing, transportation, education, and, as I have covered in some detail, employment. The new Commission for Equalities and Human Rights is potentially a major agent for change in this respect.

Public health programs relating to tobacco, alcohol, and diet have had some impact, but troubling signs remain that the message is still not getting through to young people and to some of the most socioeconomically vulnerable.

For instance, smoking has fallen from 39 percent of the population in 1980 to 26 percent in 1994, but has varied little since; 94 percent of all smokers started before the age of twenty-five, and 23 percent of all fifteen-year-olds smoke. This despite significant increases in tobacco excise duty, an advertising ban, and widespread health risk information.

Likewise, statistics on obesity and nutrition are worrying. Well over half of all British adults—twenty-four million—are either overweight or obese, as are 30 percent of children under fifteen. Among young adults, only 18 percent of women and 15 percent of men eat the recommended five portions of fruit and vegetables each day. Yet the retail revolution has given this generation access to a variety of fresh produce that would have been unimaginable thirty years ago.

In the UK, some powerful cultural factors militate against the success of health campaigns. Facetious references to "the nanny state" reinforce the message that the government somehow has no business trying to influence our behavior for our own good. The fashion, media, and film industries continue, despite advertising bans, to depict smoking as a normal, indeed stylish activity, usually in connection with celebrities. When a popular TV chef in the UK campaigns for better school food, he is applauded, because he's attacking the government's record, but when the minister for public health launches a campaign to promote the eating of fruit (including demonstrations on how to tackle some of the more unusual fruits), she is ridiculed in the press.

Under significant pressure from food and health campaigners, the major supermarket chains in the UK have greatly improved labeling (with "traffic light" symbols indicating salt, fat, fiber, and the like), with promotion of better nutrition, a "five portions per day" message, and availability of a wider range of fruit and vegetables. Unfortunately, costs remain outside the scope of some target groups.

These negative trends will have to be reversed if the current generation of under-fifteens are to enjoy the same life expectancy as their parents, let alone exceed it. Or will we continue to see today's baby boomers as the single golden generation to enjoy health and a standard of living that future generations will not be able to emulate? It is up to all of us to make sure this is not the outcome for those of us fortunate enough to live in our prosperous countries.

CHAPTER

HEALTHY AGING IN THE UNITED STATES

JEANETTE C. TAKAMURA

Since the turn of the twentieth century in 1900, the health and longevity of adults in the United States have improved significantly, as have the health and longevity of their counterparts in the developed world. In 1900, the average life expectancy at birth in the United States was forty-seven years, and people aged sixty-five and over numbered 3.1 million, 4 percent of the total population. By the turn of the twenty-first century, the average life expectancy nationwide was 76.9 years, and not only had the number of older adults soared to 35 million (by 2004 it had reached 36.3 million), but the percentage of total population had increased dramatically, to 13 percent. As in many other countries, the fastest-growing segment of the older adult population for several decades has been composed of people aged eighty-five and older. Between 1900 and 2000, this segment multiplied thirty-four times in size. However, the most dramatic rise in the number of older adults aged sixty-five and over in the United States will occur in the near future. As the baby boomers (those born between 1946 and 1964) reach that age, from 2011 to 2029, they will account for nearly seventy-six million older Americans, with a great likelihood of more centenarians than ever before.

This chapter discusses the longevity of a very diverse U.S. aging population, examines the phenomenon of healthy aging in the United States, and identifies some of the policies and programs that have enabled the improved health status of older

Americans as a group. It concludes by speculating about the health status of future generations of older people in the United States, most notably the baby boomers.

THE LONGEVITY OF OLDER AMERICANS

Although the longevity of older Americans can be examined against that of their counterparts in other developed nations, comparisons based on national averages can be misleading. The United States, unlike most nations in the world, is a country with a very heterogeneous population. A review particularly of within-population differences—differences by gender, race and ethnicity, economic status, and religious affiliation, for example—is essential if older Americans are to be accurately represented and understood.

Gender differentials in aging and longevity have been consistently noted in the United States and in nations around the world. In the United States in 2000, of those aged sixty-five and over, there were 1.43 women for each man. Among those aged eighty-five and over in 2000, the gender ratio of women to men was significantly more dramatic, at 2.46 to 1. Racial and ethnic diversity distinguishes the older adult population in the United States from many of its sister countries. During the civil rights era of the 1960s, when identity politics were at their height, minority racial and ethnic groups redefined themselves, striving for unified voices. *Black* or *African American* became the appellations for the descendants of people captured in Africa for the slave trade that provided forced labor in the United States between 1776 and 1865. The indigenous peoples of the lower forty-eight states and Alaska became known as American Indian/Alaska Natives, and citizens who could trace their ancestral roots to an Asian country or a Pacific island or nation were initially categorized and counted by the census as Asian Americans/Pacific Islanders. Today, Native Hawaiians and Other Pacific Islanders is a category separate from Asian Americans. Finally, the rubric *Hispanic* came to represent people of Latin American or Spanish descent whose ancestral community of origin is Spanish-speaking. These overarching rubrics—Black or African American, American Indian/Alaska Native, Asian American, Native Hawaiian and Other Pacific Islanders, and Hispanic—imprecisely suggest the homogenization of peoples with roots in many nations, kingdoms, and tribes.

Of the more than 36.3 million Americans who were at least sixty-five in 2004, over 18 percent were minority elders. In 2005, approximately 84 percent of older Americans were white, 8.2 percent were African American, 0.4 percent was American Indian/Alaskan Native, 2.9 percent were Asian American/Pacific Islander, and 6 percent were Hispanic (U.S. Census, 2000). White older Americans formed the largest segment of the United States population aged sixty-five and over and had much lower poverty rates than did African Americans, Hispanics, and American Indians/Alaskan Natives.

By 2020, nearly 24 percent of all elderly Americans will be members of ethnic or racial minority groups. This percentage is expected to rise to just under 40 percent of the U.S. population aged sixty-five and over by 2050 (U.S. Census, 2000). At mid-century, elderly whites will likely account for 61 percent (fifty-three million) of all older

Americans, African American elders will be 12 percent (ten million), Asian Americans/ Pacific Islanders will equal approximately 8 percent (seven million) of all older Americans, and the percentage of elderly Hispanics will rise dramatically to 18 percent (fifteen million).

When comparisons are made of the average longevity of older Americans who are African American, American Indian/Aleut Native, Asian American, Native Hawaiian and Other Pacific Islander, and Hispanic, data on their health status and risks can be illuminating. In 2003, the U.S. population had an average life expectancy of 77.5 at birth, with men averaging 74.8 and women 80.1. White men could anticipate a life expectancy on average of 75.3, white women 80.5. In comparison, African Americans had at-birth life expectancies of 69.0 years for men and 76.1 for women. The life expectancy of Hispanic women is 83. The at-birth life expectancy of Asian American women is nearly 87; for Asian American men it is 80. Native Hawaiian and Other Pacific Islanders do not fare as well.

At age sixty-five, American men have an average life expectancy of 16.8 years; women at sixty-five have a considerably longer average life expectancy (19.8 years). White men at age sixty-five can expect to live an average of an additional 16.8 years and white women an additional 19.8 years. By comparison, older African American men at age sixty-five have a potential life expectancy of an additional 14.9 years, compared with an additional 18.5 years for older African American women. At age sixty-five, Hispanic and Asian American men and women have life expectancies three to four years longer than those of white American men and women. Male Native American life expectancy at age sixty-five is eighteen years; Native American women at the same age have a life expectancy of twenty-three years.

Murray and colleagues (2006) recently reported a comprehensive analysis of U.S. mortality disparities by race and county. Their study of national U.S. Census and National Center for Health Statistics data for the twenty-nine-year period from 1982 to 2001 revealed huge variations in life expectancy when race, location of county, population density, race-specific county level per capita income, and cumulative homicide rate are considered.

The Murray team surfaced "Eight Americas," each representing subpopulations composed of millions of residents and distinguished by unique race-county, population density, income, and homicide rate configurations. The eight distinctive Americas for which life expectancy disparities are noteworthy are "Asians, northland low-income rural whites, Middle America, low-income whites in Appalachia and the Mississippi Valley, western Native Americans, black Middle America, low-income southern rural blacks, and high-risk urban blacks" (p. 6). Most dramatic among the disparities is the twenty-one-year spread in life expectancy that separates Asian women (5.6 million women) from high-risk urban black men (3.4 million men); the latter group's mortality disparity is attributable to a higher incidence of chronic illnesses and injuries linked to violence and other causes.

Murray's analysis also suggests that the observed disparities are not new, but were apparent the late 1980s as well (Murray and others, 2006). If we accept these findings, efforts by U.S. public health agencies and programs to address health disparities by targeting preventive interventions to specific populations would be advised to use comparable research to inform, strengthen, and devise culturally appropriate, subpopulation-specific methodologies.

There is widespread consensus about environmental factors that have generated significant improvements in the longevity of the overall U.S. population. Until the early years of the 1800s, infant and childhood mortality rates (to age five) were as high as 50 percent, with average life expectancies typically hovering at thirty years. From the latter part of the nineteenth century through the twentieth century, much was accomplished to enable greater numbers of people to live longer, healthier lives, including public health measures adopted by cities and towns to improve sanitation, clean drinking water, and better nutrition; immunizations against childhood and communicable diseases (chicken pox, measles, polio, mumps, diphtheria, for example); public education; and safety measures in the workplace. Consequently, infant and childhood adversities and mortality among America's young, in particular, declined significantly in the first half of the twentieth century.

Policy and program interventions to reduce toxic and risk-laden environmental (including occupational health and safety), sociobehavioral, and other factors continue to top the agendas of many public health, child welfare, labor, and global ecology advocacy organizations. This is essential, as a significant number of children are disadvantaged by the cumulative effects of poor health, social exclusion, poverty, poor nutrition, family disorganization, and other difficulties. Unfortunately, these young people are more likely to face physical and mental health risks in adulthood and their older years.

Since the mid-twentieth century, improvements in life expectancy have been most noteworthy in the later decades of the human life span. In fact, centenarians have registered an astounding annual growth rate (8 percent) in the United States. Super-centenarians are also increasing in number at a significant rate, manifesting "demographic selection" and remarkable hardiness and resilience against cardiovascular, Parkinson's, and other diseases typically more prevalent in the advanced years (Perls, Kunkel, and Puca, 2002). In both of these oldest-of-older-American groups, women outnumber men, although gendered differentials in health must be considered carefully, as older women's longer lives are often marked by years of reduced mobility, hearing and visual impairments, and chronic illnesses, and concomitantly by comparatively strong and supportive social networks.

Research to understand why some people, whether in the United States or elsewhere, live to become centenarians and super centenarians (110 years and older) has pursued the biological and genetic basis of aging and of "exceptional longevity." Some theories suggest that centenarians may be genetically predisposed to escaping or surviving major illnesses or to delaying the onset of illnesses that can lead to death or disability.

It appears unlikely that environmental factors have played a major role in extending longevity and decelerating morbidity post-1950 (Perls, Kunkel, and Puca, 2002).

Stronger explanations can probably be found by recognizing the important impact of, on one hand, medical and drug interventions produced by biomedical and related research, and on the other, improved access to health care spurred by national policies. Unfortunately, employer-sponsored health-care plans are now on the wane, and Medicare and Medicaid, which have afforded many older Americans access to health care since their enactment in 1965, may undergo significant changes and be less protective in the decades ahead.

Conventional wisdom might presume a strong association between socioeconomic status and health risk and thus life expectancy in the United States. Yet the statistics on life expectancies for Hispanics and Asian Americans appear to fly in the face of presumptions that socioeconomic status, access to health care, and expectable length of life are necessarily linked. Rather, the lifestyles of some members of these two ethnic groups may include salubrious dimensions that are yet to be identified. Research to tease out explanations of the health status and the longevity of diverse populations is sorely needed.

HEALTHY AGING IN THE UNITED STATES

Until the last three decades of the twentieth century, aging was commonly regarded as synonymous with decline, illness, and senility. Thanks to several extensive longitudinal studies and to federally funded biomedical, psychological, and sociobehavioral research, many faulty conceptions of normal aging have been dispelled. We know now that rates of individual aging vary and thus that biological and chronological ages do not necessarily correspond. We also no longer perceive Alzheimer's and other dementias to be inevitable diseases inherent in the aging process. Moreover, the trajectories of diseases and conditions prevalent in old age are less apt to be shrouded in misconceptions, the efficacy of various preventive health behaviors has been documented, and preventive and other health regimens have been broadly disseminated. Finally, care options for families of elders have been legitimized and supported at the local, state, and national levels. In line with this, both formal professional and informal family caregivers of older Americans are relying increasingly on clinically tested treatments and interventions.

Our understanding of the phenomenon of healthy aging in the United States has grown thanks to major longitudinal studies that have tracked relatively large samples of primarily white adults and examined their physiological and psychological health from the 1950s to the present. For example, the Duke Longitudinal Studies found that social and psychological functioning tends to be stable in older people. Duke data also suggested that health and physical functioning can often improve and that aging processes tend to vary individually. The Baltimore Longitudinal Study found that diet, physical activity, and other lifestyle factors affect physiological health and changes in health status. The Framingham Heart Study and the Ni-Hon-San Heart Study have also offered rich insights into many of the determinants of health over the life course.

Today, in addition to private industry, federal departments and agencies are engaged in health-related research and public health education programs that inform and support healthy aging. Those involved include the National Institutes of Health (NIH), the Centers for Disease Control and Prevention (CDC), and the Food and Drug Agency (FDA), all within the Department of Health and Human Services; the National Aeronautical and Space Agency (NASA); and the Department of Agriculture. Based on research to date, the approaches widely prescribed for optimal health promotion in the United States include simple diets with low fat and low salt content, moderate consumption of alcohol such as red wine (purportedly because of the properties of resveratrol, flavonoids, and other antioxidants), avoidance of tobacco and smoking cessation, vigorous physical activity, annual pneumococcal and influenza immunizations, fall and injury prevention, routine wearing of seat belts in automobiles, and maintaining a positive attitude toward life. In contrast, in some developed countries and in many developing ones, alcohol and smoking consumption and transportation safety are not yet primary public health targets.

Seventy-five percent of premature deaths in the aged sixty-five and over population are due to heart disease, stroke, cancer, arthritis, diabetes, and obesity. Nearly 50 percent of all disabilities among older Americans can be attributed to chronic conditions. Among people aged sixty-five and over, 80 percent have one or more chronic illnesses; the majority of these may be prevented through adherence to a healthy lifestyle. Because chronic illness is the leading cause of death and of costly disabilities among older Americans, health promotion and preventive health behaviors are a high priority for the "aging network" of federal, state, and local agencies; tribal organizations; service agencies and providers; and national aging organizations.

A true picture of the health of older Americans must factor in health disparities that distinguish older people of color and older people who are poor from white and middle-class elders. According to a Kaiser Family Foundation report, elderly African Americans are more than twice as likely as elderly white Americans to die from heart conditions, possibly because of significant differences in access to care and the quality of care received (Kaiser Family Foundation, 1999). Similarly, Medicare-eligible African American women are less likely to be screened via mammography for breast cancer. If health disparities in the United States are to be accurately documented and effectively addressed, research must focus on diverse elders and their health risks, their needs, access to appropriate health care, and the development of culturally appropriate, sociobehavioral interventions.

POLICIES AND PROGRAMS

Policies and programs instituted over the last two centuries in local communities and states to protect and promote the public health of all Americans have contributed to overall improvements in health status and in life expectancy. Several federal policies, typically implemented in collaboration with states and localities, deserve mention. The Safe Drinking Water Act of 1974, the primary federal law to ensure the safety of water for human consumption, is an important example. Food safety provisions and national dietary guidelines—the latter published since 1980 by the U.S. Department of Agriculture in collaboration with the U.S. Department of Health and Human Services— are also aimed at public health protection and promotion. Programs addressing the use of safety belts, emergency medical services, and drunk-driving laws are all led by the National Highway Traffic Safety Administration in the U.S. Department of Transportation. Another important law, the Occupational Safety and Health Act of 1970, has resulted in significant decreases in workplace fatalities and declines in occupational injury and illness rates.

Although the foregoing are essential to protect the public's health, one of the most forceful social policies to curb and prevent impoverishment among older Americans and thus support access to health care, the ability to afford healthier diets, and social engagement remains the Social Security Act of 1935. Social Security benefits keep a significant number of older women, who are at greater risk of financial vulnerability than older men, out of the clutches of poverty.

A bundle of policies and programs enacted in the 1960s during the Johnson administration have enabled healthy aging. Some ensured civil rights and affirmative action and, along with these, equal access and opportunity for diverse populations with longstanding histories of marginalization in the United States. Two entitlement programs—Medicare and Medicaid—and the Older Americans Act (OAA) discretionary programs were enacted in 1965. The federal Medicare program helps with acute and hospital care costs, and federal and matching state dollars fund Medicaid's coverage of certain long-term care costs for people with limited incomes. Home-delivered and community-based meals programs for frail and vulnerable older people, family caregiver support services and options, long-term care ombudsmen, and other services are funded through the OAA, but historically appropriations for OAA programs have been modest. Although Medicare, Medicaid, and the OAA provide important protection, a comprehensive national health and long-term care policy has remained elusive.

National health goals and objectives are articulated in Healthy People 2010, the promotional responsibility for which lies in the Office of the U.S. Surgeon General. They focus and involve state and local public health systems in their implementation. Several leading health indicators, all with implications for healthy aging, are part of the foci of Healthy People 2010. These include level of physical activity, overweight and obesity, tobacco use, substance abuse, responsible sexual behavior, mental health, injury and violence, environmental quality, immunization, and access to health care. Among these, overweight and obesity problems plague almost two out of three Americans. Overweight and obesity-linked illnesses such as heart disease and diabetes cause one out of eight deaths in the United States and cost billions of dollars (Carmona, 2003). Although a configuration of genetic, environmental, social, and metabolic causes are probably at the root of weight problems, older Americans are simply not physically active enough. Thus, research is ongoing to identify and translate specific evidence-based interventions and methods into community-based physical activity programs. It appears that physical activity is positively correlated with education and income, but negatively correlated with gender, non-white race and ethnicity, weight, smoking, age, and rural residency. Again, research on minority populations is sparse at best, and the construction of cost-effective, responsive, culturally appropriate programs that could eliminate disparities among racial and ethnic groups requires reliable, valid evidence.

THE FUTURE

The baby boomers will number between seventy-six and seventy-seven million, constituting the largest population of older Americans ever. This is a widely diverse "generation," with the Beatles and the Vietnam War defining the leading-edge boomers and the marriage of Prince Charles and Diana and the introduction of Pac-Man and MTV distinguishing the tail-end boomers. For these Americans, the seventh decade of life may truly become the new middle age. If current trends continue, "active aging," with continued engagement in economically and socially rewarding activities, will become even more commonplace. Science will inevitably play a larger role in the creation and definition of health, indirectly appropriating the opportunity to maintain youthfulness in aging selectively among those who can afford special interventions and lifestyles. In such a context, "healthy aging" may take on new meanings in the United States.

REFERENCES

Carmona, Richard. Testimony of the Surgeon General Before the Subcommittee on Education Reform, Committee on Education and the Workforce, United States House of Representatives on "The Obesity Crisis in America," July 16, 2003.

The Henry J. Kaiser Family Foundation. *Key Facts: Race, Ethnicity, and Medical Care.* Menlo Park, Calif: Kaiser Family Foundation, Oct. 1999.

Murray, C.J.L., and others. "Eight Americas: Investigating Mortality Disparities Across Races, Counties, and Race-Counties in the United States." *PLoS Medicine*, 2006, September, *3*(9), e260 and corrections in *PloS Medicine*, 2006, Dec. 26, *3*(12), e.545.

Perls, T., Kunkel, L. M., and Puca, A. A. "The Genetics of Exceptional Human Longevity." *Journal of the American Geriatrics Society*, 2002, *50*, 359–368.

PART

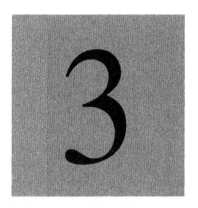

COUNTRIES FACING RAPID POPULATION AGING IN THE NEXT TWENTY TO THIRTY YEARS

CHAPTER

17

HEALTH AND AGING IN AFRICA

NANA ARABA APT

Africa, like the rest of the world, is growing older. The number of aging people living on the continent is increasing rapidly (United Nations, 2005). The increase in numbers of those who require care to achieve an acceptable quality of life has occurred at the same time as the strength of traditional social welfare system—the extended family—has begun to wane (Caldwell, 1968; Shuman, 1991), and the continent, ravaged by an HIV/AIDS epidemic, is unable to meet the drug costs. However, HIV's impact in Africa goes beyond the cost of drugs. Those of reproductive age who are dying are leaving behind young orphaned children in the care of aging parents who may need care themselves. In addition, there is the general increase in the dependency ratio as the numbers of those in the productive and reproductive ages are reduced. Furthermore, young people's attitudes towards filial care are changing (Aboderin, 2001)as economic imbalances become more and more a feature of Africa's development scene. All of these factors have implications for the health and well-being of older people in Africa. Urbanization, migration, and modernization of economies have placed great strains on the extended family system. There are signs that this traditional social welfare system no longer offers older people the customary care and social protection they previously enjoyed.

Living to a ripe old age is something new in Africa. Improvements in nutrition, environmental health, and prophylactics and antibiotics have ensured that many more African children survive childhood and move on to adult years and old age. Aging of the population—a worldwide phenomenon addressed in this book—has its own drawbacks for Africa, as it is generating social and economic crises never before encountered in traditional history. The current average proportion of older people in the African population is still low; this has encouraged the view that aging is not an issue of concern. But Africa is aging rapidly, and although the aging population appears insignificant now, its numbers are nevertheless rising faster than any other age group (United Nations, 2005). Rural populations are aging even more rapidly, as young people migrate to the cities and towns for better life alternatives or are stricken with HIV/AIDS. Older people left behind and, often caring for their sick children, are forced to take on increased economic and household responsibilities, which take a heavy toll on their health (HelpAge International, 2006).

Many national governments in Africa have not tackled the issue of how to develop an appropriate social welfare policy for their aging populations. Typically, social welfare has a low priority, and the contribution of the family to social welfare has largely been neglected. Policy thinking has barely commenced on how better to harness the energies and resources of the family and the community in resolving the social needs of aging individuals and groups. But more than in any other regions of the world, in Africa older generations are living in a world that has undergone the fastest and greatest social and economic changes in history. Not only will there be increasingly larger numbers of older people in this region, but they will also have great educational, health, and other social needs, which must be studied and met if a major human aging catastrophe is to be avoided in the near future. Their educational needs, for example, range from literacy to technical training, through civic and political education to banking and enterprise skills.

This chapter considers aging and health in Africa in this context of rapid social change, poverty in aging, increased burdens, and the marginalization of older people.

HEALTH OF THE AGING

The goal of health maintenance is to enable older people to maintain their self-esteem and physical and mental well-being, to facilitate their continued participation in society, and to recognize their valuable contribution to their families and communities. In this respect, life satisfaction is an indicator for health and social well-being. Are older people in Africa satisfied with their present status and living conditions? Increasingly, in Africa, the indicators show a trend away from the traditional perceptions of elders' life satisfaction.

When elderly Nigerians were asked "What sort of things give you status today?" the least mentioned "things" were children and family—the traditional status norm (Ekpenong, Oyeneye, and Peil, 1987, pp. 16–17). The majority of Nigerian elders are said to be pessimistic about modern circumstances and about the present and future life situations of old people. The authors concluded that even though elderly Nigerians continue their traditional roles, these roles are now less important to an increasingly materialistic society.

Elderly Temne of Sierra Leone, also in West Africa, assess themselves as a "short changed generation" (Dorjhan, 1989). They had "paid their dues" when they were young but their turn for payoff was taken from them through social change. Of elderly Samians of Kenya, in East Africa, Cattell (1989, p. 233) observed that "their influence has been devalued, displaced and replaced" and a significant basis of their respect has been eroded. Cattell further observed that many Samians identify education as the crucial element in this change and emphasized that this lack has reduced respect for them, the support and care given to them and advice sought from them. Now, they explained, one needs new knowledge, which "old persons, especially women lack" (p. 236). In rural Mozambique, an elderly man sums it all up in a philosophical reflection about life: "Now it's just a question of living because it's other people's time" (Da Silva, 1999, p. 30).

The challenge for countries and communities in sub-Saharan Africa in terms of older people's health is to provide conditions that promote quality of life and enhance their ability to work and live independently as long as possible. Health begins with well-being. The well-being of old people is not synonymous with health provision, yet much of the limited research and policy work on aging has been concerned with health institutions rather than the social realities of the old. Even in economic terms in sub-Saharan Africa, economic activities do not stop at any given age. In many African countries, between 74 percent and 91 percent of people over sixty-five continue to work (International Labour Organization, 2000). The World Bank (1994) presents old age as an eventual crisis in economic terms, but policy makers in Africa need to look critically at overall issues of dependency rather than assuming that the problem relates only to older people.

Health must begin with the preservation of older people's economic and social productivity, especially that of older women. An important indicator of well-being is the poverty status of a given population. Poverty in turn is an indicator of the health status of the population. In sub-Saharan Africa in particular, poverty in old age usually reflects poor economic and education status earlier in life, and women are more affected than men. This disadvantages women who also face discrimination in the modern workforce. Lack of education presents as large a barrier as physiological constraint, if not a larger one, to the social and economic participation of older people in Africa. An increase in the number of generations in a fast-changing world necessarily accentuates the educational distance between the younger and older generations (Apt, 1996) if education is viewed purely as the preserve of youth. A lifetime approach to education, which equips older generations with new skills, minimizes this distance.

Within the context of the rights of people of age, we should be concerned, at least in part, with the social status of the older people in society. Increasingly, to a large extent, this segment is experiencing a lack of abilities and declining social power. To that extent, the health of older people in Africa presents a concern about the broader issue of social justice and fundamental human rights. Therefore, any strategy for health maintenance of older people in Africa will be meaningful only if older people are brought back into the mainstream and then rehabilitated. In Africa, both policy makers and ordinary people are clearly struggling to cope with the challenges of a moderniz-ing *and* aging world that places destructive pressures on indigenous social welfare arrangements. Indigenous welfare nevertheless must be retained if we are to avert a social welfare crisis. Presently, within the struggle new patterns of interaction are developing that retain linkages with customary arrangements while adapting to the increasingly monetized world. The search by older people for a prolonged economic life in a monetizing society is one such adaptation that ought to be studied and refined.

AGING IN AFRICA: CRITICAL ISSUES

Aligned to health and aging are the following critical issues that must be considered in the context of human rights.

HIV/AIDS

Worldwide, over thirty-six million people are living with HIV/AIDS, more than two thirds of them in sub-Saharan Africa (The Joint United Nations Programme on HIV/AIDS and World Health Organization, 2004). Contrary to popular misconceptions, HIV/AIDS is not widespread in all African countries. However, in 2004 alone, 2.3 million Africans died of AIDS and AIDS-related illnesses (The Joint United Nations Programme on HIV/AIDS and World Health Organization, 2004). United Nations esti-mates show that at least two million infected adults live in each of these four African countries: Ethiopia, Kenya, Nigeria, and South Africa. In five African countries—Botswana, Lesotho, Swaziland, Zambia, and Zimbabwe—at least one in five adults has HIV or AIDS (United Nations, 2001).

Most of the deaths caused by AIDS occur in younger age groups; the loss of these young lives disproportionately affects productivity and economic growth and the social fabric of family and society. Some thirteen million children have been orphaned because their parents died of AIDS. Ethiopia, Nigeria, and Uganda each have more than 900,000 AIDS orphans. Three other countries—Kenya, United Republic of Tanzania, and Zimbabwe—all have at least half a million orphans due to the AIDS pandemic. The number of AIDS orphans will continue to grow in countries where HIV is still gathering momentum.

It is crucial to note older people's own critical overload with the care of children and grandchildren, especially those dying from AIDS or orphaned by AIDS. Older people are forced to assume dual roles of caregiver and breadwinner for the family at a time in their lives when they might not expect to shoulder this responsibility and when, as is the case in many African countries, their main source of income would tra-ditionally be from their children. A striking feature of AIDS orphan care in Africa is the proportion of older women who are responsible for them. It is largely women who fill this role, as "family care" in Africa generally means care provided by women. By observation, quite a large number of Africans infected with HIV/AIDS live in abject poverty, and upon the death of economically active breadwinners no resources are left behind for caregivers who are generally old and disadvantaged. More often than other age groups, older people—in particular older women—suffer from the economic consequences associated with HIV/AIDS. In the vast majority of African countries, where old age pensions are mostly available only to formal sector employees and where the majority of people work on the land, older people mainly rely on family resources. Caring for people with AIDS and grandchildren who are orphaned by the disease includes the provision of medical care and emotional support, and replacing income lost when their children, the wage earners, fall sick.

For caregivers of adult children with AIDS, above all their experience is one of loneliness and social isolation from friends and families, as they are stigmatized and discriminated against (HelpAge International, 2006). This burden can be especially heavy for older people if they themselves have health problems and are economically dependant on their family members. In the context of their role as caregivers of orphans of HIV/AIDS victims, it is essential that older people's poverty be understood in respect to their health so that HIV/AIDS actions are developed that can meet their needs.

Urbanization and Migration

Urbanization and migration are often cited both separately and jointly as contributing to a change in values: in the past, older people were sustained by a close-knit, age-integrated African society. Urbanization brings changes in the family unit and kinship networks that can have both beneficial and adverse consequences for the health and well-being of the older members (Kinsella, 2001). Urbanization generates changes in the socioeconomic profile of a workforce, as workers—mostly young, in the African context—shift from predominantly agricultural work to industrial and services employment. Concern about the well-being of the old, left behind in rural Africa while the young and able-bodied seek better prospects in urban centers, was articulated well by African delegates at the first World Assembly on Ageing in Vienna in 1982. Urbanization and family dispersal have thus had a negative effect on the pattern of balanced exchange between generations (Apt, 1992; Van der Geest, 1997). Urban living means that the old and the young no longer inhabit the same dwelling and the family unit is increasingly a nuclear one. Thus, older people's lives are characterized by growing inadequacy of family support, poverty and material deprivation, ill heath, and marginalization from family care and modern health services.

Changing Family Structures

The exodus of young people from rural areas to the cities in Africa raises the proportion of older people in the rural proportion. Traditional family support systems for frail elderly may decrease as younger family members living abroad or in urban areas may provide money but are unlikely to be physically present to provide health care for ailing family members. How then shall we make policy that designs intergenerational support back into mainstream social relations so that older people are not marginalized and put at risk by the urbanization process? Public assistance institutions are developed in some countries to provide the caregiving functions that the family is unable to fulfill in modern times. Translating that experience in the developed world to developing countries, however, has proved less than satisfactory. This has unfolded in a variety of ways, but its principal emphasis has been on strategies of community development and participation: to try to close the wide gap that exists between the deprived and the disadvantaged, on the one hand, and existing institutional structures on the other. The implementation of those strategies has often been problematic, particularly for the aging who are often in a double bind: being part of depressed communities of the urban or rural poor and also regarded as passive recipients of care within those communities.

Social Protection

There are no universal pension systems in most African countries. For lack of education and modern skills, jobs in the formal sector are out of the reach of older people, who also face discrimination in access to credit facilities, literacy education, and skills training—all of which thwart their attempts to earn better income. Besides, social security systems in some countries are under pressure because of the structural adjustment programs introduced to reform their stagnant economies. The less older people are able to rely on traditional care systems, which are rapidly waning, the more they must rely on their own income. Adequate food, housing, and health care are essential if African people are to enjoy their older age, but the attainability of these essentials depends heavily on material security. All over Africa many people are aging poor. Poverty not only inhibits the full enjoyment of social and civic rights but also is a major determinant of social exclusion, discrimination, and ill health. The problem of households headed by older people—many of whom are grandparents with primary childrearing responsibility—who have no pension and no community resources, urgently needs policy action.

Gender and Aging

The relationship between gender, aging, and health is of particular significance in Africa. Social policy development, whether by donors or governments, must explicitly concern itself with this issue. In many African societies, women have unequal and inadequate access to basic services, food, and good nutrition. They have no rights to land ownership, and widowed and divorced women suffer from degradation and extreme deprivation. In most African countries, women have little or no formal education. Although there may now be more equality with regard to education in urban areas, the gravest disadvantage of older women in modern Africa is that they lack education. This fact has many consequences for aging. Older women are less likely to participate fully or benefit from national development efforts. and they are more likely to be poorer in old age. Education is an important variable in human well-being in Africa.

It is related to health status and health practices, fertility and mortality behavior, occupation, income, access to credit, and political awareness and participation. Although informal education is very important, most of the higher-level skills and training that are related to these variables are strongly influenced by formal education. The level of participation in social and political activities, openness to social change, and acceptance of new ideas are all influenced by formal education. For the present generation of older women in Africa, family life has undergone rapid change in their lifetime, and the hope for a secure old age surrounded by their children and grandchildren is no longer a reality. Older women's mental health is on the wane. HelpAge Ghana, an age care organization in Ghana on whose board I serve, has adopted the geriatric ward of the country's largest psychiatric hospital, which is overflowing with older women patients diagnosed for depression.

For many older women in this region, health problems began from a very early age, when they were circumcised. Some girls are forced into early marriages to men three times their age and reluctantly become mothers. All these factors have a disproportionate impact on women's health when they age. Those without children and able relatives are most vulnerable. Increasingly, to a large extent, this population is experiencing lack of abilities and declining social power. To address their poverty, we must give consideration to creating income opportunities for them. The aging of African societies necessitates a change in the traditional gender arrangements, whereby a woman's financial position was mediated through her male partner. Programs and policies that endow women with social and economic resources at the point of widowhood will enable women to negotiate for better care and services within their own kinship structures.

In sum, the aging of women in Africa, as compared with men, raises the issue of developing appropriate forms of education, training, and financial assistance based on gender. Social policy on aging in Africa must address older women's need to both increase their financial security and take an active part in public life. Gender and aging should immediately be addressed as part of poverty alleviation strategies throughout Africa.

CONCLUSION: THE ECONOMIC EMPOWERMENT MODEL FOR HEALTH AND AGING IN AFRICA

Africa ended the millennium poorer than it was in 1990 (United Nations Development Programme, 2003). Of the fifty-three countries represented in this region, twenty-three are poorer than they were in 1975. A full 50 percent of the people live on less than $2 per day, and over 50 percent live on less than $1 per day. Bad governance, corruption, and ethnic wars continue to deplete scarce resources. Africa has the worst human development indicators in the world (United Nations Development Programme, 2003). It has the lowest primary school enrollment (only 60 percent of children), only 50 percent of the population have access to improved water sources, and Africa has twenty of the worst-performing health systems in the world. HIV erodes capacity for economic growth in Africa. From 1992 to 2002, South Africa lost $7 billion annually, and in eleven African countries annual GDP dropped by 1.1 percent (International Labour Organization, 2000). In addition to the African burden of malaria and TB, HIV destroys national capital in respect to health and education and exacts high economic costs in terms of medical care and lost earnings, which particularly affects older people, as the most economically active sector of the population also tends to have the highest rate of infection.

Africa is thus aging at a time when its resources are most depleted.

This presents challenges to a region with a critical mass of children and youth whose needs are yet to be adequately met. How to share the national budget equitably between the young and the old requires policies and strategies that value older people's societal contributions. Economic empowerment of older people is crucial to their health and well-being. Empowerment is not only about rights but also about obligations. The empowerment of older people and their development of mutual support systems is not a matter for older people alone. Enabling conditions must be created so that older people have the maximum autonomy and less pressure on scarce social resources. This area needs extensive study. For example, providing leverage funding for mutual support schemes should be the more sustainable alternative to a blanket social security provision. Tout (1989) discusses precisely these issues in his proposed new approach to the problems of older people in developing countries. Mutual support, however, should be viewed not simply as the cheaper option but in terms of the active participation benefits it brings. Mutual support offers the opportunity for enhanced sociability, greater bargaining power across the generations, and greater security in the context of shrinking kinship structures and resources. Therefore, developing an empowerment perspective—a movement away from the "aging as deterioration" medical paradigm of the developed regions—enables older people to define an active part for themselves in social and economic life. Similarly, mutual support structures, well used in traditional African societies, provide older people with more control over their own lives.

Social protection is gradually emerging as one of the main strategies in poverty reduction in Africa. The African Union's Ouagadougou Plan of Action 2004 commits member states to improving the living conditions of older people through better social protection services, including improved pensions, health care, and other schemes (HelpAge International, 2006). Cash transfers and pensions can serve to meet the basic needs of the poor, such as food, health care, and shelter. The right to social protection ought to take center stage in Africa's development plans, with appropriate legislation and resources such as that now being considered in Tanzania, Uganda, and Gambia (HelpAge International 2006). South Africa is one country in Africa where social protection is a right that people can claim in court.

In modern Africa it is the acquisition of resources that earns the status of the sacred or the valued. In a society envisaged in the twenty-first century, with increasing numbers of people living into old age in Africa, great age is less likely to be valued without an accompanying resource base. Because old age is increasingly associated with diminishing returns, it is likely to be viewed as both a societal and a familial burden. Burdens generate anxiety and ill health. Policy thinking on how to better harness the energies and resources of the family and the community in resolving the social needs of individuals and groups has barely begun. If the family is to be expected to continue to serve as the primary safety net it once was, we must know more about how social changes have affected the family's ability to undertake such responsibilities.

These are the challenges that call for clear policy directives to ensure the well-being of the rising population of older people in this millennium. Concerns about population growth, basic health problems and health care provision, mortality and morbidity rates, and infectious diseases—especially the HIV/AIDS pandemic—have dominated the collective attention in most African countries. But there is still an urgent need to increase knowledge and awareness of aging issues throughout Africa. Africa needs to think about aging issues, and not necessarily about issues of health care, which has been the developed region's failing model for addressing the needs of this growing population. Rather, we need more well-researched information on which to base meaningful aging policies that recognize the social needs of family members as a whole. The generations must be assisted to support each other in a meaningful manner that leaves none overburdened. This was Africa's strength in decades past, and this should constitute its greatest strength in the future, through appropriate culturally ingrained health policies that address

- How to promote healthy aging and affordable community integrated social-care systems that are age-friendly

- How to ensure the general well-being of older people in the framework of the family without overloading it because of lack of resources

- How to reduce poverty in old age and combat negative attitudes toward older people

- How to maintain intergenerational links

- How to contain HIV/AIDS so that older people are not unduly stressed by responsibilities

It is essential that we develop comprehensive and culture-sensitive strategies that will ensure a humane society for all in Africa, regardless of age. This received a lot of attention at the conference of the African Gerontological Society (AGES) held in Accra, Ghana in 2002. The need for research on aging in Africa was high on the list of recommended actions. There is a huge research gap to be filled. The recently established African Research on Aging Network (AFRAN) is definitely a step in the right direction. We need to develop appropriate methodologies and collect better descriptive data on the social and economic support systems around aging in Africa. And there is also a need for a radical review of the policy options open to governments, development agencies, and communities to tackle the social and economic requirements of massive demographic change. Until such time as Africa can boast of having readily available information for policymakers and the public at large to be useful in shaping a new paradigm (Africa's own paradigm) for an aging world, let us not equate aging with illness.

REFERENCES

Aboderin, I. "Decline and Normative Shifts in Family Support for Older Persons in Ghana: Implications for Policy." Paper presented at the Annual DAS conference, Manchester, Sept. 10–12, 2001.

Apt, N. A. "Changing Family Patterns and Their Impact on Ageing in Africa." In *Social Security and Changing Family Structures,* Studies and Research No. 29. Geneva: International Social Security Association, 1992.

Apt, N. A. *Coping with Old Age in a Changing Africa: Social Change and the Elderly Ghanaian.* Aldershot, UK: Avebury, 1996.

Caldwell, J. C. *Population and Family Change in Africa.* Canberra: Canberra University Press, 1968.

Cattell, M. "Knowledge and Social Change in Samia, Western Kenya." *Journal of Cross-Cultural Gerontology,* 1989, *4*(8), 233.

Da Silva, T. "Disaster, Migration and Older Persons in Mozambique." In *Ageing in Changing Societies,* Workshop Report of the African Gerontological Society, Nairobi, Kenya, 1999.

Dorjahn, V. R. "Where Do the Old Folks Live? The Residence of the Temne of Sierra Leone." *Journal of Cross-Cultural Gerontology,* 1989, *44*(3), 272–275.

Ekpeyong, S., Oyeneye, O., and Peil, M. "Health Problems of Elderly Nigerians." *Social Science Medicine,* 1987, 24.

International Labour Organization. *World Labour Report 2000.* Geneva: International Labour Organization, 2000.

Kinsella, K. "Urban and Rural Dimensions of Global Population Ageing: An Overview." *Journal of Rural Health,* 2001, *17*(4), 315.

Shuman, T. K. "Support of the Elder: The Changing Urban Family and Its Implications for the Elderly." *Ageing and Urbanization,* 279–287. New York: United Nations, 1991.

Tout, K. *Ageing in Developing Countries.* Oxford: Oxford University Press, 1989.

United Nations. *World Population Prospects: The 2002 Revision.* Population Division, Department of Economic and Social Affairs, New York, 2005.

The Joint United Nations Programme on HIV/AIDS (UNAIDS) and World Health Organization. AIDS Epidemic Update. Geneva: The Joint United Nations Programme on HIV/AIDS (UNAIDS) and World Health Organization, Dec. 2004.

United Nations Development Programme (UNDP). *Human Development Report 2001.* New York: United Nations, 2001.

United Nations Development Programme (UNDP). *Human Development Report 2003.* New York: United Nations, 2003.

Van der Geest, S. "Between Respect and Reciprocity: Managing Old Age in Rural Ghana." *Southern African Journal of Gerontology,* 1997, *6*(2), 20–25.

World Bank. *Averting the Old Age Crisis.* Washington, D.C.: World Bank, 1994.

CHAPTER

18

AGING OF POPULATIONS: IS CHINA'S PATTERN UNIQUE?

LINCOLN CHEN AND LINGLING ZHANG

An elderly Westerner has lived in a mortgaged house throughout the adult years, eventually selling the house to raise money for old-age social security. A Chinese elder saved for a lifetime and finally, in old age, purchased a new house. Because he will not sell a house he has saved a lifetime to acquire, he becomes economically insecure in old age.

—A CHINESE OFFICIAL

Population aging is a global phenomenon. The social, economic, and ethical dilemmas associated with population aging are no longer unique to the industrialized world but have spread rapidly throughout the developing world. With the demographic and health transitions experienced over the past century, Western industrialized countries have long been coping with the consequences of aging (Laslett, 1991). Similar but more recent transitions in most developing societies have rapidly ushered in societal aging in previously low-income countries. In all societies, the transition from a youthful to an elderly age structure will dominate the demography of the twenty-first century.

China, the most populous country in the world, has been dramatically aging, as its proportion of people over age sixty crossed the 10 percent international standard threshold in 1999 (Lee, 2004). Indeed, China is now aging faster than any other country (*Beijing Review*, 2005). However, China's demographic policies and the pace of its economic development are both recent and dramatic, generating unprecedented aging challenges surpassing those of the developed countries.

Figure 18.1 shows the projected proportion of the elderly (aged sixty-five and over) in China, Japan, the United States, and India (Arriaga and Banister, 1985;

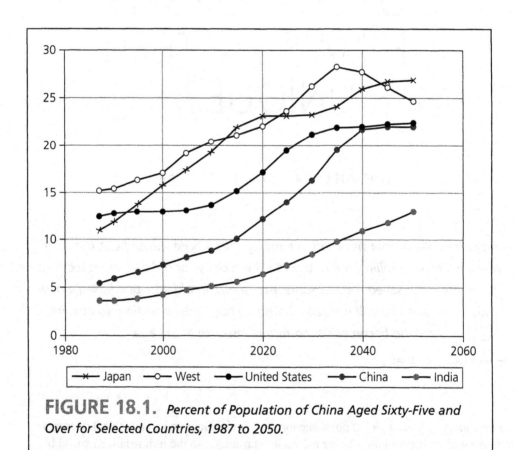

FIGURE 18.1. *Percent of Population of China Aged Sixty-Five and Over for Selected Countries, 1987 to 2050.*

Source: Banister, 1990.

Banister, 1990). In the United States, the of elderly population, which constitutes about 12 percent of the total population, is projected to increase to more than 20 percent by the middle of the twenty-first century. Like the United States, Japan also has an elderly population of 12 percent, but it is projected to increase to more than 25 percent by 2050. China, currently at about 7 percent, will see a similar increase to 25 percent. The rapid graying of China's population naturally raises concerns over the care of the elderly, dependency burdens on the economy, and spiraling medical costs.

This chapter will argue that the aging of populations involves not just the elderly but also the entire society. We will also assert that although aging in China shares many attributes with that in Western industrialized countries, some of the causes and implications of China's aging are distinctive, requiring an "Asian approach" to the region's unique demographic future.

ASIAN DEMOGRAPHY

The basic parameters of population aging are illustrated by China's age structure, as shown in Figure 18.2. Population aging may be defined as the proportion of the population aged sixty-five and over out of the total population. Thus, by definition, the process and problems of aging cannot focus entirely on the elderly. Aging also involves at least two other age groups: productive adults and children. Adults are responsible for economic productivity and caring for future and past generations, and it is usually the

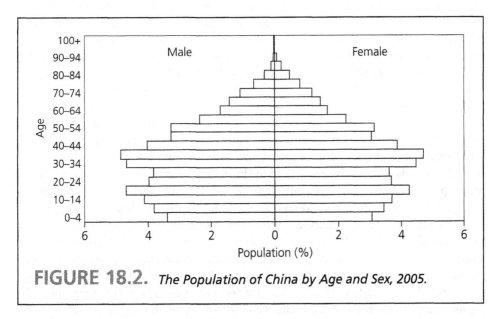

FIGURE 18.2. *The Population of China by Age and Sex, 2005.*

Source: United Nations Population Division, 2005.

size of cohorts of children that determines the proportion of the elderly in an entire population. As we will explain, women also play especially significant demographic and social roles in population aging (Lock, 1993). It is also important to underscore that population aging must address the distribution of age groups among the elderly themselves. The proportion of the very old (those over seventy-five or eighty) has a significant effect on such aging issues as the functional capacity of the elderly to care for themselves and the intensity and duration of caretaking required from family members and the society at large.

The demographic mechanisms that determine how a population ages involve both mortality and fertility, which can be indicated as a *rectangular survival curve*. A fully rectangular curve graphically depicts an optimization of human survivorship: all live births enjoy a full life without any mortality before all die at some biologically maximum age, such as one hundred years. In the rectangular, the survival curve of a country can demonstrate the progressive shift of curves toward the optimal rectangular position and how far such optimization has been realized. This shift has the effect of increasing both the proportion of the elderly as well as the very old among the aged.

Contrary to natural expectation, however, such a survivorship shift in comparison to fertility has only a modest effect on the proportion of population over sixty-five years. This is because demographically the aging of population is more powerfully influenced by a society's birth rate than by its death rate. Figure 18.3 demonstrates the power of fertility, rather than mortality, in influencing the age distribution of human populations. Using the West model life tables, Mosley, Bobadilla, and Jamison (1993) show the age distribution of population according to different levels of births and deaths (Coale and Demeny, 1983). The age distributions of models A and B are youthful, whereas distributions C and D are elderly. The differences between A/B and C/D are the assumptions of a total fertility of 8 in the former and a total fertility of 3 in the latter curves. High fertility thus is associated with a youthful population structure, and low fertility is associated with population aging. Although patterns A and B have similar high fertility levels, one has a life expectancy of seventy-five years in comparison with the other of forty-five years; a similar difference in life expectancy characterizes C and D. These curves demonstrate that changes of life expectancy have less effect on the age structure of populations than does total fertility. The age distribution of populations is exquisitely sensitive to the birth rate, because as smaller birth cohorts grow up to be children and then adults, they constitute much smaller proportions of the total population than did the children of earlier, high-fertility periods.

From these data and analyses, three distinctive aspects of aging in Asia are highlighted. First, rapid economic growth in China is being accompanied by sharply lower birth rates. The consequence is very rapid population aging—a recent demographic phenomenon in Asian countries that throughout their history have experienced high fertility. Asia's economic success, therefore, is breeding uniquely Asian aging problems. Second, the velocity of these demographic changes is

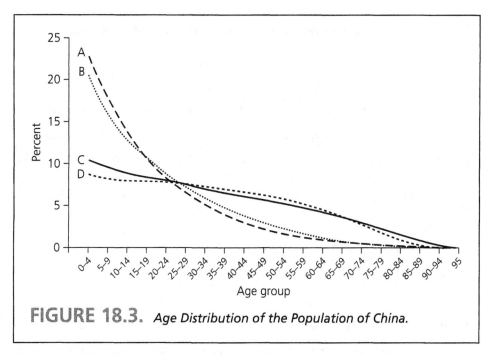

FIGURE 18.3. *Age Distribution of the Population of China.*

Source: Mosley, Bobadilla, and Jamison, 1993.

extremely rapid, perhaps the fastest in human history. Population aging in China is taking place over twenty-five years, in comparison to the one-hundred-year time frame experienced by Western societies (Ogawa, 1988; Zeng, Zhang, and Peng, 1990). The consequent social and economic dislocation in Asia is much more dramatic. Third, because aging is influenced more by fertility than by mortality, the dramatic birth declines in Asian societies are having unprecedented effects. The Chinese policy of a one-child family will have powerful, largely unanticipated effects. The absolute number of the aged in China, for example, is projected to increase from 77 million in 1982 to about 300 million by 2025 to 430 million by 2050 (Banister, 1990).

The urban and rural differentials in China's aging are prominent. Sixty percent of China's population resides in rural areas. As of this writing, the aging process in the urban population is faster and ahead of the rural population, but the rural elderly population is much larger (see Table 18.1). Given the massive rural-to-urban migration—mainly of working-age people—the urban aging process will be slowed down, even as the rural aging process accelerates. Therefore, although fertility in rural areas of China is much higher than in urban areas, aging problems will be more serious in rural China (Zeng and Vaupel, 1989).

TABLE 18.1. Urban and Rural Elderly over Sixty-Five in 1998, 2001, and 2004.

		1998			2001			2004		
	Category	Total	Male	Female	Total	Male	Female	Total	Male	Female
Urban[a]	Number	33,875	16,263	17,614	35,783	17,166	18,617	45,073	21,682	23,394
	%	2.72	2.57	2.88	2.93	2.76	3.11	3.60	3.40	3.80
Rural	Number	58,521	27,116	31,408	59,843	28,230	31,615	62,227	29,789	32,438
	%	4.70	4.29	5.14	4.90	4.53	5.29	4.97	4.68	5.27

Source: China Population Statistics Yearbooks 1999, 2002, and 2005.

[a]Urban: including city and town.

FAMILY AND SOCIETY IN ASIA

The aging of populations affects all members of society, not just the elderly. In Asian countries such as China and Japan, the ideal family structure has been the so-called *three-generation family*—children, parents, and grandparents residing in the same household (Government of Japan, 1984, 1986). Some call this an *extended family*, but it is more properly termed a *stem-family*, because as married children establish independent households, grandparents usually remain with the family of the eldest male child (Croll, 1990). Nuclearization of the stem-family has been under way in China for much of this century. Historically in China, the three-generation household was common (Kono, 1990). The average family size in China has been relatively stable throughout the country's history (Liang, 1980). In the early parts of the twentieth century, about two-thirds of the households were three-generational, but today only about one-fifth of families live in three-generation households. Table 18.2 shows the generational structure of families in China in 1982 (Zhang, 1990). Despite government policies to encourage home-based residential care of the elderly, this secular shift toward nuclearization characterizes the population of both China and Japan.

Lifecycle events and timing are also affected by population aging: less time is spent in childbearing and childrearing activities and more in married life, coresidence in three-generational households, and under elderly care. The Japanese demographer Shigemi Kono (1990) estimated that although in 1920, coresidence in three-generational homes averaged ten years, by 1980 it averaged twenty-four years. Even more noteworthy, home-based care of the elderly averaged five years in 1920 but had increased to eighteen years by the 1980s.

TABLE 18.2. **Comparison of Generational Structure of Families in 1982.**

Region	One Generation	Two Generation	Three Generations
Whole Country	13.78	67.46	18.76
North	16.22	67.89	15.89
Northeast	13.24	72.03	14.73
East	15.22	66.82	17.96
Mid-South	12.58	65.65	21.77
Southwest	12.29	68.43	19.28
Northwest	11.44	67.91	20.65

Source: Zhang, 1990.

These family and lifecycle changes powerfully affect all family members, but particularly women, who are expected to manage the upbringing of children and the care of the elderly. As societies shift from high to low fertility, and thus from a youthful to an elderly population, it is women who are being asked to shift their nurturing from children to the elderly (Lock, 1993). Women's work outside of the home becomes incompatible with such extensions in the duration of coresidence and of elderly care. Will Chinese women be willing to forsake work and career opportunities outside of the home? Will Chinese women accept such sacrifices into the future? If not, what social alternatives will be made available through state assistance?

If the elderly are the worse-off segment in the population, than elderly *women* have the worse situation among the worse-offs. They have lower health status, on average, than both elderly men and the elderly as a whole. They are hit by a higher prevalence of chronic diseases than are elderly men. And they are more vulnerable to the diseases of the elderly. Research indicates that women are more likely than men to have depression (Etaugh, 2003). Elderly women who are living alone are at especially high risk.

With low fertility, less interaction is possible among siblings, cousins, uncles, aunts, nephews, and nieces. With fewer collateral relatives around, the socialization of children may also change. Children will increasingly grow up in a family context of vertical kinship relations: child-parents-grandparents. What kind of psychosocial effects will this verticalization of family relationships have on children? Will it result in more individualistic adults, unaccustomed to the sharing and mutuality of complex

family relations? Moreover, in some Asian countries like China, there is strong preference for boys who provide old-age support of parents. Excessive parental spoiling of
boys has already led to the coining of the term *little emperor* in China, not to mention
the concomitant neglect and abuse of girls.

Given the lack of familial preference for girls, however, some evidence shows that
as sons increasingly neglect their traditional filial duty, daughters are more and more
likely to become the main caretakers for their elderly parents (Yan, 2003). But facing
the reality of more ancestral relatives, which compose a 4-2-1 family structure (four
grandparents, two parents, one child), it is a matter not of willingness to take care of the
elderly at home but of the capacity for home care. Nursing homes—called "old people's homes" in China—used to be for childless elderly people in both urban and rural
areas. Their number is quite limited. But as the demand for elder care is escalating,
many more nursing homes are being established. As of the end of 2001, the number of
homes for the elderly plus orphanages and elderly apartments had reached 40,741,
accommodating 810,000 elderly (China Civil Affairs Statistical Yearbook, 2002).

GOVERNMENT POLICIES

Two categories of government policies to address population aging merit scrutiny:
socioeconomic and medical (see box). In socioeconomic policies, two of the demographic solutions are probably not feasible, either in Asia or in Western countries. The
return of a "baby boom" seems very unlikely, although the demographic future is
impossible to predict. Nor can we expect societal acceptance of a large-scale
importation of labor aimed at increasing the number of productive adults in the society. Large-scale immigration is hotly debated in the developed countries, and some
Asian countries like China may find it difficult to attract the necessary numbers.

A more promising approach is to focus on what Laslett (1991) has called the *third
age*. In all industrialized societies with low fertility, a third age is emerging—the
fifties, sixties, and seventies, or the years between the age when one's children's
achieve independence and one's old age (which is increasingly termed the *fourth age*).
People reaching the third age want more flexible retirement systems, meaningful
activities, and social and intellectual stimulation. Laslett therefore proposes social
policies to develop flexible retirement systems and social sports clubs. He also recom-
mends "gray universities" to give the elderly a second chance at relearning in a rapidly
changing world. China has about 17,000 schools eligible to meet this need, with more
than 1.5 million students throughout the country. At these schools, the elderly may
learn calligraphy, painting, foreign languages, computer, history, cooking, meditation,
and so on (China Civil Affairs Statistical Yearbook, 2002).

Most socioeconomic policies focus appropriately on pensions and social security
systems. These are not simple matters. In all societies, the economic support of the
elderly can be very expensive. The welfare states of the Western economies are all
burdened by growing social obligations. It has been estimated that in forty years
Germany will devote about a third of its income to meeting the needs of the elderly

GOVERNMENTAL SOCIOECONOMIC AND MEDICAL POLICIES TO ADDRESS POPULATION AGING

Socioeconomic Policies

Increasing fertility through a new baby boom

Augmenting the working adult population through labor immigration

Understanding and management of the third age

Optimizing social security and pension systems

Medical Policies

Increasing medical science investigation into and understanding of the biology of longevity

Preventing chronic and degenerative diseases

Anticipating the perennial emergence of new threats

Planning for allocation of medical care resources

Improving health research capacity and promoting recognition of its importance

Medical and Cultural Ethics

Conserving Asian moral and spiritual values toward the elderly

Developing unique Asian ethical approaches

(Zeng, Zhang, and Peng, 1990). The wealthier developed countries, such as Germany, the United States, and Japan, may be able to afford the massive transfer of income from productive adults to the elderly, even if considerable sacrifice is required. But what will happen in Asian countries like China, where annual per capita income today is $1,740 (World Bank, 2005)? There is also the growing dilemma of intergenerational inequity, as today's elderly receive unprecedented support from a large cohort of productive adults. Because of declining fertility, these same cohorts will not receive in return a similar level of benefits when they themselves become elderly. Perhaps the major lesson from Europe and North America is not to rely on a single source of revenues to support the elderly. Multiple sources of income must be tapped—from the retired person's own savings and from the family, the community, and local and national government.

Medical policies must involve the medical professions, the pharmaceutical industry, and government working together with the public. In such cooperative approaches, we cannot make assumptions about longevity, because the biology of aging remains uncharted scientific territory (Comfort, 1979). We do not yet know, for example, the fixed life span for humans. Studies have shown that all species display biologic aging after reaching maximum body size at biologic maturity. Thereafter, decrements of cellular function appear inevitable. The problem is that we do not know how the pace of such aging is influenced by environmental and genetic factors. Recent epidemiologic studies are documenting the unprecedented advances in longevity among the elderly (Laslett, 1991). In the past two decades, remarkable advances have been observed. Such is the velocity of longevity gains that some have projected that the average life expectancy, now around 80 years, will reach 150 years by the year 2100!

Nor do we have complete solutions in medical policies. It makes sense to pursue inexpensive prevention of costly, yet preventable diseases such as heart disease, stroke, and cancer—yet to do so will simply expose populations to other, perhaps more intractable conditions. This poses powerful ethical dilemmas concerning the allocation of medical resources. The resolutions must be culturally specific because they involve the values of a society. The only conclusion relevant to all societies, yet too often neglected by policymakers, is that a strong health research system is absolutely vital for solving old health threats and combating new ones—a perennial challenge of humankind.

Ultimately, the policy challenge is moral and ethical. Chinese cultures influenced by Confucianism accord respect, prestige, and power to the elderly in home and society. Many in China and Asia worry that with population aging and family nuclearization, Western "individualism" and moral decay may overwhelm Asian cultures. How can the Chinese and Asians retain their spiritual values in the face of population aging? Can we shape a unique Asian cultural response to population aging? It may be useful to note here that Europe before the Industrial Revolution also held the elderly in great esteem but disregarded this tradition when it became "inconvenient" (Laslett, 1991). Will this happen too in China and Asia?

REFERENCES

Arriaga, E., and Banister, J. "The Implications of China's Rapid Fertility Decline." In *International Population Conference, Florence 1985, 2*, 168–172. Liege, Belgium: International Union for the Scientific Study of Population, 1985.

Banister, J. "Implications of the Aging of China's Population." In Y. Zeng, C. Zhang, and S. Peng (eds.), *Changing Family Structure and Population Aging in China*. Beijing: Peking University Press, 1990.

Beijing Review, "How to Cope with Aging?" Feb. 17, 2005, 13.

China Civil Affairs Statistical Yearbook, 2002.

China Population Statistics Yearbooks. China Statistics Press, 1999, 2002, 2005.

Coale, A. J., and Demeny, P. *Regional Model Life Tables,* 2nd ed. New York: Academic Press, 1983.

Comfort, A. *The Biology of Senescence,* 3rd ed. New York: Elsevier North Holland, 1979.

Croll, E. J. "The Aggregate Family: Households and Kin Support in Rural China." In Y. Zeng, C. Zhang, and S. Peng (eds.), *Changing Family Structure and Population Aging in China.* Beijing: Peking University Press, 1990.

Etaugh, C. A. *The Psychology of Women,* Beijing: Peking University Press, 2003.

Government of Japan, Institute of Population Problems, Ministry of Health and Welfare. Report on the Field Survey of the Family Life Course and Change in the Household Structure. Tokyo: Ministry of Health and Welfare, 1986.

Government of Japan, Japan Population Commission. *The Population and Society of Japan.* Tokyo: Tokyo Kerzai Shimpo-sha, 1984.

Kono, S. "Changes in the Family Life Cycle and the Issues of the Three-Generation Household in Japan." In Y. Zeng, C. Zhang, and S. Peng (eds.), *Changing Family Structure and Population Aging in China.* Beijing: Peking University Press, 1990.

Laslett, P. *A Fresh Map of Life: The Emergence of the Third Age.* Cambridge, Mass.: Harvard University Press, 1991.

Lee, L. "The Current State of Public Health in China." *Annual Review of Public Health,* 2004, *25,* 327–39.

Liang, F. *Historical Statistics of Household, Farmlands and Land Taxes.* Shanghai: Shanghai People's Press, 1980.

Lock, M. *Encounters with Aging: Mythologies of Menopause in Japan and North America.* Berkeley, Calif.: University of California Press, 1993.

Mosley, W. H., Bobadilla, J. L., and Jamison, D. T. "The Health Transition: Implications for Health Policy in Developing Countries." In D. T. Jamison, W. H. Mosley, A. R. Measham, and J. L. Bobadilla (eds.), *Disease Control in Developing Countries.* New York: Oxford Medical Publications, 1993.

Ogawa, N. "Population Aging and Medical Demand: The Case of Japan." In *Economic and Social Implications of Population Aging.* Proceedings of the International Symposium on Population Structure and Development, Tokyo, 254–275. New York: United Nations, 1988.

World Bank. China Data Profile, 2005. [http:www.worldbank.org/].

United Nations Population Division, 2005. [http://esa.un.org/unpp/].

Yan, Y. "Support for the Elderly and the Crisis of Filial Piety." In *Private Life Under Socialism: Love, Intimacy, and Family Change in a Chinese Village 1949–1999.* Stanford, Calif.: Stanford University Press, 2003.

Zeng, Y., Zhang, C., and Peng, S. *Changing Family Structure and Population Aging in China.* Beijing: Peking University Press, 1990.

Zeng, Y., and Vaupel, J. "The Impact of Urbanization and Delayed Childbearing on Population Growth and Aging in China." *Population and Development Review,* Sept. 1989, *15*(3), 425–445.

Zhang, C. "Family Size and Structure and Their Trends in China." In Y. Zeng, C. Zhang, and S. Peng (eds.), *Changing Family Structure and Population Aging in China.* Beijing: Peking University Press, 1990.

CHAPTER

HEALTH AND AGING IN INDIA

SHARAD D. GOKHALE

Population aging is a global challenge for the twenty-first century. Because of increased longevity, India's population aged sixty years and over increases by about eight lakhs (eight hundred thousand) every month. By 2025, there will be over 800 million older people—two-thirds of them in developing countries, and the majority of them women.

The population of India aged sixty and over numbered about 57 million in 1991 and 82 million in 2004, and it will be 177 million by 2025 and 324 million by 2040. Declining mortality and increasing life expectancy has led India's life expectancy to increase by about thirty years since independence. This is good news, but it also presents a tremendous challenge. In India, fifty-two million older people live on less than a dollar a day. Eighty percent of the older people have no regular income. Eighty percent of the old people live in the rural areas. Ninety percent are from the unorganized sector and have no social security, no pension, no provident fund or gratuity, and no medical coverage. Of India's aging population, 55 percent are women, and a staggering twenty million elderly women are widows.

The vast majority of older women are housewives who depend completely on their family for survival. In the rural areas, 70 percent of the older women work as agriculture laborers. Widowhood in India is a disadvantage, especially to the older women for whom it is a loss of social status.

HEALTH AND THE ELDERLY IN INDIA

The growth rate of the total population in India is 1.93 percent; the growth rate of the elderly population is 3.01 percent. Further, the number of the oldest old is growing much faster than that of the young old. This means that the population aged eighty and over is growing rapidly. Some important aspects of aging in India are the rapid feminization of aging, rural poverty, and inadequate health insurance and social security. Presently, India is passing through the last phase of demographic transition—that is, low mortality and low fertility. Life expectancy at age sixty is around sixteen years for males and eighteen years for females.

Experience shows that health services, if delivered well, can improve outcomes for even the poorest groups. A health program in the Gadhchiroli district in India reduced neonatal mortality rates by 62 percent. But the availability of good health services tends to vary inversely with need. Those who need such services the most often get the least. Poor groups and regions have less access to sanitation and vector control. Illness pushes households into poverty, through lost wages, high spending for catastrophic illness, and repeated treatment for other illness. Poor nutrition practices, careless handling of water and waste, and inadequate care for the ill are major contributors to poor health.

In India, older people often live with their children in extended families. The average size of the household is four to six people in most societies. The traditional extended family system is changing. Consequently, the social safety net and support provided by family structures are increasingly unavailable to many older people. The challenge is to strengthen the family and community support. Strengthening the primary health centers is now a priority. It is not possible to achieve poverty reduction without the explicit inclusion of older people.

If we cannot find answers to these problems today, we must return to the solutions offered by our tradition and culture. At present, family network, religious societies, village councils, and senior citizen clubs form part of this support network.

THE NATIONAL POLICY ON OLDER PERSONS

The well-being of older people has been mandated in the Constitution of India. Article 41, a Directive Principle of State Policy, has directed that the State shall, within the limits of its economic capacity and development, make effective provision for securing the right to public assistance in old age. Other provisions direct the State to improve the quality of life of its senior citizens.

India's National Policy on Older Persons (NPOP) of the Ministry of Social Justice and Empowerment seeks to assure the elderly that they are valued members of society and that their concerns are national concerns. The government anticipates extending the level of support for financial security, health care, shelter, and welfare for wider coverage. The government, private funds, NGOs, the community, and the family all will provide for the vulnerable elderly.

THE NPOP ON HEALTH CARE AND NUTRITION

The NPOP also states that the health care needs of the older people will be given high priority. The goal should be good affordable health services, very heavily subsidized for the poor, with a graded system of user charges for others. It will be necessary to have a judicious mix of (1) public health services, (2) health insurance, (3) health services provided by nonprofit organizations including trusts and charities, and (4) private medical care. Although the first of these will require greater state participation, the second category will need to be promoted by the state; the third category given some assistance, concessions, and relief; and the fourth regulated by an association of providers of private care.

The primary health care system will be the basic structure of public health care. It will be strengthened and oriented to be able to meet the health care needs of older people. The public health services—preventive, curative, restorative, and rehabilitative—will be considerably expanded and strengthened, and geriatric care facilities provided at secondary and tertiary levels. This will entail much larger public sector outlays, proper distribution of services in rural and urban areas, and much better health administration and delivery systems.

The development of health insurance will be given high priority to cater to the needs of different income segments of the population and make provision for varying contributions and benefits. Packages catering to the lower income groups will be entitled to state subsidy. Various concessions in health insurance will be given, coverage will be enlarged, and insurance will be made more affordable.

Trusts, charitable societies, and volunteer agencies will be promoted and assisted by way of grants, and tax relief and land at subsidized rates will be made available for providing free beds, medicines, and treatment to the indigent elderly.

Organizations representing private hospitals and nursing homes will be requested to direct their members to offer a discount to older patients. Private general practitioners will be given opportunities for orientation in geriatric care.

Public hospitals will be directed to ensure that elderly patients are not subjected to long waits and visits to different counters for medical tests and treatment. They will endeavor to provide separate counters and convenient appointments on specified days. Geriatric wards will be set up in the public hospitals.

Medical and paramedical personnel in primary, secondary, and tertiary health care facilities will be given training and orientation in health care of the elderly. Facilities for specialization in geriatric medicine will be provided in the medical colleges. Training in nursing care will include geriatric care. The elderly have difficulty gaining access to and making use of health services because of distance and the lack of escorts and transportation. These difficulties will be addressed through mobile health services, special camps, and ambulance services by charitable institutions and nonprofit health care organizations. Hospitals will be encouraged to have a separate welfare fund, which will receive donations and grants for providing free treatment and medicines to poor elderly patients.

The old who are chronically ill and deprived of family support, will need hospices supported or assisted by the state and public charity and volunteer organizations. These are also needed to provide care for chronically ill elderly patients who are abandoned at public hospitals. Assistance will be given to geriatric care societies for the production and distribution of instructional material on self-care by older people. Preparation and distribution of easy-to-follow guidance on health and nursing care of older people for the use of family caregivers will also be supported.

Older people and their families will be given access to educational material on nutritional needs in old age, such as the right kinds of food to eat and the foods to avoid. Diet plans and recipes will be disseminated that suit the tastes of different regions, are nutritious, tasty, and affordable, fit into the dietary pattern of the family and the community, and can be prepared from the locally available vegetables, cereals, and fruits.

The concept of healthy aging will be promoted. We need to educate older people and their families that diseases are not a corollary of advancing age nor is a particular chronological age the starting point for decline in health status.

Health education programs will be strengthened by making use of mass media, folk media, and other communication channels that reach out to different segments of the population. The capacity to cope with illness and manage home care will be strengthened. Programs will be developed to educate and inform the younger generation about forming lifestyle habits that will help them have a healthy life in later years. Programs on yoga, meditation, and methods of relaxation will be developed and disseminated to the public.

Mental health services will be expanded and strengthened. Families will be given counseling facilities and information on the care and treatment of older people with mental health problems.

Nongovernmental organizations will be encouraged and assisted through grants, training and orientation of their personnel, and various concessions and relief to provide ambulatory services, day care, and health care to complement the efforts of the state.

CHANGING TRENDS: SCIENCE AND TECHNOLOGY IN HEALTH SERVICES

The field of population aging was dominated by demographic considerations in the second half of the last century. This was followed by a vigorous debate on social and economic security for the elderly. Then the focus shifted to health research, which included research in spirituality.

In India, the battle against aging is being waged on two fronts. On the first, scientists are searching for disease-specific therapies aimed at curing, controlling, or preventing a particular disease. On a second front, researchers are seeking answers to a more fundamental mystery that has the potential to produce therapies for a vast array of diseases, particularly those related to aging, from Alzheimer's and Parkinson's to arthritis, heart disease, and stroke.

Unfortunately, sometimes serious research in medicine, including in Ayurveda, is being mistakenly characterized as "anti-aging medicine." For example, sometimes it is claimed that Ashwagandha and Vajikaran and its appropriate interventions can slow, stop, or even reverse the aging process. This is only partially true. As the eminent American geriatrician Dr. Robert Butler said, in an address to a meeting of presidents of International Longevity Centers (ILCs), "Let us adopt the term *longevity medicine.*" Longevity medicine concerns extending life within genetically determined limits. The term applies to all means that would extend healthy life, including health promotion and disease prevention.

Research in subjects like blood pressure, bone density, blood sugar, heart condition, and so on, has developed only recently in India. This research is in the areas of genetics, stem cell research, and the biochemistry of aging, brain cells, and DNA.

The beginning of the twenty-first century saw medical and social research pursuing the question "why do we age?" Is the process of aging determined by genetics, impact of the environment, lifestyle, or something to do with the mind and spiritual attitude? Such issues as lifestyle, philosophy of life, understanding of life and death, religion, and spirituality were raised at the last General Assembly of the UN in Madrid and also at the Congress on Alternative Medicine organized by the International Association for the Study of Traditional Asian Medicine (IASTAM) and the International Longevity Center of India (ILC-I). This has created a feeling of urgency around research in genetics and the spiritual aspects of aging. For this purpose, the government of India has set up an organization called AYUSH (Life). Dr. R. A. Mashelkar, the director-general of the Council of Scientific and Industrial Research of India (CSIR) and a leading scientist of India, spoke of an experiment initiated by the institute:

> I believe that this is where the Golden Triangle can play a critical role. But how do you create the Golden Triangle? This issue is simple. In the past, if you look at modern medicine and modern science, they have always talked to each other. The two have always worked in harmony. But, if you look at modern medicine and traditional medicine, they have not talked to each other. The doctors and "vaidyas" (traditional ayurvedic practitioners) do not interact. Therefore, I think it is time that we start doing things differently and that is why I started an experiment in CSIR about five years ago. We brought 19 laboratories and more than 20 universities together. We got people like Arya Vaidyashala at Kotakkal and others together, and tried to see what we can learn from each other and get new clues for drug discovery and development. The kind of new breakthroughs that are taking place and the new leads that we are getting are amazing, and this includes the diseases of the old. Whether it is Alzheimer's or Parkinson's, the results are truly encouraging [Mashelkar, 2005].

SPIRITUALITY: A KEY TO LONGEVITY

India is an ancient country with an intense spiritual and religious perspective. This rich heritage provides us with a treasure-house of spiritual knowledge.

Aging is a natural process of physical and psychological change. Some individuals equate it with disease and disability; others take it with philosophical resignation and live with it. Some want to prolong our years, but we should hope to prolong the quality of life, not mere existence. Due to the loneliness and isolation that often accompany old age, some see it as a curse, but I take it as a celebration because these are really bonus years. Aging is an opportunity to look inward and be useful to society, discard selfish ambition but retain motivation.

It can be terribly tempting to think the problem of aging is so huge that nothing can possibly have any effect on the rate of aging and this can be resolved only by God or the government! It is a crisis concerning the way we think about aging, a crisis that is physical, psychological, and spiritual. Unless our philosophy of life, culture, values, and understanding of what is true and what is false about aging become grounded in reality, we may not discover the distinction between mortal existence and life with a purpose. Most modern research and studies in demography and gerontology deal too often with superficial symptoms. It is a pity we have not adequately researched the human mind and its functions.

NEED FOR RESEARCH IN SPIRITUALITY

This tendency to deal only with the superficial is rooted in our thinking: that what is quantifiable and what we can see and touch is reality and anything beyond this is not real. Since the time of the Renaissance, this paradigm of thought has dominated the western mind, and now it is nearly universal. According to this view, the only things that are real are those that can be quantified; that is, those which can be grasped by the application of mathematical techniques. Everything else, everything that cannot be caught in the net of numbers, is unreal.

According to this pragmatic view, all qualities and all considerations based on feelings—sentiments like love, affection, values, culture, beauty, and purpose of life—are not considered to be real and true because they cannot be quantified by the physical sciences. Extending this logic, anything that has to do with the soul or God is regarded as untrue or irrelevant.

If we want to understand the real nature of aging, of life itself, then we must free ourselves from this dogma. Only then will we be able to meet the challenges of life.

Spirituality is not a flight from the ethical responsibility of the material world, but a rhythm of withdrawal—harmony in doing and at the same time keeping oneself aloof from it. It is only this attitude—of being active in life and at the same time not expecting anything from it—that will return the elderly to the real life of doing and help them to be useful not only to themselves and their families, but also to the community at large. It is not running away from the reality of life. It is being involved but at the same time remaining aloof. It is doing your duty without expecting the fruits of your labor. It is like the lotus leaf, which is immersed in water and yet does not get wet.

To be spiritual is not to reject reason but to go beyond it, to think so hard that thinking becomes knowing. The greatest thinkers of the world unite in asking us to know the self. St. Augustine writes: "Lord, I went wandering like a strayed sheep seeking thee with anxious reasoning without, whilst thou wast within me . . ." Sometimes we must make a detour around the world to get back to the self. What is our true self? While our bodily organization and psychological capacities undergo changes, while our thoughts gather like clouds in the sky and disperse again, the self is never lost. It is present and yet distinct from all. The fundamental truth of spirituality is to understand what the real self is.

In conclusion, one can safely say that aging becomes a celebration and an experience of happiness if one comes to the realization that the true meaning of life is *Karma phala tyaga*—doing one's duty without being attached to it, engaging oneself in life without any expectations from it. This will make us divinely happy and satisfied. Thus spirituality is the key to coping with aging. With the help of this philosophy, the years in the eventide of our lives are not a curse but become a celebration of life.

Many of the elders in India follow this philosophy of spirituality. It is the path that leads them on to peaceful and satisfying golden years of their lives.

Spirituality is to be experienced and not treated as mere knowledge. The great wise man of China, Confucius, said, " To know that you do not know, is the beginning of knowledge." In this spirit, if we take the first step to knowing that we do not know, it will lift us up to the experience of spiritual ecstasy—and that is our goal in the long pilgrimage of life.

REFERENCE

Mashelkar, R. A. Inaugural Address, Frontiers of Research in Longevity Medicine Workshop, Pune, August 24, 2005. In *Frontiers of Research in Longevity Medicine*. Pune, India: International Longevity Center, 2005.

CHAPTER

HEALTH AND AGING IN THE EASTERN MEDITERRANEAN REGION

MOHAMED H. EL-BANOUBY

The Eastern Mediterranean region has a strategic location that connects Africa, Asia, and Europe. It also contains vast natural resources, including the world's largest oil reserves. These and other factors have contributed to a variety of regional conflicts.

As of 2007, with United States forces still in Iraq, the war begun in 2003 had led to a civil war among the Shiites, Sunnis, and Kurds, with an estimated 655,000 lives lost and a million refugees, according to a John Hopkins study (Parsons, 2006).

The civil wars in Darfur, Southern Sudan, and Somalia have caused the deaths and injury of hundreds of thousands of Africans. In Pakistan, there are two conflict fronts: one against the Taliban followers and supporters along the western borders, the other in Kashmir. The Palestinian-Israeli problem is the core conflict in the region. The series of wars between Israel and the Arabs characterize the hostility between the parties. Both President Sadat, who signed the Camp David Treaty, and Prime Minister

Rabin, who signed the Oslo Peace Accord, believed that this hostility is mainly psychological and the conflict can be solved through negotiations that will eventually lead to peace and prosperity in the region. Unfortunately, both these leaders were assassinated by native extremists.

Wars have negative effects on the economies of the participating parties. Before the eight-year Iraq-Iran war, the standard of living of the Iranians was expected to reach that of the French within five years, and the standard of living of the Iraqis was expected to reach that of the Italians within the same period. Neither of these expectations has been realized. Today, the Iranian economy is directed toward funding military preparations for protection against possible American attack and supporting anti-American militias. The Iraqi economy has been destroyed. Proper planning for economic development and welfare services is almost impossible in countries involved in or threatened by war.

IMPACT OF WAR ON THE ELDERLY

When war breaks out, all civilians suffer, but the sufferings of older people are much greater. Yet elders' positive roles are underestimated. It is the elderly who care for dependents and reassure panicking children during war. Moreover, they lend a hand in rebuilding their societies following war. Their traditional skills, experience, and knowledge are vital for coping in such critical situations.

We know that because of the aging of the population worldwide, the number of older victims of armed conflicts is rising. We also know that there are more older women than older men among the war victims. But comprehensive information regarding the impact of wars on the elderly is still lacking. That is why the WHO Eastern Mediterranean Region is conducting field research on the elderly of Southern Lebanon as of this writing.

The following are areas identified so far by recent research as presenting particular problems for the elderly during and following war:

Inability to Access Humanitarian Resources. Due to their limited mobility and lack of strength, older people cannot compete with younger persons who push others aside for food and medical services.

Loss of Income. Sources of income for the elderly can be lost. Loss of land, livestock, property, employment, or pension payments can be disastrous to the elderly and their dependents.

Isolation. Older people are often left behind to guard property when stronger family members flee as refugees. Sometimes they are abandoned for good. Their isolation increases when they are considered unproductive and consequently excluded from rehabilitation programs.

Cultural Problems. Emergency delivery and shelter arrangements may not take the local cultural norms and beliefs into consideration. In spite of women's responsibility for dependents, in certain cultures they are denied inheritance rights or employment opportunities.

Mental and Psychological Disorders. The main psychological impact of war on the elderly takes the form of posttraumatic stress syndrome and depressive illnesses. Separation from families and lack of support is particularly stressful for them.

Malnutrition. The elderly may suffer from malnutrition because of their stress illnesses, chronic diseases, vision problems, limited manual dexterity, or inability to meet the demands of physical effort.

Refugees. Refugee camps in the Eastern Mediterranean Region were first established in 1948. Young people live temporarily in these camps until they are employed; older people tend to develop chronic dependency and stay in these camps for good.

RESEARCH FINDINGS

As previous chapters have described, the population of people ages sixty and over worldwide is growing faster than any other age group. Decreasing fertility rates and increasing longevity will ensure the continued graying of the world's population. It is estimated that by 2025, about 120 countries will have reached total fertility rates below replacement level (see Table 20.1 for specific data for the Eastern Mediterranean region).

In developing countries, the population aging process took two or three decades to develop. As several leaders of the World Health Organization have pointed out, the developed world became rich before it became old; developing countries are becoming old before becoming rich. This process of rapid aging in developing countries is accompanied by dramatic changes in labor patterns and migration. It is expected that very soon most institutions of civil society in many developing countries will be overwhelmed by the social, economic, and health needs of this ever-increasing segment of the population.

There is an urgent need for the implementation of a national policy for the care of the elderly in each country. Although such policies exist in most countries, they refer to national coordinating committees administered by the country's ministry of social affairs or ministry of health. The effectiveness of existing policies and the role of national committees must be evaluated to revive and mobilize the resources available. Older people, as stakeholders, are expected to participate in the implementation of the national policy through all phases of planning, intervention, and evaluation.

The WHO Eastern Mediterranean Region, with the wide variations in the economic and demographic profiles of its member states, gives health planners a great opportunity for innovation. The basic principles of its general strategy—such as raising awareness, conducting research, and training health professionals—are the same for all member states irrespective of their social, economic, and political status.

The following demographic and socioeconomic indicators could be used for evaluating the impact of the regional strategy at the country level: aging index, median age, dependency ratio, parent-support ratio, employment, income level, life expectancy and healthy life expectancy at birth and at sixty, gender ratio, total fertility rate, marital

TABLE 20.1. Population of Older People, Life Expectancy, Per Capita Health Expenditure, Doctor-Population Ratio, and Fertility Rates in the Eastern Mediterranean Region.

Country	Life expectancy at birth (years)	Per capita health expenditure (US$)	Physicians per 1000	Population aged 60+ (%) (2000)	Population aged 60+ (%) (2025)	Fertility rates 2000–2005	Fertility rates 2025–2030
Afghanistan	44.7	8	1.9	4.7	5.2	6.8	4.7
Bahrain	73.8	565	18.5	4.7	20.4	2.3	2.1
Djibouti	44.1	41	1.6	5.5	6.2	5.8	3.9
Egypt	70.1	66	22.2	6.3	11.5	2.9	2.1
Iran	69.0	259	11.9	5.2	10.5	2.8	2.1
Iraq	63.2	44	6.3	4.6	7.5	4.8	2.3
Jordan	71.5	163	22.6	4.5	7.0	4.3	2.4
Kuwait	78.4	630	16.0	4.4	15.7	2.7	2.1
Lebanon	71.3	12	28.1	8.5	13.5	2.2	1.9
Libyan Arab Jamahiriya	69.5	246	12.1	5.5	9.9	3.3	2.1

Morocco	69.5	56	5.2	6.3	11.2	3.0	2.1
Oman	73.8	218	13.9	4.2	6.6	5.6	3.7
Pakistan	63.6	18	7.3	5.7	7.3	5.5	3.5
Palestine	72.3	138	8.3	4.9	5.6	5.1	2.8
Qatar	74.7	672	23.5	3.1	21.8	3.3	2.1
Saudi Arabia	71.4	448	15.3	4.8	7.9	5.5	3.2
Somalia	47.0	4	0.4	3.9	4.0	7.3	5.1
Sudan	56.6	13	1.7	5.4	7.9	4.5	2.3
Syrian Republic	71.5	59	14.3	4.8	7.9	3.7	2.1
Tunisia	73.0	132	8.1	8.4	13.4	2.1	2.1
Emirates	72.6	767	16.9	5.1	23.6	2.9	2.1
Yemen	62.9	21	2.2	3.5	3.6	7.6	5.4

Source: World Health Organization, 2006a.

status, urban/rural distribution, education level and literacy rate, and living arrangements (Arnaout and Kalache, 2006).

To secure adequate services for the elderly, the following must be accomplished:

- Integrated social welfare for the elderly, presented by the ministries of social affairs in cooperation with the ministries of manpower and of health

- Participation of nongovernmental organizations and good philanthropy systems

- Legislative efforts in the parliaments to protect elderly rights

- Participation of the elderly in planning for their welfare services

- Encouragement of businesses to support relevant community-based research

- Communication with relevant international organizations and institutions for problem-solving and exchange of expertise

- Efficient training and educational programs

- Good integrated health systems with computerized database profiles

The Eastern Mediterranean Region member states are not homogeneous in terms of the availability of adequate systems for the welfare services presented to the elderly. They can be classified according to three categories, described in the following sections (Gezairy, 2002).

Category I

These are countries such as the Gulf States: Bahrain, Kuwait, Oman, Qatar, Saudi Arabia, and the United Arab Emirates. These countries already have welfare services for the elderly within a reasonably adequate system. With little effort, they will reach the standard of the developed countries. The countries in this category are rich in natural resources, and their oil revenues make it possible to support and develop their welfare schemes.

Countries of this category have many features in common: language, religion, government regimes, traditions and customs. Sometimes members of one tribe are spread across the border between two countries. These countries are members of the Gulf Cooperative Council, which has succeeded through its annual meetings in solving many of their problems and settling many disputes.

The population density of these countries is generally low. Even Saudi Arabia, the highest with 18.9 million citizens, is not densely populated when we consider its relatively huge space. The least populated state is Qatar, with only 693,000 citizens. In some cases, the number of citizens is lower than the number of foreign residents.

Aside from oil production and exportation, the main source of income is commerce and petrochemical industries. Saudi Arabia gains additional income from Muslim pilgrims to the holy lands in Mecca and Medina. The average person's income in these countries is fairly high. Medical care in most of these countries is highly technical, free, and supported by strong administrative and social systems. It is ideal for the natives.

Elderly affairs in most countries of this category are supported by a basic medical-care system in which all citizens have computerized profiles. At geriatric clinics elderly receive needed services with relative ease. Free physiotherapy and rehabilitation programs for the handicapped, as well as drugs and aids, are available. Professionals at these clinics visit the elderly at home to directly present required services or, depending on the nature of each case, refer them to general or specialized hospitals. In some of the member states of the Gulf Cooperative Council, geriatric clinics and geriatric departments in public hospitals are supervised by geriatric physicians. The other states have realized the importance of this specialization.

Statistics for Category I show that its mean life expectancy in the present time is 74.0 years, with the highest in Kuwait (78.4) and the lowest in Saudi Arabia (71.4). The average annual per capita health expenditure in these countries is $550, with the Emirates highest at $767 and Oman the lowest at less than $218. The population of those aged sixty and over is expected to reach 16 percent of the total population in 2025, with a high of 23.6 percent in the United Arab Emirates and a low of 6.6 percent in Oman. The mean fertility rate for this category reached 3.7 percent in 2000–2005, with 5.5, the highest, in both Oman and Saudi Arabia and 2.3, the lowest, in Bahrain. In 2025–2030 these figures are expected to decrease. The mean fertility rate for this category is expected to reach 2.5, with 3.5, the highest, in Oman and 2.1, the lowest, in Bahrain, Kuwait, Qatar, and the United Arab Emirates. At present, the average number of physicians is seventeen for every one thousand persons in this category of countries; the highest is 23.5, in Qatar, and the lowest is 13.9, in Oman.

In some Category I countries, there has been a tendency to provide governmental integrated medical support for the elderly within their families, but officials realized that the elderly occupy a high percentage of hospital beds, which makes it difficult to handle critical cases. Therefore, they have begun to think of the long-term care institutions as a more convenient alternative.

In this group of countries, legislation that protects elderly rights is applied and observed by all parties. There are laws that secure pensions for government employees, pensions for private sector employees, exceptional pensions for the handicapped and early retirement pensions. Any behavior that hurts the elderly is punished according to the law and traditions.

The elderly with disabilities and low-income are granted Zakat and charity money. This is not limited to the elderly citizens of these countries, but is usually sent to needy Muslims worldwide. The Zakat and charity money sent abroad has recently been reduced for fear of its being received by terrorist organizations.

Recreational activities are available to the elderly free of charge. Even transportation to recreational sites is free for them. Unfortunately, rehabilitation programs for the elderly who are strong enough to perform volunteer or paid work are still in early stages.

There is good communication between the Gulf States and the international institutions concerned with elderly affairs, such as the WHO Eastern Mediterranean Region. These states have developed criteria for evaluation of the services offered to the elderly.

Category II

This category of countries includes two groups: Egypt, Jordan, Libya, Morocco, Tunisia, and Yemen (Group A) and Iran, Iraq, Lebanon, Palestine, Pakistan, and Syria (Group B). In both groups there are problems in the medical systems and problems related to the services they offer to the elderly. The only difference between the two is that in the second group, war or preparations for war dramatically consumes the budgets for health, education, and other social services.

Category II countries need to make tremendous efforts toward organization of their medical services, proper investment in human resources, solution of internal problems, and settlement of disputes with other nations. Countries that succeed in meeting these needs will step forward to join Category I and reach the standards of developed countries. Consequently, their elderly will have a better chance to be healthy and happy. Any country that fails in meeting these needs will drop to Category III, among those countries whose medical and social services are terribly poor, even on the brink of collapse.

Statistics for Category II show that the mean life expectancy is 71.1 years, with 73.0 years the highest, in Tunisia, and 69.5 the lowest, in Libya and Morocco. The mean annual per-capita health expenditure is $105 in these countries, with Libya highest, reaching $246 and Lebanon the lowest, less than $12. The average number of physicians in this category is 13.0 for every one thousand persons; the highest ratio is 28.1, in Lebanon, and the lowest is 5.2, in Morocco. The mean fertility rate for this category reached 3.1 in 2000–2005, with 4.3 the highest, in Jordan, and 2.1 the lowest, in Tunisia. The fertility rate for most countries in this category was around 2.1 percent in 2000–2005.

These countries are suffering from many problems as a result of the deterioration of services following the transition from a socialist economy to a free market economy. The following phenomena have resulted, in most countries of this category:

- Gradual erosion of the middle class

- Deterioration of educational and health services

- Prices soaring due to increased inflation

- A sharp increase in unemployment rates

- A rapid drop in the value of already low wages

As a direct result of increasing unemployment, the elderly continue to support their dependents from their already low pensions. Meanwhile, many employers offer short-term employment contracts to avoid the payment of two-thirds of the employees' social security. The disastrous result is that when they grow old, these employees will not have a pension.

Problems related to the health system structure, the medical insurance system, and the welfare services for the elderly make people resort to the private sector for better medical care, which typically costs them about 40 percent of their family income.

Problems in this domain can be solved through consideration of the following suggestions:

- Giving priority access to health services to the poor elderly

- Providing rehabilitation programs for the healthy elderly, especially those who are needy

- Activating regulations that protect elderly rights

- Including geriatric and gerontology courses in the syllabi of those who are expected to work with the elderly

- Educating primary-care physicians and family doctors in how to handle the problems of the elderly, particularly when to refer them to a geriatric department

- Providing quality medical insurance for all citizens, with special categories for the elderly

- Establishing geriatric departments in the main hospitals, supervised by a geriatric team

- Maintaining proper communication between the ministry of health and the ministry of social affairs for follow-up work with the elderly following their discharge

- Ensuring participation of nongovernmental organizations in the welfare services offered to the elderly (geriatric clubs, geriatric residence, day care and nursing institutions)

- Encouraging mosques and churches, supported by philanthropic leaders, to play an important role in caring for both the healthy and disabled elderly

- Providing coordinated support, with the participation of all parties, to families that include elderly members (in fact, most elderly persons are presently supported by their families)

- Devoting particular attention to Group B, which, as mentioned earlier, is suffering from more problems than Group A because of war or the threat of war

Category III

This category of countries includes Afghanistan, Djibouti, Somalia, and the Sudan. All are suffering from natural disasters, war, or both. Consequently, the state medical services, including those offered for the elderly, are poor. The efforts of NGOs and international humanitarian organizations are badly needed for all.

Statistics on this category show very low values. The per-capita health expenditure is roughly $25 a year in three countries, with Djibouti higher at $41. The average number of physicians is less than two for every one thousand people in these countries. The gap between the traditional health practices used in these countries and the modern scientifically based medical techniques in the developed countries is tremendous.

RECOMMENDATIONS

Novelli was quite right when he claimed that "management and leadership for improving global health, especially in an aging world, require an internationalist perspective and, ultimately, worldwide vision and worldwide solutions" (Novelli, 2005).

Each country needs to develop its own model strategy for the twenty-first century, taking into consideration its specific cultural and socioeconomic realities. Such a strategy must be community based, with the goal of achieving active aging for its elderly. The cornerstone of this strategy is the primary health care system, in cooperation with the secondary and tertiary systems.

To guarantee complementary rather than redundant efforts, all concerned parties—the ministries of health and of social affairs, as well as nongovernmental organizations and philanthropy leaders—must identify their specific roles in caring for the elderly. This could be carried out through the training of multidisciplinary teams of doctors, nurses, social workers, psychologists, and rehabilitation specialists to work cooperatively with the elderly. Educating and supporting the families of the elderly is one of the important principles to be considered, because families are responsible for giving care to most of the elderly population throughout the region.

The component strategy for the twenty-first century should include the following:

- Formulation of policy and strategy
- Agreement that the elderly have a fundamental human right to health care
- Primary health care as the cornerstone of active aging
- Strong participation of the older population in society
- Development of human resources for quality health care
- Creation and maintenance of multidisciplinary networks to facilitate care of the elderly
- Research, surveys, and studies to establish a database for evidence-based care
- Increased awareness of active aging among the population
- Evaluation of quality standards for the plan, using set indicators and experienced evaluators
- Active pursuit of the latest assistive technology for the elderly
- Efforts to increase the availability of mental health services
- Promotion of an optimistic lifestyle for the elderly

CONCLUSION

The elderly population is likely to increase rapidly in the countries of the East Mediterranean region in the next thirty years. It is therefore in the interest of all the region's societies to have the elderly participate actively in economic development.

This participation may take the form of regular jobs, freelance work, or volunteer activity, depending on individual needs, preferences, and capacities.

From a public health perspective, features commonly associated with aging include decline of physical activity, multiple pathologies, iatrogenic factors, drug interaction and medication adjustment, socioeconomic decline aggravated by war and poverty, the double burden of communicable and noncommunicable diseases, depression, and memory decline. These risks affect the quality of life of elderly and create the need for community-based health approaches. Helping older people to remain as healthy and active as possible should be regarded as a necessity rather than a luxury. This help may take the form of prevention and reduction of such burdens as avoidable disability, chronic and acute diseases, and premature mortality.

Health care in the developing countries is generally considered the responsibility of the individual. Governments that do not take this responsibility instead support and facilitate the efforts of individual citizens, throughout their lives, by providing environments in which such efforts are likely to succeed. The private sector, NGOs, philanthropic leaders, and religious and humanitarian organizations are expected to ensure that all people, including the elderly, get the health care they need. The elderly individuals should receive adequate food and proper shelter. The health care they need should be received with dignity, secure from elderly abuse and ageism. After all, they have earned this right throughout their lives.

Globalization means that we must work hard to improve the quality of life for all humans on our planet. Some countries do get together to coordinate their contributions in spite of their old political hostilities, their different ethnic origins and different languages. Unfortunately, some other countries allow their subcultures to clash violently and consequently reject the alternative of unity.

The free-market economy will continue to increase the gap between the rich countries and the poor countries. This is why national, regional, and global visions and policies must be based on cooperation, equality, and respect for all humans.

REFERENCES

Arnaout, S., and Kalache, A. "Active Aging and Promotion of the Health of Older People: Report on a Regional Consultation, Manama, Bahrain, April 26–28, 2005," EMRO, Cairo. World Health Organization, Regional Office for the Eastern Mediterranean. P4-14 WHO-EM/HSG/022/E 2006.

Gezairy, H. A. "Eastern Mediterranean Region." In C. E. Koop, C. E. Pearson, and M. R. Schwarz (eds.), *Critical Issues in Global Health*. San Francisco: Jossey-Bass, 2002.

Novelli, W. D. "Managing Health, Health Care and Aging" In W. H. Foege, N. Daulaire, R. E. Black, and C. E. Pearson (eds.), *Global Health Leadership and Management*. San Francisco: Jossey-Bass, 2005.

Parsons, T. "Updated Iraq Study Affirms Earlier Mortality Estimates." *The Johns Hopkins University Gazette*, October 16, 2006, *36*.

World Health Organization, Regional Office for the Eastern Mediterranean. "A Strategy for Active Healthy Aging and Old Age Care in the Eastern Mediterranean Region 2006–2015," EMRO, Cairo. WHO-EM/HSG/030/E 2006.

CHAPTER

21

HEALTH AND AGING IN RUSSIA

VLADIMIR KH. KHAVINSON

OLGA N. MIKHAILOVA

DEMOGRAPHIC ASPECTS OF AGING IN RUSSIA

The demographic shifts that emerged in the twentieth century and continue to develop throughout the world—Russia included—are inevitably accompanied by changes in the structure of human morbidity and hence relate directly to the present and future challenges of public health.

The change in the structure of morbidity, with the shift toward noncommunicable diseases and their increasing prevalence over communicable ones, has been designated an epidemiological transition (Napalkov, 2004).

The current commonly accepted definition of a demographic transition is a change in the type of population reproduction, whereby an initial acceleration of population growth is replaced by its deceleration, with a subsequent stabilization of the population and a change in its age structure. Demographic transition develops in a brief historical space of time and has the character of a global process. Its most important consequences are population aging and disequilibrium between the younger and older generations. Russia is entering the final stage of the demographic transition, a period in which, for many reasons, increasing demands on the system of social protection and public health are inevitable (Napalkov, 2004). Between the All-Union census of the population in 1989 and the one in 2002, the average age of Russian citizens increased by three years, to 37.7 years. The dependency ratio index continues to grow as well. Eighty-nine million (61.3 percent) of the population are of working age (males aged sixteen to fifty-nine, females aged sixteen to fifty-four); 26.3 million (18.1 percent) are younger than sixteen, and 29.8 million (20.5 percent) are over working age.

One striking characteristic of the age structure of the Russian population is an imbalance between the male and female populations (see Table 21.1). Moreover, gender-related differences in mortality are significant in Russia. This leads to a significant gender imbalance in the aged population, the values of which are much higher for the female population.

Approximately one-fourth of Russia's population resides in the rural areas, so it is important to consider the differences between urban and rural population, both from the viewpoint of the best care for the needs of the elderly citizens and for the

TABLE 21.1. **Number of Males per 1,000 Females in Russia and Selected European Countries, 2002.**

Country	Number of Males per 1,000 Females		
	60+ years	65+	80+
France	732	681	453
Germany	705	617	348
Italy	744	696	485
Spain	755	717	503
Sweden	784	735	541
United Kingdom	764	712	464
Poland	665	616	431
Ukraine	561	490	301
Russia	531	458	251

Source: United Nations, 2006.

optimization of budget expenditures. The indices of aging appeared to be highest in the female population of rural areas.

Alongside one uniform demographic situation across Russia—that is, low birth rate and high mortality rate throughout all eighty-nine regions grouped in seven federal districts (FDs)—we observe significant differences in demographic indices between districts. This in its turn generates differences in age structure and indices of population aging. The computation shows the lowest indices of population aging in the Far Eastern Federal District and the highest in the Central Federal District (Safarova, 2005) (see Table 21.2).

Thus, while speaking of social policy, one must take into consideration the heterogeneity of aging processes throughout Russia.

The following aging characteristics have been considered, computed, and compared for all regions of the Russian Federation: the share of population aged sixty and over, aging index, old-age dependency ratio, parent support ratio, and total dependency ratio (see Table 21.3) (Age-Sex and Marital Structure, 2004; Elderly People in the Russian Federation, 2002). It should be mentioned that only a small part of the Russian population (4.6 percent) shows extremely low aging indices; for more than half of the population (the Central FD, the North West FD, the Privolzhsky FD) these indices are higher than average for Russia (Safarova, 2005).

According to the projection of the State Committee of the Russian Federation on Statistics, for the period to 2016 the population of the Russian Federation will continue to decrease. The positive net migration will not compensate for the natural decline of the population. By 2016, the size of the resident population of Russia will be 134 million people, having decreased by 11.6 million people or by 8 percent compared with the beginning of 2000 (Vishnevsky, 2004).

Moreover, a shorter life expectancy for men compared with women is a characteristic of Russia's sociodemographic development. As a result, the number of single elderly people, most of whom are women, keeps growing.

HEALTH IN RUSSIA

Contrary to the situation in many other "graying" countries, the aging of population in Russia is not accompanied by improvements in health or life expectancy indices.

To understand the causes of low life expectancy, we must keep in mind that, according to population studies in different countries, health is determined 45 to 55 percent by lifestyle (nutrition, working and living conditions, other material factors), 17 to 20 percent by the environment and climate, 18 to 20 percent by genetic human biology, and 8 to 10 percent by the public health care system (Voitenko, 1991). In Russia, neither environment, nor material factors or income per capita, nor the health care system contribute to longevity.

The General Assembly of the Russian Academy of Medical Sciences (RAMS), which took place on October 4, 2006, stated that in recent years the medicodemographic processes in Russia have taken a catastrophic turn (Resolution of the

TABLE 21.2. Main Demographic Indices for Russia and Its Federal Districts (FD), 2002 and 2004.

INDICATOR	TFR		Life Expectancy at Birth						Rate of Migration (per 10,000 of population)	
			2002			2004				
REGION	2002	2004	Male and Female	Male	Female	Male and Female	Male	Female	2002	2004
RUSSIA	1.286	1.340	64.95	58.68	71.90	65.27	58.89	72.30	4	7
The Central FD	1.146	1.218	65.60	59.28	72.58	66.14	59.77	73.12	16	35
The North West FD	1.210	1.251	63.84	57.47	71.00	63.76	57.12	71.26	–0.2	9
The South FD	1.378	1.510	67.24	61.42	73.39	67.92	62.16	73.94	10	–0.4
The Privolzhsky FD	1.314	1.335	65.15	58.69	72.29	65.22	58.59	72.57	–1	–2
The Urals FD	1.355	1.392	64.63	58.40	71.55	65.07	58.69	72.10	–1	4
The Siberian FD	1.363	1.394	63.05	56.79	70.12	63.27	56.87	70.45	–6	–11
The Far East FD	1.392	1.466	62.64	56.70	69.65	62.36	56.32	69.52	–15	–31

Source: Safarova, 2005.

TABLE 21.3. **Dependency Ratio and Aging Characteristics for Russia and Its Federal Districts (FD), 2002.**

INDICATOR			Dependency Ratio		
Region	60+ Proportion %	Aging Index	Old-age Dependency Ratio	Dependency Ratio	Parent Support Ratio
RUSSIA	18.5	112.8	28.4	53.5	4.7
The Central FD	21.4	155.3	33.0	54.3	5.5
The North West FD	18.8	128.9	28.3	50.2	4.4
The South FD	17.6	91.4	28.0	58.6	5.1
The Privolzhsky FD	18.9	112.4	29.3	55.3	4.9
The Urals FD	16.1	94.7	24.1	49.6	3.8
The Siberian FD	16.2	92.2	24.5	51.2	3.7
The Far East FD	13.2	73.7	19.1	45.0	2.2

Note: Computation based on the 2002 census.

Source: Safarova, 2005.

XVII [80] Session . . . , 2006). As stated in the Resolution, mortality indices in nearly all age groups significantly surpass those in economically developed countries. In the working-age population, this is 8.2 percent—two to four times higher than in economically developed countries. Life expectancy for men did not exceed fifty-six years in several regions of Russia in a recent five-year period; overall in Russia it is about fifty-nine years, which is fifteen to twenty years less than in Japan, Sweden, Great Britain, France, Germany, and the United States. As for deaths, among the leading causes are cardiovascular and cancer diseases at 56.7 percent, traumas at 12.5 percent, and poisoning and other consequences of adverse external effects at 13.7 percent. The citizens of Russia typically die from malignant tumors fifteen to twenty years earlier than do residents of Europe and the United States. In addition, the General Assembly of the RAMS stated that these comparatively extremely high death rates persist in spite of significant advances in modern medicine that, if available, can save lives and preserve working ability for the majority of those patients who now perish from cardiovascular, cancer, oncohematologic, communicable, endocrine, and other diseases, as well as heavy traumas and poisoning. It was emphasized that the risk of death from the majority of diseases depends largely on the availability, timeliness, and adequacy of medical aid. However, high-technology methods are introduced into the Russian health care system very slowly. Governmental funding of expensive medical technologies is inadequate for the needs of the population. As a result, many patients die for lack of access to modern medical care (Resolution of the XVII [80] Session . . . , 2006).

Physical health unequivocally has a direct effect on elderly people's capability to be involved in the society's life. A mere 22 percent of Russia's elderly people are considered effectively healthy (Elderly People in the Russian Federation, 2002). We must admit that the Russian public health sector was largely neglected by the government throughout the post-Soviet years; as a result, the already aging system was more severely hit by recent economic reforms than any other public sector. Perhaps the most notable achievement of the Soviet system was the state disease-prevention policy, which included mass regular checkup campaigns. The government allocated lavish funding for annual medical monitoring and primary care at schools, factories, and offices, which helped diagnose various disorders at early stages. The disease prevention system was the first to collapse when the state funding started to dry up in the 1990s.

After almost fifteen years of neglect, health has finally gotten the attention of the government, and in September 2005 President Vladimir Putin announced an ambitious plan to spend billions of rubles on improvements to the health sector. The plan is focusing on bringing improvements to the so-called primary section of the public health sector by raising salaries of general practitioners and nurses in municipal and rural clinics, equipping ambulances and clinics with modern diagnostic equipment, and restoring the system of disease prevention.

In 1999, the Ministry of Health of the Russian Federation introduced a set of measures to improve administration of health services to elderly people. The measures are aimed at expanding the scale and improving the quality of medical care and sociomedical services, preventing premature aging, and intensifying gerontological studies (Elderly People in the Russian Federation, 2002). Today, elderly people receive medical treatment at multifunctional therapeutic and disease prevention institutions including 18,300 outpatient clinics; 10,800 inpatient institutions; 50 specialized centers with 15,000 beds between them, to provide medical treatment to elderly patients; and over 100 nursing homes.

The Geront Foundation created for the purpose embraces the following subdivisions: premature aging prevention, diabetes mellitus school, groups for people with hearing impairments, and an association for Alzheimer's disease.

The geriatric center opened in Saint Petersburg in 1994 is an example of a promising organizational model combining health care and social services. Every day the center caters to around one thousand elderly patients receiving outpatient clinic and inpatient hospital services; nearly one hundred additional patients are processed by the center's sociomedical examination board. The center arranges for consulting physician visits to patients in their homes, individualized consultations for elderly patients and their families, visits by social workers to patients' homes, and assistance for older persons being admitted to inpatient social services institutions.

The sociomedical department is yet another new type of institution providing sociomedical services to elderly people in their homes. A total of 1,273 departments of this type, staffed by over 6,000 nurses, have been opened across the country.

As stated previously, the aging of the population necessitates reorganization of the health care system. This is related to the change in the structure of morbidity with the shift toward noncommunicable diseases. The majority of people suffering chronic noncommunicable diseases need extended and expensive treatment, special attendance and social care and rehabilitation measures; the needs become even more complicated when the patient becomes an invalid. Napalkov (2004) describes this in the case of cancer. He notes that in the final decades of the twentieth century the incidence of malignant tumors and resulting mortality increased by over 23 percent worldwide. A similar trend was observed in Russia: in the period from 1992 to 2001 the index of mortality from malignant tumors rose from 271.8 to 313.9 per 100,000 population, an increase in morbidity of over 16 percent. The analysis of data presented by Population Cancer Registers confirms the opinion that cancer is largely an affliction of elderly people. The comparison of total indices of aging for one year, according to the St. Petersburg Population Register revealed that cancer incidence among males aged eighty and over is 180 times that of males aged under fifteen. In the analogous female groups the difference is 150 times.

We should face the necessity of focusing on prevention of age-related diseases and increasing expenditures for the purpose. The cost for preventive measures will be well justified when compared with the cost of treatment, servicing, and maintenance.

PERSPECTIVES OF FUNDAMENTAL GERONTOLOGY IN PREVENTION OF AGE-RELATED DISEASES

Experimental gerontology has methods for increasing the individual life span of different kinds of animals by 20 to 40 percent. However, even the most efficient means for prolonging life span—that is, *geroprotectors*—may be ineffective if social reforms and healthy lifestyle habits are neglected. The UN Research Agenda on Aging for the Twenty-first Century understandably regards healthy aging as an absolute priority. The development of means to prevent premature aging is a key to the implementation of these programs.

As we know, there are two scenarios of aging: physiological (natural) and pathologic (premature). Physiological aging is a natural part of active longevity, whereas premature aging provokes pathologies and diseases (Korkushko, Khavinson, Shatilo, and Antonjuk-Scheglova, 2006). In the vast majority of the population (90 to 95 percent), the process of aging develops according to the premature (accelerated) type. Diseases typical for the second half of human life (atherosclerosis, ischemic heart disease, hypertension, cancer, diabetes mellitus, and the like) accelerate the development of age-related alterations in the organism and cause premature aging and death before the individual reaches the specific limit of the biological life span.

Figure 21.1 displays the main desirable directions for prevention with respect to premature aging risk factors.

Experimental studies confirm the importance of evaluating geroprotectors and introducing them into clinical practice. As experiments have shown, regulatory peptides synthesis in the organism decreases with aging, together with the changes in the sensitivity to them of target cells (Korkushko, Khavinson, Shatilo, and Antonjuk-Scheglova, 2006). Peptides regulate the process of protein biosynthesis in cells through gene expression (Korkushko, Khavinson, Butenko, and Shatilo, 2002). Peptide regulation disorders induce alterations in the functional state of cells, and on the molecular level there is a decline of gene expression and protein synthesis. Disorders in peptide regulation of gene expression are supposed to lead to a gradual decrease in organism functions (Korkushko, Khavinson, Butenko, and Shatilo, 2002). Premature aging prevention with peptides isolated from different animal organs and tissues or constructed by means of direct synthesis seems to be one of the prospective physiological approaches to the problem.

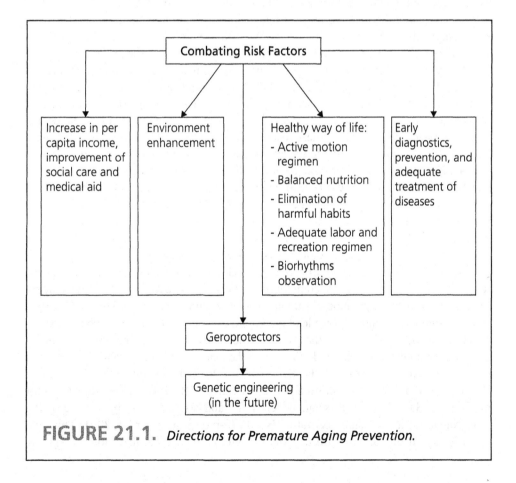

FIGURE 21.1. *Directions for Premature Aging Prevention.*

In clinical studies, the geroprotective effect of a preparation can actually be registered only if, under its effect, there is a lowering of biological or functional age, increase in physical and mental capacity, normalization of metabolism parameters and immunity and neuron endocrine regulation, and increase in the adaptive abilities of the organism.

Experimental studies reveal that the older the subject when the substance is administered, the less effect the substance will be at preventing age-related changes and tumors. Thus it advisable to prescribe geroprotectors at the earliest signs of aging, which often appear around thirty-five to thirty-nine.

Decrease in the functional potential of vitally important systems and decline of the organism's adaptive abilities and its capacity for resisting pathogenic factors are prerequisites to the use of geroprotectors.

The regulatory effect of geroprotectors on the main functions of the organism is one of the currently available means for improving the quality of life and extending the active life span, as well as for prevention of premature aging. The elaboration of this approach was begun in 1971 at the Military Medical Academy (Saint Petersburg). Since 1992 it has been continued at the Saint Petersburg Institute of Bioregulation and Gerontology of the North-Western Branch of the Russian Academy of Medical Sciences. To date, thirty bioregulators have been designed for application as medicinal substances and biologically active food supplements. All of these preparations are natural or synthesized peptides and are capable of restoring many functions of the organism.

The results of thirty years of experimental and clinical studies of the bioregulators conducted in the leading medical research institutions in Russia and abroad have demonstrated their high efficiency. Experimental data document an increase, under the effect of bioregulators, in the average life span of animals and normalization of the biochemical and physiological indices. These results have been verified by the results of clinical studies. Clinical studies conducted from 1992 to 2004 in two leading geronotological centers, Kiev Institute of Gerontology of the Ukrainian Academy of Medical Sciences and Saint Petersburg Institute of Bioregulation and Gerontology. Both showed that course application of peptide bioregulators in elderly and old people led to the restoration of the main physiological functions and an increase in mental and physical working capacity, as well as a twofold decrease in the level of sickness and death rate (Korkushko, Khavinson, Shatilo, and Antonjuk-Scheglova, 2006).

Based on these findings, a draft was developed at the Saint Petersburg Institute of Bioregulation and Gerontology, "Program for prevention of premature aging and occupational life extension for the population of Russia." The program was considered by the Commission on Promoting Healthy Lifestyle of the Public Chamber of the Russian Federation.

It should be mentioned that the goals and mechanisms for realizing this program are in keeping with the principles and priorities of the concept of demographic development of the Russian Federation for the period up to 2015, based on the Decree of the President of the Russian Federation No. 24 of January 10, 2000, "About the Concept of National Safety of the Russian Federation," and approved by the Decree of the Government of the Russian Federation No. 1270-p of September 24, 2001. This program is also in full accord with the Madrid International Plan of Action on Ageing, adopted at the Second World Assembly on Ageing in Madrid in April, 2002, at which representatives of 159 countries stated the importance of research on aging and age-related issues, and medical preventive and rehabilitation measures as an important instrument in the formulation of policies and programs on aging.

Among the Madrid Plan's 239 recommendations for action, seven are directed to the scientists working in the field of aging. The Madrid Plan emphasizes the central role of research in the actions on aging on both national and international level. The Madrid Plan also identifies the decisive elements (see box) for its successful implementation on the national level. The research component is clearly crucial to the Plan.

It is notable that Russia and Russian gerontologists participated in the implementation of Madrid Plan of Action and took part in the preparation of the Research Agenda on Ageing for the 21st Century (working meetings in New York, 1999, Salsomaggiore, 2000, and Barcelona, 2003) ("Elderly People in the Russian Federation," 2002) and in organizing of the symposium "What Fundamental Studies in Biology Tell Us About Ageing Today" in the World Gerontological Forum, Valencia, 2002. The Second European Congress of Biogerontology, which took place in Saint Petersburg, Russia, in 2000, was conducted in the framework of the Research Agenda on Ageing for the 21st Century (Andrews and others, 2001). The VI European Congress of the International Association of Gerontology and Geriatrics, in Saint Petersburg in 2007, also follows the framework of this Agenda. The journal *Advances in Gerontology,* issued by the Gerontological Society of the Russian Academy of Sciences, was the first in the world to publish the Research Agenda (Age-Sex and Marital Structure, 2004). Also important for the implementation of the Madrid Plan of Action were the state report on the status of elderly citizens in the Russian Federation (Karelova, 2003b) and the National Report "Elderly People in the Russian Federation: Situation, Problems, and Prospects," prepared for the Second World Assembly on Ageing in Madrid ("Elderly People . . . ," 2002).

DECISIVE ELEMENTS OF THE IMPLEMENTATION OF THE MADRID PLAN OF ACTION ON THE NATIONAL LEVEL

- Creating effective organizations for older persons

- Providing instruction, education, and research in the field of aging

- Collecting and analyzing national data, such as obtaining data disaggregated by sex and age for planning, monitoring, and estimating the implementation of the Plan

- Independent and unbiased observation of Plan implementation

- Mobilizing resources by organizations representing the older people or supporting them by, among other things, increasing the benefits for such organizations

However, the proposed project of state social policy in relation to elderly citizens, to be pursued by the Ministry of Labor and Social Development of the Russian Federation in 1999 for the period until 2005, later postponed to 2010, then to 2015, now still remains just a proposal (Karelova, 2003a). Unfortunately, the project plans neglected such important tasks as development of gerontological science and training for social gerontologists and health care workers.

THE SOCIAL ASPECT OF AGING

Raising the retirement age seems to be the easiest instrument to reduce the number of retirees and expenditures of the pension system and increase the workforce, and thus tax revenues, thereby replenishing funds used for the pension payments. The following arguments are used to advance this approach:

- Russia's retirement age is one of the lowest in the world: fifty-five for women and sixty for men. It was introduced in 1932 when many workers retired because of disability, and it has not been changed since that time, although the character and conditions of labor have changed significantly (Zakharov and Rakhmanova, 1997).

- The Russian population is growing older: in 1939 the share of men aged sixty and over was 6.7 percent; in 1959, 9.0 percent; and by 2002, it had more than doubled, to 18.5 percent (Age-Sex and Marital Structure, 2004). The old-age dependency ratio also has increased: in 1939 there were 164 retirees per 1,000 workers; in 1959, 202 retirees; and in 2002, 335 retirees.

The development of the pension system in Russia in the twenty-first century was triggered by legislation approved in 2000–2002. These legislative acts were realized mainly on the organizational and technological basis of the Russian Federal Pension Fund, thus altering the structure of pension system and the sources of and rules for its funding. At the same time, several years' experience with these legislative acts in force shows us that the pension system of Russia needs to be further developed, because of factors characteristic of pension systems in all socially developed countries—mainly, the tendency of the society's demographic development.

Calculations show that the budget of the Russian Federation may lose 440 billion rubles in 2010 and 1.7 trillion rubles in 2020 through a gross domestic product deficit due to the lack of workers. On average, the budget will lose more than one trillion rubles (in present-day rates) annually in the years 2011–2020 (Rybakovsky, 2006). According to expert calculations, the economic loss just from health loss in the Russian population in 1999 totals approximately 65 billion U.S. dollars (Roik, 2006).

At the Lisbon Forum in 2000, the EU leaders took on the task of increasing the level of employment among citizens aged fifty-five to sixty-four from the 42 percent of a year previous to 50 percent (Kolesnik, in press). To achieve this increase, it is important to support or improve the health reserves of people in this age group. Moreover, to attain these ends, elderly citizens must be sufficiently motivated.

The number of old-age retirees (that is, citizens who mastered a profession and have been working, as a rule, for at least twenty to twenty-five years) equals one-third of the total economically active population. Pensioners are often regarded as people who are only consuming the society's resources; this overlooks the fact that older people possess approximately one-half of the total professional knowledge held by the currently working population.

We must keep in mind that significant amounts of resources were invested in the education and career training of old-age pensioners, and these investments were repaid during the period of their active work. The professional skills and experience of these Russian citizens could find a "second life" if we were to establish a system of for conveying their professional knowledge to the younger workers. The establishment of such a system is vital for pensioners themselves as well as for the government and the society. It is also noteworthy that many pensioners have experience in handling crisis situations, which is presently necessary for the working population (Kolesnik, in press).

REFERENCES

Age-Sex and Marital Structure. *Results of All-Russian Census 2002*, Vol. 2. Moscow: "Statistika Rossii," 2004.

Andrews, G. R., and others. "The United Nations Research Agenda on Ageing for the 21st Century." *Advances in Gerontology*, 2001, *7*, 7–25.

Demographic Yearbook of Russia 2005. Moscow: The State Committee on Statistics of the Russian Federation (Rosstat), 2005.

Elderly People in the Russian Federation: Situation, Problems, and Prospects (national report). Moscow: Human Rights Publishers, 2002.

Karelova, G. N. (ed.). Concept of State Social Policy in Relation to Elderly Citizens for the Period of up to 2015: Social Work for Elderly People's Professionalism, Partnership, Responsibility. Proceedings of the All-Russia Congress of Social Workers. Saratov: 2003a, 201–213.

Karelova, G. N. (ed.). State Report on the Status of Elderly Citizens in the Russian Federation. Saratov: 2003b, 21–47.

Kolesnik, A. P. Concerning Alteration of the Paradigm of Pension Assurance (in press).

Korkushko, O.V., Khavinson, V. K., Butenko, G. M., and Shatilo, V. B. "Peptide Preparations of Thymus and Pineal Gland for Prevention of Premature Aging." Saint Petersburg: NAUKA, 2002.

Korkushko, O. V., Khavinson, V. K., Shatilo, V. B., and Antonjuk-Scheglova, G. M. "Geroprotective Effect of the Pineal Peptide Epithalamin in Elderly People with Premature Ageing." *Bulletin of Experimental Biology and Medicine*, 2006, *142*(9), 328–332.

Napalkov, N. P. "Cancer and Demographic Transition." *Problems in Oncology*, 2004, *50*(2), 127–144.

Resolution of the XVII (80) Session of the General Meeting of the Russian Academy of Medical Sciences, October 4, 2006.

Roik, V. D. "Demographic Problems in the Modern World: Phenomenon of the Graying Population: New Global Challenge." *Social Herald of Pension and Social Funds*, 2006, 1–2, 68.

Rybakovsky, L. Strategy of Demographic Development of Russia in the 21st Century. *Social and Demographic Policy*, 2006, *1*, 42.

Safarova, G. L. Demographic Aspects of Russian Population Aging. *Native Notes (Otechestvennye Zapiski)*, 2005, 3, 110–123.

United Nations. Demographic Yearbook of Russia 2006; World Population Ageing (1950–2050). New York: United Nations, 2006.

Vishnevsky, A. (ed.). Population of Russia: Tenth Annual Demographic Report. Moscow: Knizhny Dom Universitet, 2004.

Voitenko, V. P. Health of the Healthy: Introduction to Sanology. Kiev: 1991.

CHAPTER

22

HEALTH AND AGING IN LATIN AMERICA AND THE CARIBBEAN

ENRIQUE VEGA

There is no doubt that Latin America and the Caribbean have been aging rapidly. But even more noteworthy is that this aging process will increase exponentially in the coming years. Today it can be said that the populations of all the countries in the region are aging, although there are marked differences among them.

In 2006, 9 percent of Latin America's population was aged sixty and over, or just over fifty million people. While the population in general is growing by 1.5 percent annually, the population over sixty is growing at a rate of 3.5 percent annually. This demographic shift means that by around 2050, 24 percent of the population—some two hundred million people—will be older adults. Beyond being a symbol of demographic maturity, this aging process is a specific product of the social advances and progress in health in the region. However, it is also clear that the aging of its population is one of the biggest challenges that Latin American and Caribbean society must face during this century.

WHAT CHARACTERIZES THE AGING OF LATIN AMERICA AND THE CARIBBEAN?

The population of our region ages in a distinctive manner; we can find common characteristics but also an important diversity. These characteristics can be demonstrated in four fundamental aspects.

The Emergence of Aging

The demographic causes of aging are the same in all the region's countries. The evolution of those trends in Latin America has been interesting and distinctive from that in other regions. Although mortality is always of secondary importance in determining the causes of the aging process, in our case there was a point in the early 1970s when there was a small increase in the elderly population as mortality declined and there were consequent rapid increases in life expectancy at birth and in the numbers of older adults. Notwithstanding this development, it is the decline in the fertility rate that has been the main cause of the aging of the region, perhaps with the distinction that this decline in fertility occurred recently, but abruptly, and has since held steady.

Diverse Transitions

One characteristic of Latin America's aging process is its diversity. There are countries in our region that correspond to each group in the demographic transition. While more than 15 percent of the population in Barbados, Cuba, Argentina, and Uruguay is over sixty, and those countries are now considered demographically old countries, only 6 percent of the population in Haiti, Bolivia, and Guatemala is over sixty, making these three the youngest countries in the Hemisphere. The nations of the Caribbean, where older adults make up 11 percent of the population, have the oldest populations of any developing region in the world. Yet within the Caribbean, Haiti's population is one of the youngest and its life expectancy at birth one of the shortest in the developing world.

A Rapid Transition

The demographic transition in our region has occurred very rapidly, as indicated by the absolute figures for the growth of the elderly population. Whereas in 1950 there were 5.5 million older adults in Latin America and the Caribbean, a half a century later that figure had increased to more than 40 million. From 2000 onward, the figure will double every twenty-five years—that is, there will be some hundred million older adults in the region in 2025 and almost two hundred million in 2050.

Relation to Economic Development

The decline in mortality in the western hemisphere has been associated with improvements in related socioeconomic and health status. However, the social and economic situation has also been a factor in keeping mortality figures very high, albeit in the early stages of life. The improvement should have been greater during this period, and it has not brought the anticipated results.

In terms of fertility, there is a major difference from the European experience: the decline in Latin American fertility, having taken hold, has held steady despite significant variations in the regional economy and times of severe crisis. The clearest consequence of this has been a progressive and rapid aging shift that has not been associated with a particularly favorable economic situation like that of Europe or North America.

A GREATER OPPORTUNITY TO REACH OLD AGE

The possibility of reaching old age has clearly increased. Today, 73.8 percent of people born in the world will live beyond sixty and almost 34 percent beyond eighty. The major inequities of the world are very evident in this regard. While only 48 percent of Africans will reach old age and only 16.9 percent will reach eighty, twice as many Europeans (83.4 percent) will surpass the age of sixty and 42.3 percent will reach eighty.

In Latin America, more than 75 percent of the people born today will live to the age of sixty and 40 percent beyond eighty. In the twenty-five years from 1975 to 2000, life expectancy in Latin America and the Caribbean increased by seventeen years. The life expectancy of the region's people who are sixty years old in 2006 is nineteen years for men and twenty-three years for women.

Greater longevity is essentially due to significant reductions in mortality, beginning in the 1940s, stemming from better public medical and health care, with a consequent decline in deaths from infectious diseases and in the early stages of life.

STEPS WE CAN TAKE TO INCREASE LIFE EXPECTANCY IN THE REGION

In the final decades of the twentieth century, proportional mortality among older persons had greater significance in terms of the years of life to be gained, especially in developed and developing countries. A comparison of the mortality burden in the elderly population in Latin America and the Caribbean in the 1980s and 1990s, which examined the gap between the ages of sixty and eighty-five (years of life lost or years of life to be gained), showed that six to nine potential years of life could be gained by Zreducing mortality in this age group (La Carga de Mortalidad en los Adultos Mayores, 2003).

It was even possible to look for the specific causes of the lost years and how they contribute to years of potential life lost (YPLL). The risk of dying from infectious causes accounted for 0.5 YPLL—half of that from respiratory infections. Cancer accounted for the loss of 1.7 YPLL of men and 1.2 YPLL of women over age sixty. Even though there has been a reduction in the risk of dying from cardiovascular diseases over the past decade, these diseases continue to be the greatest cause of YPLL for those over sixty: 3.5 YPLL for men and 2.9 YPLL for women. For women, diabetes mellitus accounted for more YPLL (0.58) than the sum of the negative contributions of infectious causes (0.39) and external causes (0.14). Diabetes in men accounted for 0.48 YPLL (La Carga de Mortalidad en los Adultos Mayores, 2003).

Significant steps could be taken to increase life expectancy in older persons. Many of these are related to identified risk factors. Among these steps, primary and secondary prevention can have a major impact on survival, even among the elderly.

HEALTH IN OLDER PEOPLE

Given the increase in life expectancy, one of the greatest challenges for public health is to provide an adequate quality of life for this age group in terms of human development. In this regard, as with socioeconomic status, the differences between the developed and developing world are much more evident than those seen in the increase in life expectancy. In the developing world, the increase in the length of life has not been accompanied by comparable improvements in economic, social, and health conditions. In the case of Latin America and the Caribbean, which has some of the greatest inequities of any region of the world, these differences are glaringly apparent.

HEALTH OF OLDER PEOPLE IN THE REGION TODAY

Evaluating the health of older adults can be a complex process, approachable from many different angles. Recent research in the region has provided interesting results in terms of understanding the health and well-being of older adults.

Self-reporting on health has been shown to be a valuable indicator—even a prognosticator—of health status. Whereas in the United States only 22.7 percent of people over sixty-five and only 32.2 percent of those aged seventy-five and over report having fair or poor health, in Latin America the majority report having fair or poor health: 58 percent of women and 51 percent of men. In the United States and Canada, women more frequently report having excellent or good health, whereas in Latin America women reported worse health than did men—a result of older women having longer life expectancy but under socioeconomic conditions that make them very likely to be dependent on others.

Functional independence, or autonomy, in the activities of daily living (ADLs) is a health indicator for older adults. It can be evaluated by reporting the extent to which basic activities of daily living (BADLs) are performed, including using the toilet, bathing and dressing oneself, getting in and out of bed, eating, and controlling bodily functions. The evaluation of ADLs is complemented with what are called instrumental activities of daily living (IADLs), which are more complex and represent greater independence in a more concrete social environment. These activities include managing money, shopping, transportation, cooking, and medicines. ADLs are a very concrete expression of the quality of life of older adults.

Even though the U.S. census in 2000 reported some fourteen million older adults with at least one disability, studies consistently show a decline in the prevalence of disabilities in the United States. The situation in Latin America and the Caribbean is another story. The Health, Well-Being and Aging study (known as SABE—Salud y

Bienestar de las Personas Mayores) found a high proportion of persons with at least one affected ADL; 20 percent of respondents had limitations in BADLs, and that number increased to 26 percent among people over seventy. (The SABE study, conducted in 2001 by the Panamerican Health Organization [PAHO] with the collaboration of many national and international institutions in the region, sampled more than ten thousand people representative of population groups aged sixty and over living in communities in seven Latin American capitals: Buenos Aires, Argentina; Santiago, Chile; Bridgetown, Barbados; Havana, Cuba; Mexico City, Mexico; Sao Paulo, Brazil; and Montevideo, Uruguay.) There were significant differences between the genders, predominantly functional limitations in women. As was to be expected, functional dependency increased with age. One in every two men and two of every three women surveyed by the study reported a disability.

Two out of three older adults in Latin America and the Caribbean reported having one of six chronic diseases commonly associated with that age group (hypertension, diabetes, heart disease, cerebrovascular disease, joint problems, and chronic pulmonary disease). Although the figures are high, they deal only with known diagnoses, and if the study is compared with other research, the figures suggest a high level of underdiagnosis in some instances.

The prevalence of hypertension in 46 percent of the sample represents some forty-eight million older adults with hypertension in the region; of those, two-thirds are women. The diagnosis of diabetes varied widely: in some cities it was above 22 percent and in others around 10 percent. Underdiagnosis may be a plausible explanation for these differences. The risk of a heart ailment was reported by 20 percent of women and 18 percent of men. Nearly half of the women in the region suffer from arthritis, with a significant impact on their ability to function.

The presence of risk factors in older adults in Latin America and the Caribbean is very high, even among the youngest groups in the sample (aged sixty to sixty-nine). Two out of every three respondents in this group had at least two risk factors among those cited (smoking, overweight, or lack of rigorous physical activity): 61 percent were overweight, and of those, half were obese; three out of every four did not engage in any vigorous physical activity; and one out of every four men smoked.

Regarding other risk factors that are less often reported but have an immense impact on mortality and disability, the results were no better: 30 percent of those surveyed by the SABE study had suffered at least one fall in the year preceding the study, making it possible to assume that almost thirteen million people in the region could have that problem.

The fragility and dependency of older adults is related very strongly to emotional and mental disorders. The prevalence of cognitive deterioration exceeded 20 percent in the cities studied by SABE. The level was lower in the study's younger age groups, among whom there was a strong correlation with low educational levels: almost half of those affected in this group were found to have low levels of schooling. Interesting results also were found in terms of emotional status: the average proportion of people in the study with symptoms of depression exceeded 18 percent, with the highest levels in the younger age groups and among women. Among respondents who had at least two chronic conditions, 24 percent suffered from depression. An extremely important point is that only 5 percent of the people surveyed who reported suffering from depression had received treatment with antidepressants.

OTHER FACTORS AFFECTING THE HEALTH OF OLDER ADULTS

There is no doubt that poverty and discrimination adversely affect the health of older adults. Slightly less than 50 percent of those surveyed in the SABE study said that they did not have sufficient resources to meet their daily needs. Other studies show that 33 percent of the elderly in urban areas and 50 percent in rural areas live in poverty. In some countries, as many as 70 percent of older adults live in poverty. According to figures from the Economic Commission for Latin America and the Caribbean (ECLAC), one-third of persons aged sixty-five and over do not have retirement benefits, pensions, or gainful employment (Guzmán, 2002).

In developed regions, literacy has become universal in all countries, with few exceptions. But in developing countries in 2000, approximately half of people aged sixty and over were illiterate. Only 30 percent of women and 60 percent of men in this group knew how to read and write. In Latin America and the Caribbean, older adults have levels of schooling lower than the rest of the population, with very high levels of illiteracy that reach 80 percent in rural areas in some countries.

The SABE study examined the relationship between educational levels of older adults and their health. Those with less education more frequently reported their health as fair or poor and had harmful habits such as smoking and a lack of physical inactivity. This finding was twice as high among people with lower educational levels.

CARE OF THE ELDERLY

One interesting area of study addressed who cares for older persons in the region, taking into account their high demand for services due to their health status. In the region, it is families—especially women (90 percent)—that provide most of the care for older people. These caregivers, usually over age fifty, are subject to very high levels of stress, with 60 percent of them saying that they "cannot do any more" and slightly more than 80 percent reporting problems "meeting expenses." However, in most countries there are few programs to support these caregivers.

The issue of health services coverage for the elderly is far from resolved. Those who have access still do not receive quality services, due in particular to the lack of training among service providers. Despite the agreements resulting from the Second World Assembly on Ageing in Madrid, Spain, and the Intergovernmental Regional Conference on Ageing in Santiago, Chile, the fragmentation of services impedes continuous adequate care for older adults, and adequate recovery from health problems for this group has not been guaranteed.

The relationship between older adults and health services was also studied. Forty percent of those surveyed by SABE who suffered from hypertension had not had a primary care consultation in the last twelve months. Only 27 percent of women reported having had a mammogram in the last two years, and 80 percent of respondents reported having unmet dental needs. According to the research, 69 percent of older adults were not vaccinated against influenza. Only 2 percent of the countries have health promotion goals for people aged sixty and over.

The real situation in terms of long-term care in the region is quite unknown, although studies under way—especially in the Southern Cone (that part of South America south of the Tropic of Capricorn)—will provide important data in the years ahead, especially on institutions devoted to long-term care. In particular, the monitoring of mistreatment and abuse of people who are institutionalized—and thus their human rights—is one area that has been examined very little and should be vigorously addressed. It is therefore essential that more research and surveillance be carried out on the health problems of older adults, their access to health services, and the quality of this coverage.

The foregoing statistics pose a major challenge for health care providers who do not have the capacity necessary to tackle this challenge. Today, families provide most of the care for older adults, but they will be unable to continue doing so unless they receive support from society and the institutions that provide social and health services.

The 2002 Madrid International Plan of Action on Ageing cited the improvement of the health and well-being of older persons as one of its three priority directions. It also recognized that the aging of the developing world is occurring in a context of insufficient economic resources and programs and services of inadequate quality. The lack of coordination among the sectors in providing comprehensive and sustainable national and local programs for the elderly is an unresolved issue in Latin America.

How will health providers of the region address a phenomenon of such magnitude with so little of the resources that the developed countries traditionally spend on such matters?

As part of the final agreements of the World Assembly on Ageing, it was decided to create a mechanism to guarantee adequate monitoring of the Madrid Plan by the member states. It was also decided that each region of the world would create its own monitoring mechanism, taking into account its specific realities and needs.

In our area, following this guideline, a United Nations Inter-Agency Group on Ageing in Latin America and the Caribbean was created. It proposed a regional implementation strategy discussed and approved by the Intergovernmental Regional Conference on Ageing in Santiago in November 2003.

Prior to that conference, experts from the region had met in Panama City, Panama to devise the monitoring strategy for Priority Direction II ("advancing health and well-being into old age") and to develop a coherent proposal on this topic for Santiago. The Inter-Agency Group has taken on the task of defining the indicators that will make it possible to evaluate this process. The Pan American Health Organization has taken a leadership role in this process for Priority Direction II. The Aging and Health Program of this organization is working on a proposal for a performance evaluation system for health systems that responds to the priorities of older adults. The goal is to improve the health of people throughout life and to promote the democratization of longevity.

To establish and improve this evaluation system, a framework has been proposed that takes four components into account: the definition of public health system functions to promote health and well-being in old age, standards to evaluate the functions defined, performance indicators, and outcome indicators.

There are great disparities in the region in the availability and allocation of technical and human resources, both among and within countries. Also, the people who provide, design, implement, and direct health programs and services at all levels usually have not received the necessary training to address the growing list of needs. Without these human resources, it will be impossible to tackle the challenge posed by aging. It is essential to train human resources capable of providing the care that these people need and designing and operating health programs and services that address the health problems of older adults in the economic and social context of the region, making the limited resources available more effective and efficient.

An example of a successful strategy in this area is the creation of the Latin American Academy of Medicine for Older Adults (Academia Latinoamericana de Medicina del Adulto Mayor—ALMA). Established in 2002, ALMA is a leader and a primary reference source for promoting excellence in all aspects of geriatric care at all levels of care in Latin America. Given the importance of health care for older adults, ALMA has placed special emphasis on this area of fundamental responsibility. With a view to combining academic excellence in geriatrics with leadership in public health, ALMA conducts evidence-based training in geriatrics, promotes research among countries on issues of public health and aging, provides policy analysis on issues that affect access to and the quality of health care for older adults, and advocates and contributes to the development of a health workforce trained to care for older adults.

Despite the rapid aging of the region, the coming years will provide a significant window of opportunity for appropriate interventions to ensure that the aging of the population, however formidable a challenge, does not become a factor that could contribute to the collapse of health and social security systems in Latin America and the Caribbean.

REFERENCES

Guzmán, J. M. *Envejecimiento y desarrollo en América Latina y el Caribe*. Santiago, Chile: Centro Latino-americano y Caribeño de Demografía (CELADE), División de Población, 2002.

He, W., Sengupta, M., Velkoff, V. A., and DeBarros, K. A. U.S. Census Bureau, Current Population Reports, P23–209, 65+ in the United States: 2005. Washington, D.C.: U.S. Government Printing Office, 2005.

La Carga de Mortalidad en los Adultos Mayores. *Informe Técnico*. Unidad de Gobernabilidad & Políticas DPM/GPP/PG Salud del Adulto Mayor AD/THS/MH, Washington, D.C., Sept. 2003.

Las Personas Mayores en América Latina y el Caribe: Diagnóstico Sobre la Situación y Las Políticas. Conferencia Regional Intergubernamental Sobre Envejecimiento: Hacia una Estrategia Regional de Implementación para

América Latina y el Caribe del Plan de Acción Internacional de Madrid Sobre el Envejecimiento. CEPAL, Oct. 2003.

Menéndez, J., and others. *Enfermedades Crónicas y Limitación Funcional en Adultos Mayores: Estudio Comparativo en Siete Ciudades de América Latina y el Caribe. Rev. Panam.Salud Pública,* 2005, *17*(5/6), 353–61.

Merck Institute and the Panamerican Health Organization. The State of Aging and Health in Latin America and the Caribbean Report. Merck Institute and the Panamerican Health Organization, 2003.

Salud de las Américas. Organización Panamericana de la Salud Publicación Científico Técnica. Edición 2002.

Segunda Asamblea Mundial Sobre el Envejecimiento. Informe de la A/CONF.197/9. Publicación de las Naciones Unidas. Número de Venta: S. 02.IV.4, 2002.

World Health Report 2004 Statistical Annex. World Population Aging 1950–2005. Population Division. Department of Economic and Social Affairs. New York: United Nations, 2002. [http://www.who.int/whr/2004/annex/en/print.html].

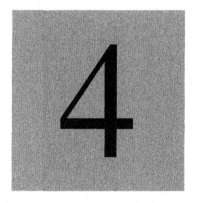

LEADERS IN RESEARCH AND INNOVATIVE PROGRAMS

CHAPTER

23

THE BIOLOGY OF AGING: CURRENT RESEARCH AND EXPECTED FUTURE GAINS

GEORGE M. MARTIN AND JOSHUA LEDERBERG

Interest in research on the biology of aging has surged during the last few decades, particularly regarding its most basic aspects, such as the role of genes in the modulation of life span and susceptibility to late-life disorders. This is graphically illustrated in Figure 23.1, which contrasts the continuing substantial rate of increase in the scientific literature (Medline) on genetics and aging with the recent apparent plateau in the rate of publications dealing with genetics and birth defects.

What accounts for biologists' growing interest in the nature of aging processes? First of all, powerful new methodologies (Sioud, 2006) have become available that have led to an acceleration of progress in all of the biological sciences. Second, there has been a gradual growth of funding by the National Institute on Aging, established in 1976 with a mandate to include a portfolio of research and training grants on the biology of aging and to provide well-standardized resources, such as banks of cells

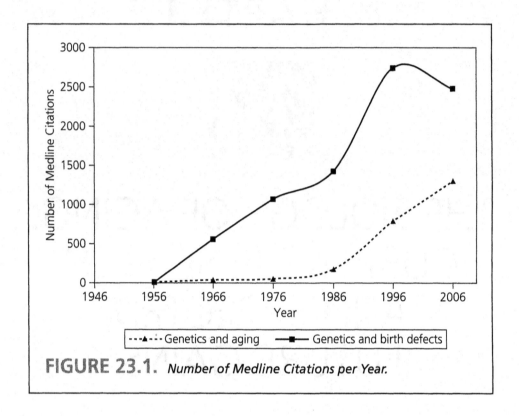

FIGURE 23.1. *Number of Medline Citations per Year.*

lines and genetically defined strains of rodents free of major infectious agents and with well-characterized life tables. This national public effort has been supplemented by nonprofit granting agencies dedicated to the advancement of basic research on the biology of aging, notably the American Federation for Aging Research and the Ellison Medical Foundation. Moreover, given the fact that the number-one risk factor for most geriatric disorders is biological aging, organizations dedicated to specific late-life disorders, such as the Alzheimer's Association, have provided substantial and relevant support for our common mission. Third, scientists have become increasingly aware of the medical, social, and economic implications of major demographic shifts toward aging societies in the populations of the developed societies (and, before long, among the developing societies). Fourth, there has been a recent breakthrough in basic research using model organisms that are amenable to genetic analysis and also have comparatively short life spans.

This research has provided strong evidence that there exists at least one common biochemical genetic pathway that can be experimentally modified in organisms as diverse as yeast, worms, fruit flies, and mice to extend both health span and life span (reviewed by Sinclair and Guarente, 2006). That such common "public" mechanisms of aging exist had been suggested by seventy years of research showing that a simple environmental manipulation—dietary restriction—can increase the life spans and health spans of a wide range of organisms (Masoro, 2005). A number of laboratories are now trying to reconcile these two general results, asking whether they are comparable at the cellular and molecular levels of organization.

BIOLOGICAL CONCEPTIONS OF AGING

Plant biologists often use the term *aging* to describe all changes in structure and function, from birth to death. However, most biogerontologists (biologists who do research on aging) use the term *aging* to refer to the deleterious, nonadaptive changes in structure and function that gradually and insidiously unfold soon after the peak of reproductive activity. This is not to say that the way in which an organism develops has nothing to do with how it ages. Clearly, how well an organism is built will have a lot to do with how long it continues to function well. It is also apparent that not every change in structure and function is deleterious; some are adaptive compensations, including alterations in behavior (Martin, 1997).

The timing of these various life history events is best understood by evolutionary biological theory (Austad, 1997; Rose, 1991). Species that evolve in ecological settings with extreme hazards (such as numerous predators, uncertain food and water supplies, harsh changes in climate, dangerous terrain, and potentially lethal infectious agents and their vectors) have to "get the job done fast." That job, of course, is reproduction. Such species therefore can be expected to have a rapid rate of development, with early sexual maturity and numerous progeny over a comparatively short period of time. Given such a scenario, there is no selective pressure for nature to invent enhanced mechanisms to ensure long periods of robustness. The energetic expense account is better used for reproduction. "Good" varieties of genes (alleles) will appear by mutation from time to time, but given the age-structured populations of most animal species, any allele that may have contributed to the enhancement of late-life survival of a rare individual will have had little chance of contributing significantly to the subsequent generations, as these alleles will have been greatly outnumbered by the vastly more common alleles in the general population dominated by members of the younger cohorts.

The same would of course be true of any "bad" gene that did not reach some threshold of phenotypic effect until comparatively late in the life span. Nature would have little opportunity to select against such genes—hence the difficulty of purging populations from such mutations as those associated with diseases such as Huntington's disease. Given changing ecologies, however, different life-history trajectories can be expected to evolve. There is experimental evidence to support that conjecture, given certain conditions (Austad, 1993).

There have been a number of challenges to the overall picture we have presented. For example, some species of fish continue to enjoy apparently indefinite growth (Patnaik, Mahapatro, and Jena, 1994). As such, they would be expected to be more resistant to predators as they age. The patterns of selection with age are therefore likely to be quite unusual (Baudisch, 2005). Some anthropologists and economists, as well as most laymen, will argue that genes are indeed selected in grandparents who provide support for their children and grandchildren (Kaplan and Robson, 2002; Lee, 2003). There is no denying that this has occurred in modern times and that it might be measurable in contemporary "primitive" tribes, but we are the result of natural selection that produced our species long ago, at a time when it seems likely that very few grandparents would have survived, although there is little direct fossil evidence to document such a conclusion.

One aspect of the biology of aging is clear to all biogerontologists: the enormous plasticity of life spans and, by inference, intrinsic rates of aging. Among mammals, typical strains of laboratory mice live for up to three to four years, while some species of whales, as judged by indirect chemical assays, can survive for over two hundred years (George and others, 1999). Such plasticity provides a degree of optimism for the potential to intervene in processes of aging. As described in the discussion that follows, however, there are also a large number of "private" mechanisms of aging— mechanisms that apply to particular individuals or pedigrees. This is particularly apparent in our own species, which is subject to considerable variation in its genetics and environment. It is also apparent that Lady Luck plays a large role in how we age, as we shall see.

THE ROLES OF NATURE, NURTURE, AND CHANCE IN LONGEVITY

Studies of the longevities of human twins, particularly those in the Scandinavian countries, have provided estimates of the role of heredity. Readers may be surprised that genes explain only about a quarter to a third of the variability of longevity in our species (reviewed by Finch and Tanzi, 1997). We do not know how much of the residual variation is due to chance events and how much to environmental impacts. Research with model organisms lead us to suspect that chance events have the largest impact; *Caenorhabditis elegans*, a roundworm, provides a robust example. Laboratory isolates of these worms are genetically identical, and they can be aged under exceedingly well-controlled environments (suspension cultures free of bacteria). Despite this excellent control of genes and environment, numerous experiments have documented enormous variability in how long such worms can live (Vanfleteren, De, and Braeckman, 1998). The same phenomena have been repeatedly observed for inbred strains of fruit flies, mice, rats, hamsters, and other species. Some recent research hints at an important role for random changes in the regulation of gene expression, presumably related to chemical modifications that are "on top of" the genetic material (Rea and others, 2005). These were originally referred to as *epinucleic* events (Lederberg, 1958), but are now usually referred to as *epigenetic* alterations.

There is no doubt, however, that environmental agents can greatly affect the pace of aging, at least for some aspects of aging. The best example is cigarette smoke, which has deleterious effects on virtually all body systems (Bernhard, Moser, Backovic, and Wick, 2006). Cigarette smoke contains about four thousand chemical agents, including numerous carcinogenic substances (Burns, 1991). Many of these compounds cause gene mutations, but here too one sees a role for chance events. There can be two genetically identical individuals with comparable exposures to mutagenic substances, but the genome of one may sustain "hits" in varieties of genes that are keys to the development of cancers, whereas the other may sustain most of the "hits" in less important segments of DNA, such as pseudogenes.

CLASSES OF GENE ACTION THAT MODULATE RATES OF AGING

The evolutionary theory of why we age, briefly referred to earlier, provides guides to how we age. One group of such gene actions has been termed *longevity assurance genes* (Hodes, McCormick, and Pruzan, 1996). They include many genes involved in the repair of damaged DNA and the protection of macromolecules from oxidative damage. The latter class of genes is relevant to what is arguably the leading current hypothesis for how we age: the accumulation of oxidatively altered proteins, lipids, DNA, and RNA, particularly those found within mitochondria—the cell organelle that generates the major flux of reactive oxygen species (Wallace, 2005). Research on rare human genetic disorders (progeroid syndromes) that appear to accelerate the rates of onset and progression of many features of aging has shown that they often result from failures to protect the genetic material from mutations and rearrangements, indicating the importance of the normal copies of such genes in the maintenance of genomic stability; that is, their importance as longevity assurance genes (Martin, 2005).

A second major class of gene action responsible for senescent phenotypes is called *antagonistic pleiotropy* (Rose, 1991; Williams, 1957). This refers to a situation in which a variety of gene, although selected because of its beneficial effect on the organism during the early stages of its life history, has bad effects late in the life course. One example often cited by biogerontologists relates to the observation that many types of human cells gradually lose the ability to replicate because the enzyme (telomerase) that is necessary to copy terminal portions of the chromosomes (telomeres) is greatly down-regulated in the course of early development (Shay and Wright, 2000). This is thought to have evolved as a mechanism for the suppression of cancers during the early period of life. Late in life, however, when fully replicatively senescent cells begin to accumulate in tissues, they can have the paradoxical effect of contributing to tumor progression as a result of factors secreted by these cells that change the properties of the connective tissues and stimulate the growth of nearby epithelial cells (Campisi, 2005). There is now good evidence that replicatively senescent cells do indeed accumulate in the skin of aging primates and that these cells show foci of DNA damage (Jeyapalan, Ferreira, Sedivy, and Herbig, 2006).

A third class of gene action predicted by the evolutionary theory, called *mutation accumulation* (Medawar, 1957), involves mutations whose phenotypic effects do not reach a significant threshold until after the peak of reproduction, when physiological assays show declines in function of many body systems. Nature therefore cannot effectively select against such mutations, and they can accumulate in certain pedigrees, creating the "private" mechanisms of aging just referred to. While individually rare, there are potentially vast numbers of such mutations. Three such genetic loci have already been documented as bearing dominant mutations leading to Alzheimer's disease (reviewed by Tanzi and Bertram, 2005). Although referred to as early onset cases, these forms of dementia typically unfold in late middle age and thus usually will have escaped the force of natural selection. Recent research has revealed a growing list of genes whose mutations can lead to forms of Parkinson's disease (Hardy and others, 2006).

WHAT THE FUTURE HOLDS

For the immediate future, given the very recent decline in research funding by the National Institutes of Health (Zerhouni, 2006), the pace of biomedical research may well decline somewhat and we may lose young investigators to other occupations. This is quite unfortunate, as the opportunities for progress have been growing exponentially, as evidenced, for example, by the data of Figure 23.1. Some scientists have made extraordinary claims, suggesting that we are now close to the stage of engineering very substantial enhancements of life spans and health spans (de Grey, 2005). Most biogerontologists do not agree with such claims, given the fact that we remain ignorant of the detailed mechanisms of aging. Moreover, interventions typically come with tradeoffs. For example, let's assume that it will be possible in the not-too-distant future to develop drugs that mimic the effects of dietary restriction in rodents. First of all, we do not yet know if dietary restriction will have comparable effects in human subjects. Second, given the marked genetic heterogeneity of our species, there is likely to be substantial variability in the response to any such intervention ("one man's meat is another man's poison"). Third, not all subjects will be happy about a tradeoff that involves a decrease or cessation of reproduction or a possible effect on libido.

Nonetheless, there are some encouraging developments that could lead to interventions in particularly susceptible individuals. There is, for example, considerable interest in a recent publication indicating that large doses of a polyphenolic compound found in red wine (resveratrol, trans-3,5,4'-trihydroxystilbene) can normalize the patterns of gene expression, improve the insulin sensitivities, and increase the life spans of overfed, obese mice (Baur and others, 2006). At least one biotechnology company is said to be now actively pursuing the synthesis of related compounds that might have greater specific activities. Meanwhile, we do not recommend drinking the amount of red wine (some three hundred glasses per day) needed to match the dose of resveratrol used in these experiments with mice!

There is also reason to celebrate the emergence of the field of regenerative medicine. A particularly exciting recent finding has been the observation that defects in the repair of skeletal muscles of aging mice are due not to a deficiency of muscle satellite cells (the stem cells of skeletal muscle), but to a deficiency in the microenvironments of such cells. The deficiency could be corrected by a circulating factor or factors found in young animals (Conboy and others, 2005). The implications for therapy are substantial, particularly if this obtains for many types of stem cells, as one might be able to develop small molecular weight compounds that could "awaken" the stem cells in older individuals.

CONCLUSIONS

We can conclude that there has been striking progress in our understanding of basic mechanisms of aging, but that we are still a long way from applying this knowledge for the "engineering" of unusually long and healthy life spans. There are both common ("public") and unusual ("private") ways to age. Any future attempts at intervention must take this into account.

REFERENCES

Austad, S. N. "Retarded Senescence in an Insular Population of Virginia Possums (*Didelphis virginiana*)." *Journal of Zoology* (London), 1993, *229*, 695–708.

Austad, S. N. *Why We Age: What Science Is Discovering About the Body's Journey Through Life*. New York: Wiley, 1997.

Baudisch, A. "Hamilton's Indicators of the Force of Selection." *Proceedings of the National Academy of Sciences of the United States of America*, 2005, *102*, 8263–8268.

Baur, J. A., and others. "Resveratrol Improves Health and Survival of Mice on a High-Calorie Diet." *Nature*, 2006, *444*, 337–342.

Bernhard, D., Moser, C., Backovic, A., and Wick, G. "Cigarette Smoke—An Aging Accelerator?" *Experimental Gerontology*, 2006, *42*, 160–165.

Burns, D. M. "Cigarettes and Cigarette Smoking." *Clinics in Chest Medicine*, 1991, *12*, 631–642.

Campisi, J. 2005. "Aging, Tumor Suppression and Cancer: High-Wire Act!" *Mechanisms of Ageing and Development*, 2005, *126*, 51–58.

Conboy, I. M., and others. "Rejuvenation of Aged Progenitor Cells by Exposure to a Young Systemic Environment." *Nature*, 2005, *433*, 760–764.

de Grey, A. D. "The SENS Challenge: 20,000 U.S. Dollars Says the Foreseeable Defeat of Aging Is Not Laughable." *Rejuvenation Research*, 2005, *8*, 207–210.

Finch, C. E., and Tanzi, R. E. "Genetics of Aging." *Science*, 1997, *278*, 407–411.

George, J. C., and others. "Age and Growth Estimates of Bowhead Whales (*Balaena mysticetus*) via Aspartic Acid Racemization." *Canadian Journal of Zoology*, 1999, *77*, 571–580.

Hardy, J., and others. "Genetics of Parkinson's Disease and Parkinsonism." *Annals of Neurology*, 2006, *60*, 389–398.

Hodes, R. J., Mc Cormick, A. M., and Pruzan, M. "Longevity Assurance Genes: How Do They Influence Aging and Life Span?" *Journal of the American Geriatrics Society*, 1996, *44*, 988–991.

Jeyapalan, J. C., Ferreira, M., Sedivy, J. M., and Herbig, U. "Accumulation of Senescent Cells in Mitotic Tissue of Aging Primates." *Mechanisms of Ageing and Development*, 2006, *128*, 36–44.

Kaplan, H. S. and Robson, A. J. "The Emergence of Humans: The Coevolution of Intelligence and Longevity with Intergenerational Transfers." *Proceedings of the National Academy of Sciences of the United States of America*, 2002, *99*, 10221–10226.

Lederberg, J. "Genetic Approaches to Somatic Cell Variation: Summary Comment." *Journal of Cellular and Comparative Physiology*, 1958, *52*(Supp. 1), 383–401.

Lee, R. D. "Rethinking the Evolutionary Theory of Aging: Transfers, Not Births, Shape Senescence in Social Species." *Proceedings of the National Academy of Sciences of the United States of America,* 2003, *100,* 9637–9642.

Martin, G. M. "Genetics and the Pathobiology of Ageing." *Philosophical Transactions of the Royal Society of London. Series B, Biological Sciences,* 1997, *352,* 1773–1780.

Martin, G. M. "Genetic Modulation of Senescent Phenotypes in *Homo sapiens.*" *Cell,* 2005, *120,* 523–532.

Masoro, E. J. 2005. "Overview of Caloric Restriction and Ageing." *Mechanisms of Ageing and Development, 126,* 913–922.

Medawar, P. B. "An Unsolved Problem of Biology." In P. B. Medawar (ed.), *The Uniqueness of the Individual,* 44–70. London: Methuenand, 1957.

Patnaik, B. K., Mahapatro, N., and Jena, B. S. "Ageing in Fishes." *Gerontology,* 1994, *40,* 113–132.

Rea, S. L., and others. "A Stress-Sensitive Reporter Predicts Longevity in Isogenic Populations of *Caenorhabditis elegans.*" *Nature Genetics,* 2005, *37,* 894–898.

Rose, M. R. *Evolutionary Biology of Aging.* New York: Oxford University Press, 1991.

Shay, J. W., and Wright, W. E. "Hayflick, His Limit, and Cellular Ageing." *Nature Reviews. Molecular Cell Biology,* 2000, *1,* 72–76.

Sinclair, D. A., and Guarente, L. "Unlocking the Secrets of Longevity Genes." *Scientific American,* 2006, *294,* 48–7.

Sioud, M. "Main Approaches to Target Discovery and Validation." *Methods in Molecular Biology,* 2006, *360,* 1–12.

Tanzi, R. E., and Bertram, L. "Twenty Years of the Alzheimer's Disease Amyloid Hypothesis: A Genetic Perspective." *Cell,* 2005, *120,* 545–555.

Vanfleteren, J. R., De, V. A., and Braeckman, B. P. "Two-Parameter Logistic and Weibull Equations Provide Better Fits to Survival Data from Isogenic Populations of *Caenorhabditis elegans* in Axenic Culture Than Does the Gompertz Model." *Journals of Gerontology, Series A, Biological Sciences and Medical Sciences,* 1998, *53,* B393–B403.

Wallace, D. C. "A Mitochondrial Paradigm of Metabolic and Degenerative Diseases, Aging, and Cancer: A Dawn for Evolutionary Medicine." *Annual Review of Genetics,* 2005, *39,* 359–407.

Williams, G. C. "Pleiotropy, Natural Selection, and the Evolution of Senescence." *Evolution,* 1957, *11,* 398–411.

Zerhouni, E. A. "Research Funding: NIH in the Post-Doubling Era: Realities and Strategies." *Science,* 2006, *314,* 1088–1090.

CHAPTER

EXCEPTIONAL LONGEVITY

THOMAS PERLS AND DELLARA F. TERRY

TWO PEOPLE, TWO DIFFERENT PATHS

Nola Ochs and Fred Fogarty have both achieved exceptionally old age, but along very different paths.

Nola Ochs

Nola Ochs, a member of Fort Hays State College's senior class, made history in 2007 when she finished her bachelor's degree. Ochs, who turned ninety-five in November 2006, became the oldest person to graduate from this college. Having witnessed the 1918 flu pandemic, both world wars, the Dust Bowl, the Depression, the rise and fall of communism in Eastern Europe, and the advent of the air, electronics, and computer ages, Ochs has been a firsthand source of information about nearly a century of scientific, political, economic, and social changes for her classmates at Fort Hays. She's also living testimony to the contribution a healthy lifestyle can make to longevity and vitality.

"I don't come from a particularly long lived family," says Ochs, whose youthful voice belies her age. Except for a bout with breast cancer, which was successfully treated in 1983, and mild hypertension that's responded well to drugs, Ochs has had no health problems to speak of. She sees a family practitioner, but her checkups tend to be brief. "Because there's not a problem, we don't have a lot to talk about," she says.

A full-time student at Fort Hays, Ochs lives in an apartment on campus and walks regularly. During school breaks and on occasional weekends, she drives twenty-six miles to her farm. Her husband died in 1972 and three of her sons, who own farms nearby, take care of her place while she's away. "I thought I'd go home more often, but I'm too busy with course work," says Ochs. On Sundays, she attends church and catches up with her friends who aren't students.

Ochs considers her longevity and vitality blessings, but allows that her healthy, life-long habits may also figure into the equation. She's always eaten a healthy diet, maintained a healthy weight, exercised regularly, and stayed socially and intellectually engaged.

Born in 1911 in rural Illinois in a home with neither running water nor electricity, Ochs was the first of three children. Her parents were farmers. When she was two months old, the family moved to northwestern Nebraska, where her younger sister and brother were born. "Because my brother was younger than me by several years, I helped my father on the farm early on, while my sister helped my mother around the house," she recalls.

Shortly after Ochs turned sixteen, her family moved again, to Hodgman County, Kansas, where she finished high school and began teaching—but she had to stop four years later, when she married Vernon Ochs, a local wheat farmer. "That was a condition of getting the job—you had to stop when you got married because they didn't want the teacher to be pregnant in the school," she explains.

So Ochs went back to farming, working alongside her husband and, later, their four sons, "Farm work is hard work but I enjoyed it; even now I like to do yard work," she says. In addition to physical work, she's always enjoyed intellectual challenges, and she started taking classes at a nearby community college after the boys were on their own. One of her first courses was an agribusiness marketing class. She applied much of what she learned to the management of the family farm. One course led to another, and one day a professor on campus told her that she needed only to take an algebra class to finish her associate's degree. She did—and immediately enrolled at a local four-year college to work on her bachelor's degree. The school closed that same year, but Ochs, undeterred, transferred to Fort Hays. "I enjoy being on campus and I've always enjoyed learning situations," she says.

Once she's earned her bachelor's, will she apply to grad school? No, says Ochs, who also loves to travel. "I'm going to seek employment on a cruise ship as a story-teller," she explains, laughing. "You know, there are so many opportunities today that we can do most anything that appeals to us. This is a great time to be ninety-five; I'm really enjoying it."

Frank Fogarty

Frank Fogarty isn't one of those people who has always done what you're supposed to do to live a long and healthy life. He smoked half a pack of cigarettes a day for ten years when he was a young man. He indulged in a couple of plugs of chewing tobacco here and there. For a long time, he smoked a pipe or two daily. He wasn't much of a fruit and vegetable eater, either—until he started working at a produce shop and was sent home with the stuff. That was about a decade ago, when he was ninety. On July 22, 2007, Fogarty turned one hundred.

As we'll discuss later in this chapter, considerable research suggests that heredity plays a role in longevity and is a particularly important factor in determining who lives to extreme old age. That certainly seems to be the case in Fogarty's family: his grandfather lived to 108, a sister to 101. Another sister is 97; a third is 93.

Forgarty has had a few health problems. At sixty-five he needed hip replacement surgery, and shortly afterward it was discovered that he had high blood pressure. He takes medication for that, for an enlarged prostate, and to prevent seizures: the first seizure he had at age ninety-four prompted his physician to prescribe medication, and Fogarty hasn't had a seizure since. He is quite fit, sharp, and independent at one hundred. Every day he rides a stationary bike for fifteen minutes and performs a series of strength-training exercises that his doctor recommended. Since his second wife died two years ago, he's lived alone in their home in Gloversville, a town in upstate New York. An aide comes each morning and afternoon to help him with chores around the house and with shopping, since he no longer drives. Other than that, he manages on his own.

Born in Ireland's County Galway in 1907, Fogarty—one of seventeen children—was independent early on. When he was young, his parents owned a small grocery store. After the English closed the shop during the Irish War of Independence—"I saw a lot of trouble then," he says—his parents bought some land and raised much of their own food. "Ireland was a very, very poor country when I was young," he says. "There was always enough to eat when I was growing up—but not like today." Breakfast was oatmeal. Other meals were heavy on potatoes and meat. "We'd kill a pig and eat it," Fogarty recalls. "And for Christmas we had goose."

Fogarty's diet may have been less than ideal, but he always got plenty of exercise—usually on the job. At nineteen, he left Ireland for Windsor, Canada, and soon after that made the short trip to nearby Detroit, Michigan, where he worked on an assembly line at the Ford Motor Company. He earned $8 a day. After two years at Ford, he took a job as a domestic servant in the home of a wealthy Grosse Pointe, Michigan, family before making a final move to Gloversville in 1932.

In its heyday, the town, with its multitude of glove factories, made one of every three pair of gloves manufactured worldwide. A year after settling in Gloversville, Fogarty married, and he and his wife opened their own company, Fogarty Embroidery, which embroidered gloves. In 1938 the couple had a son, John, their only child, who recently retired from a career as a chemical engineer. After closing the glove shop in 1966, Fogarty started a well-drilling business that he ran until 1997. That year, the year he turned ninety, he started working at his neighbors' produce shop. In 2005, he fell and broke his tailbone, and though he made a complete recovery, he decided, finally, to give retirement a try.

"If you want to live long, well . . . you've got to exercise and keep busy," advises Fogarty, who still has an extremely active social life, often visiting, dining with, and going out with friends. Of course, it doesn't hurt to have good genes, as well.

THE NEW ENGLAND CENTENARIAN STUDY (NECS)

The NECS was founded in 1995 as the first population-based study of centenarians in the United States. To locate all the centenarians living in eight municipalities near Boston (with a total population of 450,000), the NECS relied primarily on local annual census records, but also Councils on Aging, local geriatricians, nursing home administrators, and media coverage of centenarian birthdays. All subjects' ages were systematically verified (predominantly by birth certificate). Although the sensitivity of the local censuses for detecting centenarians was extremely high (99 percent), the specificity was only 28 to 31 percent due to mortality, emigration, and both intentional and unintentional age misreporting. The low specificity was effectively overcome by achieving an 83-percent success rate in determining the validated age, living status (alive or dead), and current living situation (home, assisted living, or nursing home) of all potentially eligible subjects.

On a specific date, all known centenarians or their caregivers were contacted to determine if they were alive or dead, and a prevalence of forty-five centenarians (a population ratio of one centenarian per ten thousand people) was determined. Sixty-one percent lived in a nursing home or assisted living, 27 percent lived with family, and 12 percent lived alone. The study achieved a 53-percent enrollment rate of age-validated centenarians. As findings emerged, suggesting the need for larger samples of not only centenarians but also their family members and control subjects, the NECS grew to be international in scope.

CENTENARIAN DEMOGRAPHICS

According to the U.S. Census Bureau, in 1991 there were approximately thirty-seven thousand centenarians. In 2001, the estimate was forty-eight thousand, an increase of 35 percent over ten years. Among the developed countries in general, the number of centenarians is increasing at the rate of about 8 percent per year (Vaupel and others, 1998). At the turn of the twentieth century in the United States, approximately one in one hundred thousand was a centenarian; as of 2000 the ratio is about 1.2 per ten thousand (U.S. Census Bureau, 2000). As shown in Figure 24.1, the United Nations (UN) estimated that in 2000 there were 180,000 centenarians worldwide. By 2050, the report World Population Ageing 1950–2050 estimates that the number of centenarians will increase by eighteen times, to 3.2 million. Japan is projected to experience the greatest country-specific growth, from thirteen thousand in 2000 to almost one million in 2050 (one centenarian per hundred in the population) (*World Population Ageing 1950–2050 Population Division, 2006*).

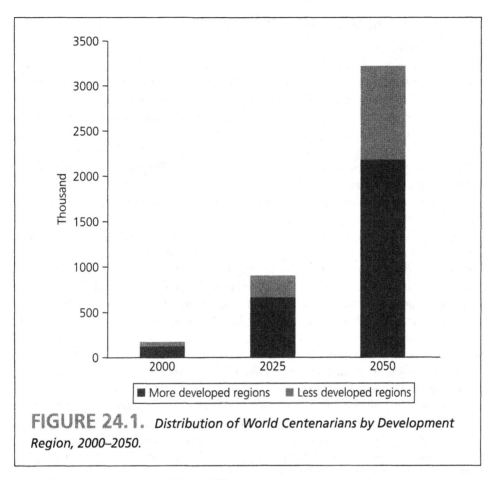

FIGURE 24.1. *Distribution of World Centenarians by Development Region, 2000–2050.*

Source: United Nations Population Division, 2001.

This dramatic increase in the number of the centenarians is likely the result of relatively recent (over the past century) public health measures that have allowed people who would have otherwise succumbed to preventable or treatable causes of childhood or premature mortality to survive to a much older age (Oeppen and Vaupel, 2002). Treatment of now readily reversible causes of death among older people is also making a significant impact. In fact, in most recent decades, reductions in mortality at the oldest ages have made significant contributions to increased survival and to the increase in the number of centenarians. As a result, many more people with favorable genetic and environmental traits are now able to achieve their maximum life expectancy (Vaupel and others, 1998). In some countries, such as China and Japan, the number of younger people relative to the older population is shrinking, which also contributes to the increasing proportion of the oldest old in the population.

MAXIMUM AVERAGE LIFE EXPECTANCY

What is the maximum life expectancy for most people? To determine this, ideally we would take a very large heterogeneous sample of people, impose maximally healthy behaviors on them in a maximally healthy environment, and see how old they live to be. Unfortunately, we are not sure what those behaviors and environments are, and it is likely that their impact on life expectancy varies substantially from one population to another and even from one individual to another. A population that might at least come close to revealing the optimal set of factors is the Seventh Day Adventists. This geographically and racially heterogeneous group has the longest average life expectancy in the United States, at eighty-eight years. This is likely due to behaviors dictated by their religion that are also conducive to good health and longevity (Fraser and Shavlik, 2001), including consuming no tobacco or alcohol (though there is evidence that regular moderate alcohol intake may be good for you), a vegetarian diet, moderate dietary intake, and regular exercise. Additionally, Seventh Day Adventists dedicate substantial time to family and religion, which may be conducive to effectively managing stress. It appears that the average life expectancy of Americans is ten years less than that of the Adventists because many Americans do not adhere to these healthy habits. This observation suggests that the majority of the variation around average life expectancy is explained by variations in people's behaviors. Along the same lines, twin studies have estimated the environmental or behavioral component of life expectancy to be around 75 percent (McGue, Vaupel, Holm, and Harvald, 1993). Note, however, that these twin studies do not estimate the heritability of living to extreme old age (that is, near or at maximum life span) because the oldest subjects in these studies are only octogenarians. Centenarians, who live an additional fifteen to twenty years beyond average life expectancy, may require more than an advantage in their habits and environment; they may require a genetic advantage that translates into a significant inherited component to exceptional longevity.

BIRTH AND OTHER COHORT-SPECIFIC DETERMINANTS OF EXCEPTIONAL LONGEVITY

Although the increase in average life expectancy over the past century seems to paint a very optimistic picture, significantly disturbing trends have emerged in the general population and in particular among socioeconomically disadvantaged groups. Olshansky and colleagues have pointed out that increasing rates of obesity, particularly among children, are leading to increased rates of age-related illnesses that could even cause a deceleration in survival rates (Olshansky and others, 2005). Although rates of smoking are markedly declining among men, this is not the case among women, teenagers, or minorities. The substantial disparity in mortality rates beyond the age of twenty between Caucasians and African Americans could be dramatically improved if we were much more effective in detecting and treating hypertension in the latter group. Hispanics experience disproportionate rates of diabetes mellitus. In East Harlem,

New York, having type 2 diabetes is nearly considered the norm rather than the exception, with many people experiencing resultant morbidities such as blindness, congestive heart failure, amputations, and kidney failure.

As described in the following section, various genetic and epidemiological studies are attempting to delineate factors and markers associated with exceptional longevity. However, over the past hundred years, humans have experienced major changes in their exposures that likely dramatically change the landscape of genetic and environmental interactions that facilitate survival to extreme old age. In the case of developed countries, a very abbreviated list, for example, would include, on the positive side, a clean water supply, increased years of education, improved obstetrical care, antibiotics and vaccines, and surgical techniques. On the negative side are a decrease in daily activities conducive to physical fitness, an increase in smoking behaviors, excessive alcohol use, marked changes in the quantities and types of food people eat, relatively recent estrogenic pollutants, and medications and over-the-counter nutraceuticals with undetected long-term side effects. Given these and many other cohort-specific exposures, it may be quite difficult to predict future longevity based on the genetic and environmental "risk" profiles of centenarians. Nonetheless, there are likely numerous factors—what we might call *robust* or *secular trend-insensitive* risk factors—that confer either beneficial effects (such as increased muscle mass for females) or detrimental effects (such as tobacco use, the apolipoprotein E ε-4 allele) (Schachter and others, 1994).

GENDER DIFFERENCES

With very few exceptions, in most populations the vast majority of centenarians are women—generally 85 percent in developed nations. An exception to the rule may be Sardinia, Italy, where the demographer Michel Poulain has reported that approximately 50 percent of centenarians, particularly those living in the mountainous region of the island, are male (Poulain and others, 2004).

Despite the fact that many more women than men achieve exceptional longevity, among centenarians the men generally have better functional status (Franceschi and others, 2000). It may be that men must be in excellent health to achieve such extreme old age. Women, on the other hand, may be more adept at living with age-associated illnesses, and thus able to achieve exceptional old age even with significant chronic disability, particularly compared to men of similar age. These observations may indicate a demographic crossover whereby women are better off than men in younger old age and men, although fewer in number, are functionally better off in extreme old age.

There are various theories why women live longer than men. Estrogen may be one cause. However, it has been noted that premenopausal women who undergo hysterectomy but not oophrectomy experience an increased risk of diastolic hypertension (Luoto, Kaprio, Reunanen, and Rutanen, 1995). Also, compared with men, women are relatively iron-deficient during the thirty to forty years in which they menstruate. Iron is a crucial catalyst in mitochondrial production of free radicals, by-products of normal metabolism. Perhaps a reduction in available iron leads to less free-radical production. For example, blood donation has been associated with reduced cardiovascular disease (CVD) risk (Meyers, Jensen, and Menitove, 2002). In addition, diets high in heme have been associated with significantly increased risk of heart disease (Qi, van Dam, Rexrode, and Hu, 2007).

Another potential female advantage that scientists have studied relates to the fact that males possess one X chromosome whereas women have two. Women thus have the prospect for somatic cell selection with advancing age, whereby the more fit of two somatic cell populations survives. Stem cell populations that give rise to highly proliferative cell populations (for example, intestinal and skin epithelium, leukocytes) would be particularly prone to such selection. The genes on the X chromosome that effect telomere length are of particular interest, in part because those cell populations that resist oxidative stress better may have longer telomeres. Increased telomere length has been associated with both improved proliferative capacity and decreased mortality (Cawthon and others, 2003).

CENTENARIANS: RARE, YET THE FASTEST-GROWING GROUP IN DEVELOPED COUNTRIES

Hypotheses for the rarity of centenarians have included the notion that surviving to extreme old age requires rare exposure(s), perhaps both genetic and environmental. However, if slower aging and delay of or escape from age-related morbidity are viewed as an evolutionary advantage (for example, to be better able to care for offspring or to be available to care for grandchildren) (Hawkes, 2004), then one would expect these genetic and environmental variations to be more common and for there to be many more centenarians.

A clue as to why centenarians are so rare comes from our study of centenarian sibships. Along with John Wilmoth, Ph.D., of the University of California, Berkley's Department of Demography, we analyzed the pedigrees of 444 centenarian families in the United States that included 2,092 siblings of centenarians (Perls, 2002). Survival was compared to 1900 birth cohort survival data from the U.S. Social Security Administration. As shown in Figure 24.2, female siblings experienced death rates at all ages that were about one-half the national level for their birth cohort; male siblings had a similar advantage at most ages, though diminished somewhat during adolescence and young adulthood.

Obviously, genetics alone cannot explain a mortality rate that is half the average of the birth cohort for the ages between twenty and one hundred years. Many behaviors and exposures that family members also have in common are likely also important, such as years of education, access to health care, dietary habits, exercise, not smoking, and other factors yet to be elucidated. It is likely that centenarians are rare because surviving to one hundred requires that a person experience a rare combination of individually common factors. For example, Nola Ochs, mentioned earlier, has generally very healthy behaviors, and perhaps her added years of education at an advanced

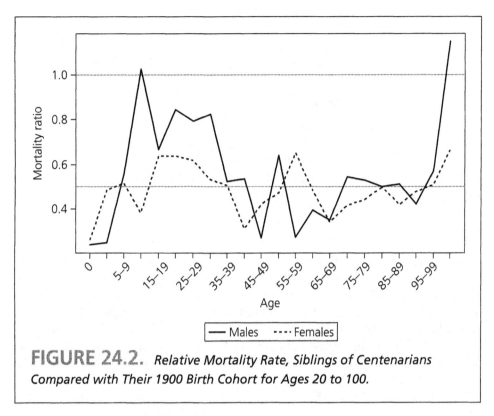

FIGURE 24.2. *Relative Mortality Rate, Siblings of Centenarians Compared with Their 1900 Birth Cohort for Ages 20 to 100.*

Source: Perls and others, 2002.

age also have played an important role. Also, in terms of genetics, she likely lacks genetic variations that predispose to premature lethal illnesses (disease genes) and perhaps has variations that relatively slow the rate of aging and decrease susceptibility to age-related illnesses (longevity enabling genes). On the other hand, our other profiled centenarian, Frank Fogarty, is a man—which makes him much less likely than a woman to live to one hundred—and he also has a long history of smoking. The impressive number of other relatives in his family also reaching one hundred and over speaks to the likelihood that he has genetic variations that are exceptionally good at combating and repairing damage by factors related to aging as well as smoking. As the cases of these two centenarians point out, a very important challenge for scientists studying exceptional longevity is the great deal of variation in the combination of factors that facilitate exceptional survival.

Figure 24.3 illustrates, in a reductionist manner, the complex interaction of disease-predisposing and longevity-enabling exposures and genetic variations that lead to different patterns of exceptional survival, which then lead to exceptional longevity. For example, based on the occurrence of the most common diseases of aging, Evert,

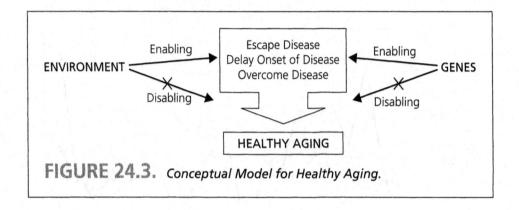

FIGURE 24.3. *Conceptual Model for Healthy Aging.*

Lawler, Bogan, and Perls (2003) noted that centenarians in the NECS sample fit into one of three categories: survivors, delayers, and escapers. In Figure 24.3, these categories are examples of different patterns of dealing with age-related diseases. Survivors were individuals diagnosed with age-related illness prior to age eighty (24 percent of the male and 43 percent of the female centenarians). Delayers were individuals who delayed the onset of age-related diseases until at least age eighty (44 percent of the male and 42 percent of the female centenarians). Escapers were individuals who attained their hundredth year of life without the diagnosis of an age-related disease (32 percent of the male and 15 percent of the female centenarians). In the case of CVD and stroke, which are typically associated with relatively high mortality risk compared with more chronic diseases such as osteoporosis, only 12 percent of subjects were survivors and the remaining 88 percent of centenarians delayed or escaped these diseases.

Why are centenarians the fastest-growing segment of industrialized countries? An analogy may be a lottery. In the past, a person needed seven numbers (or some number or "doses" of genetic and environmental factors) in the right combination to win the lottery (or to live to one hundred). But now, because of improvements in the public health, education, and medical interventions, some of those numbers need no longer be left to chance, so the odds of living to extreme old age have increased.

PURPORTED GEOGRAPHIC CLUSTERING FOR EXCEPTIONAL LONGEVITY

Several geographical areas have claimed inhabitants with extreme longevity, but after closer examination these claims have been found to be false. Vilacamba, Ecuador, almost became a tourist attraction because natives claimed their water was a fountain of youth, leading to the many super-centenarians (aged over 110 years) in that region. What about the reports of people in the Russian Caucasus living to 150 years and beyond? In fact, those purported super-centenarians were taking on the identities of their parents, aunts, and uncles (Mazes and Forman, 1979).

Still, the regions of purported exceptional longevity merit careful study. Though claims of extreme age were disproved, there still may be an unusually high prevalence of very old fit people in these regions. In the Tibetan mountains, for instance, octogenarian and nonagenarian elders reportedly herd livestock and still lead physically strenuous lives.

NATURE VERSUS NURTURE: THE RELATIVE ROLES OF GENES AND EXPOSURES

In the survival study of centenarian siblings noted earlier, the siblings had a mean age at death of seventy-seven for females and seventy for males, compared with fifty-eight and fifty-two for the general population born around the same time. Even after accounting for race and education, the net survival advantage of siblings of centenarians was found to be sixteen to seventeen years more than the general population. A similar finding of reduced mortality amongst siblings of centenarians was found in a study of 348 Okinawan families (Willcox and others, 2006). Relative survival probabilities (RSP) for the New England Centenarian Study siblings increased markedly at older ages, reflecting the cumulative effect of their mortality advantage throughout life (see Table 24.1). Compared with the U.S. 1900 birth cohort, male siblings of centenarians were 17 times as likely to attain age one hundred themselves, whereas female siblings were 8.2 times as likely (Perls, 2002).

The analysis of death rates indicates that the mortality advantage of siblings does not increase as they get older. Rather, their relative survival probability (RSP) is a cumulative measure and reflects their lifelong advantage over the general population born about the same time. Such elevated RSP values support the hypothesis that centenarian family members have genetic variations in common that are important to achieving exceptional longevity. Furthermore, mortality rates of different groups (such as gender, race, education, physical activity, socioeconomic status) converge at very old age; thus such a sustained advantage is unusual (Perls, 2002). The substantially higher RSP values for men at older ages may reflect the fact that male disease-specific mortality is significantly higher than for females at these older ages and thus the males experience a greater relative advantage from beneficial genotypes compared with women. It's also possible that an even greater and thus more rare combination of genetic and environmental factors is required for men to achieve extreme age compared to women. Either possibility could explain why men make up only 15 percent of centenarians.

Another clue supporting a strong familial role in achieving exceptional longevity emerged from our identification of six families who demonstrated exceptional clustering for extreme old age. In one family, five out of seven siblings attained the age of one hundred or older and twenty-one out of forty cousins were nonagenarians or older

TABLE 24.1. Relative Survival Probability (RSP) with 95% Confidence Intervals (CI) of Siblings of Centenarians versus U.S. 1900 Birth Cohort.

| Age | MALES | | | FEMALES | | |
	RSP	Lower 95% CI	Upper 95% CI	RSP	Lower 95% CI	Upper 95% CI
20	1.00	1.00	1.00	1.00	1.00	1.00
25	1.00	0.99	1.01	1.01	1.00	1.02
60	1.18	1.15	1.21	1.12	1.09	1.14
65	1.29	1.25	1.33	1.16	1.13	1.19
70	1.48	1.42	1.53	1.24	1.21	1.28
75	1.68	1.60	1.77	1.36	1.31	1.41
80	2.03	1.90	2.16	1.54	1.47	1.60
85	2.69	2.47	2.91	1.83	1.73	1.93
90	4.08	3.62	4.54	2.56	2.39	2.74
95	8.35	6.98	9.71	4.15	3.73	4.57
100	17.0	10.8	23.1	8.22	6.55	9.90

Source: Perls, 2002.

(Perls and others, 2000). The probability of encountering families such as these by chance is less than one per all the families that exist in the world today. Thus these family members must have factors in common with one another that facilitate such longevity.

Studies of the offspring of centenarians also support the strong familial component of living to extreme old age. Using a questionnaire-based cross-sectional study design, Dr. Dellara Terry, codirector of the NECS, led a study of the health histories of a nationwide sample of centenarian offspring (n = 176) and a comparison group of subjects (n = 166) who had at least one parent who died at age seventy-three years (the average life expectancy for that birth cohort). Compared to the referent cohort, centenarian offspring were found to have a 56-percent reduced relative prevalence of heart disease, a 66-percent reduced relative prevalence of hypertension, and a 59-percent reduced relative prevalence of diabetes after multivariate adjusted analyses that controlled for age, sex, gender, years of education, annual income, instrumental activities of daily living (IADLs) score, ethnicity, marital status, exercise, smoking, and alcohol use. Centenarian offspring did not have a lower prevalence of diseases such as cancer, stroke, dementia, osteoporosis, glaucoma, macular degeneration, depression, Parkinson's disease, thyroid disease, and chronic obstructive pulmonary disease (COPD). There may be no difference because centenarian offspring do not have differential susceptibility to these diseases or, alternatively, because of the choice of referent cohort or a function of the sample size.

Some may argue that there are differences between the two groups because the referent cohort is enriched for the early onset of CVD and CVD risk factors, not because the centenarian offspring are enriched for CVD and CVD risk factor–free survival. However, the frequencies of the referent cohort subjects reporting CVD and hypertension were nearly identical to the age-adjusted national data from the National Health Interview Survey (NHIS) (http://www.cdc.gov/nchs/data/series/sr_10/sr10_228.pdf) for individuals aged seventy-five and over: 27 percent of referent cohort members reported CVD, compared with 26.1 percent in the NHIS; 52 percent of the referent cohort members reported hypertension, compared with 55.4 percent in the NHIS. The similar rates suggest that the APL referent cohort is similar to average members of its birth cohort and that the centenarian offspring are therefore enriched for CVD-free survival.

For the centenarian offspring who did report hypertension, the age of onset was significantly older when compared to the APL referent cohort, as is demonstrated in Figure 24.4. Similar delays were noted for the age of onset of coronary heart disease, diabetes, and stroke.

Centenarian offspring also had a 62-percent risk reduction in all-cause mortality. When cause-specific mortality was examined, centenarian offspring had an 85-percent risk reduction in coronary heart disease-specific mortality and a 71-percent risk reduction in cancer-specific mortality (Terry and others, 2004). These recent findings suggest that survival to exceptional old age may involve a decreased susceptibility to CVD as well as, perhaps, a decreased susceptibility to a broad range of age-related diseases, possibly secondary to inhibition of basic contributors to aging.

The observed familial aggregation for exceptional longevity is likely because of important factors, both environmental and genetic, that family members have in common. The familial studies described here do not help us discern what proportion of this aggregation is genetic versus environmental and behavioral. Twin studies have the potential of differentiating between genetic and exposure influences and have estimated the heritability of life span to range between 25 percent and 60 percent.

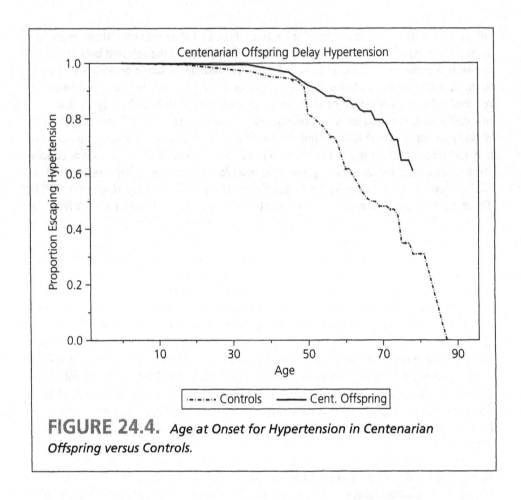

FIGURE 24.4. *Age at Onset for Hypertension in Centenarian Offspring versus Controls.*

Ljungquist and colleagues (1998), after assessing heritability in 10,505 Swedish twin pairs reared together and apart, attributed 35 percent of the variance in longevity to genetic influences and 65 percent of the variance to nonshared environmental effects. However, the oldest subjects in the twin studies were in their mid- to late eighties and the majority lived to average life expectancy.

To better address exceptional longevity, Kaare Christensen and colleagues recently analyzed survival data from Danish, Finnish, and Swedish twins born between 1870 and 1910 and found that the relative recurrence risk of reaching age ninety-two was 4.8 for monozygotic males compared to 1.8 for dizygotic males and 2.5 for monozygotic females versus 1.6 for dizygotic females (Hjelmborg and others, 2006). From these findings, the authors concluded that there might be an increasingly greater genetic component to survival at extreme ages.

GENETIC STUDIES

Collaborating with the NECS, Puca and colleagues (2001) conducted a genome-wide sibling pair linkage study to discover polymorphisms linked to EL. A group of 137 centenarians and their 171 siblings were included in a genome-wide concordant sib-pair study. Using nonparametric analysis, significant evidence for linkage was noted for a locus on chromosome 4 at D4S1564 with a maximum logarithm-of-odds score of 3.65 (P = 0.044). A detailed haplotype map was created of the chromosome 4 locus that extended over twelve million base pairs and involved the genotyping of more than one thousand single-nucleotide polymorphism (SNP) markers in two hundred centenarians and two hundred controls. The resulting genetic association study identified a haplotype marker in the microsomal transfer protein (MTP) gene as a modifier of human life span (Geesaman and others, 2003). All known SNPs for MTP and its promoter were genotyped in two hundred centenarians and two hundred young controls. After haplotype reconstruction of the area was completed, a single variant—the –493 G/T variant in the promoter of MTP—was underrepresented in the long-lived individuals, accounting for the majority of the statistical variability at the locus (~15 percent among the subjects versus 23 percent in the controls). The finding was replicated in a second set of 250 centenarians and 250 controls in the United States but not in two European populations. As MTP is rate-limiting in lipoprotein synthesis, this may affect longevity by subtly modulating this pathway. Considering that CVD is significantly delayed among the offspring of centenarians and that 88 percent of centenarians either delay or escape CVD and stroke beyond the age of eighty, it follows that the frequency of genetic polymorphisms that play a role in the risk for such diseases would be differentiated between centenarians and the general population (Evert, Lawler, Bogan, and Perls, 2003; Terry and others, 2003).

A study of Ashkenazi Jewish centenarians and their families identified another cardiovascular pathway and gene that is differentiated between centenarians and controls (Barzilai and others, 2003). Researchers noted that HDL and LDL particles were significantly larger among the centenarians and their offspring, and that particle size also differentiated between subjects with and without CVD, hypertension, and metabolic syndrome. In a candidate-gene approach, the researchers then searched the literature for genes that affect HDL and LDL particle size; genes encoding hepatic lipase and cholesteryl ester transfer protein (CETP) emerged as candidates. Comparing centenarians and their offspring against controls, levels of one variant of CETP were noted to be significantly increased among those with, or predisposed to, exceptional longevity.

Having noted the above study findings, it is important to realize that except for apolipoprotein E, most positive studies comparing centenarians and controls have demonstrated relatively modest differences in allelic frequencies. Again, it may be that centenarians are rare not because of a few rare factors, but rather because of rare combinations of genetic and environmental exposures. Furthermore, these latter observations appear to vary substantially depending on the population sample or control (or both) being studied. Even in the case of apolipoprotein E, an exception to the rule was noted in a large Korean centenarian cohort (Choi and others, 2003). Thus, not only are rare combinations likely important, but also their significance varies across populations. The difficulty in reproducing these findings speaks to the importance of ethnicity and environmental factors that can result in very different survival-related outcomes for specific genotypes.

WHAT DOES IT TAKE TO LIVE TO ONE HUNDRED?

Centenarian studies are relatively young, with formal scientifically rigorous studies beginning in the 1980s. These studies have grown and new ones have emerged as centenarians have become more common. This growth has been paralleled by development of molecular genetic techniques that are both inexpensive and powerful enough to enable genetic studies of this select cohort that may lead to insights into both environmental and genetic determinants of survival to extreme old age and maintaining good health. Although it was initially thought that centenarians were scarce because of a few rare but important determinants, more recent data suggest that there are many factors that may predispose to longevity, but the key is to attain the right combination of these factors.

An important challenge for centenarian studies is that the combination of factors that enables one person to survive to extreme old age may be quite different for another person. Replication of findings across centenarian studies will point to factors that may be important across ethnic and population lines. Studies such as the Seventh Day Adventist Health Study point to behaviors such as not smoking, regular exercise, vegetarian diet, and activities to effectively manage stress as being conducive to an average life expectancy of eighty-eight years (Fraser and Shavlik, 2001). If all of us emulated these behaviors, the result would be higher average life expectancy, perhaps into our late eighties, and fewer years spent with disability. However, how centenarians live an additional ten to fifteen years beyond age ninety is still under active investigation. As more epidemiological and genetic data become available, researchers will likely gain a better understanding of this phenomenon in the near future.

ACKNOWLEDGMENTS

We thank Barbara Loecher and the American Geriatrics Society's newsletter, *AGS News,* for providing the interviews of Nola Ochs and Frank Fogarty. We are indebted to Paola Sebastiani, Ph.D., for her insightful comments and suggestions. This work was supported by several grants from the National Institute on Aging: Characterizing Human Exceptional Longevity (Perls, 1 K24 AG025727–01A1) and the Paul B. Beeson Career Development Award: Centenarian Offspring and Vascular Disease Resistance (Terry, 1 K23AG0267754).

REFERENCES

Barzilai, N., and others. "Unique Lipoprotein Phenotype and Genotype Associated with Exceptional Longevity." *Journal of the American Medical Association*, 2003, *290*, 2030–2040.

Cawthon, R. M., and others. "Association Between Telomere Length in Blood and Mortality in People Aged 60 Years or Older." *The Lancet*, 2003, *361*, 393–395.

Choi, Y. H., and others. "Distributions of ACE and APOE Polymorphisms and Their Relations with Dementia Status in Korean Centenarians." *Journals of Gerontology. Series A, Biological Sciences and Medical Sciences*, 2003, *58*, 225–226.

Evert, J., Lawler, E., Bogan, H., and Perls, T. "Morbidity Profiles of Centenarians: Survivors, Delayers, and Escapers." *Journals of Gerontology. Series A, Biological Sciences and Medical Sciences*, 2003, *58*, 232–237.

Franceschi, C., and others. "Do Men and Women Follow Different Trajectories to Reach Extreme Longevity? Italian Multicenter Study on Centenarians (IMUSCE). *Aging (Milano)*, 2000, *12*, 77–84.

Fraser, G. E., and Shavlik, D. J. "Ten Years of Life: Is It a Matter of Choice?" *Archives of Internal Medicine*, 2001, *161*, 1645–1652.

Geesaman, B. J., and others. "Haplotype-Based Identification of a Microsomal Transfer Protein Marker Associated with the Human Lifespan." *Proceedings of the National Academy of Sciences of the United States of America*, 2003, *100*, 14115–14120.

Hawkes, K. "Human Longevity: The Grandmother Effect." *Nature*, 2004, *428*, 128–129.

Hjelmborg, J., and others. "Genetic Influence on Human Lifespan and Longevity." *Human Genetics*, 2006, *119*, 312–321.

Ljungquist, B., and others. "The Effect of Genetic Factors for Longevity: A Comparison of Identical and Fraternal Twins in the Swedish Twin Registry." *Journals of Gerontology. Series A, Biological Sciences and Medical Sciences*, 1998, *53*, M441–446.

Luoto, R., Kaprio, J., Reunanen, A., and Rutanen, E. M. "Cardiovascular Morbidity in Relation to Ovarian Function After Hysterectomy." *Obstetrics and Gynecology*, 1995, *85*, 515–522.

Mazes, R. B., and Forman, S. "Longevity and Age Exaggeration in Vilcabamba, Ecuador." *Journals of Gerontology*, 1979, *34*, 94–98.

McGue, M., Vaupel, J. W., Holm, N., and Harvald, B. "Longevity Is Moderately Heritable in a Sample of Danish Twins Born 1870–1880." *Journals of Gerontology*, 1993, *48*, B237–244.

Meyers, D. G., Jensen, K. C., and Menitove, J. E. "A Historical Cohort Study of the Effect of Lowering Body Iron Through Blood Donation on Incident Cardiac Events." *Transfusion*, 2002, *42*, 1135–1139.

Oeppen, J., and Vaupel, J. W. "Demography: Broken Limits to Life Expectancy." *Science*, 2002, *296*, 1029–1031.

Olshansky, S. J., and others. "A Potential Decline in Life Expectancy in the United States in the 21st Century." *New England Journal of Medicine*, 2005, *352*, 1138–1145.

Perls, T. T., and others. "Exceptional Familial Clustering for Extreme Longevity in Humans." *Journal of the American Geriatrics Society*, 2000, *48*, 1483–1485.

Perls, T. T., and others. "Life-Long Sustained Mortality Advantage of Siblings of Centenarians." *Proceedings of the National Academy of Sciences of the United States of America*, 2002, *99*, 8442–8447.

Poulain, M., and others. "Identification of a Geographic Area Characterized by Extreme Longevity in the Sardinia Island: The AKEA Study." *Experimental Gerontology*, 2004, *39*, 1423–1429.

Puca, A. A., and others. "A Genome-Wide Scan for Linkage to Human Exceptional Longevity Identifies a Locus on Chromosome 4." *Proceedings of the National Academy of Sciences of the United States of America*, 2001, *98*, 10505–10508.

Qi, L., van Dam, R. M., Rexrode, K., and Hu, F. B. "Heme Iron from Diet as a Risk Factor for Coronary Heart Disease in Women with Type 2 Diabetes." *Diabetes Care*, 2007, *30*, 101–106.

Schachter, F., and others. "Genetic Associations with Human Longevity at the APOE and ACE Loci." *Nature Genetics*, 1994, *6*, 29–32.

Terry, D. F., and others. "Cardiovascular Advantages Among the Offspring of Centenarians." *Journals of Gerontology. Series A, Biological Sciences and Medical Sciences*, 2003, *58*, M425–431.

Terry, D. F., and others. "Reduced All-Cause, Cardiovascular and Cancer Mortality in Centenarian Offspring." *Journal of the American Geriatrics Society*, 2004, *52*, 2074–2076.

United Nations Population Division. World Population Ageing. Department of Economic and Social Affairs. NewYork: United Nations Population Division, 2001. [http://www.un.org/esa/population/publications/worldageing19502050]. Accessed May 8, 2007.

U.S. Census Bureau CSF. Table 13. States and Puerto Rico Ranked by Population 100 Years and Over: 2000. Census 2000 PHC-T-13. Population and Ranking Tables of the Older Population for the United States, States, Puerto Rico, Places of 100,000 or More Population, and Counties, 2000.

Vaupel, J. W., and others. "Biodemographic Trajectories of Longevity." *Science*, 1998, *280*, 855–860.

Willcox, B. J., and others. "Siblings of Okinawan Centenarians Share Lifelong Mortality Advantages." *Journals of Gerontology. Series A, Biological Sciences and Medical Sciences*, 2006, 61, 345–354.

CHAPTER

CITIES, SOCIODIVERSITY, AND STRATEGY

JAIME LERNER

Every city, regardless of its size, can be an agent of change. And a positive example set by one can inspire its neighbors, helping to transform a region, a state, and a country.

But where should the efforts be targeted? What are some of the strategic issues facing cities that offer a higher potential to improve the quality of life of their citizens and of the environment?

Before examining some of these target areas, it is important to establish a fundamental concept that can connect these multiple initiatives and articulate them with the central theme of this book. When the concept of biodiversity is applied to human beings, we have this new concept: *sociodiversity*.

A city is a collective dream. To build this dream is vital. Without it, the city cannot engage the essential involvement of its inhabitants. Therefore, those responsible for the destinies of the city need to clearly draw scenarios—scenarios that are desired by the majority, capable of motivating the efforts of an entire generation. And in the drawing of these scenarios, in the construction of this dream, it is paramount to acknowledge and cherish the sociodiversity dimension that exists in our urban settlements.

As much as biodiversity is a key concern in ecological terms, sociodiversity is vital for the vigor, health, and balance of our cities. The higher the diversity of age groups, ethnic backgrounds, income levels, and talents entwined in the urban fabric—the higher the sociodiversity—the better a city will be. Therefore, the higher the awareness of this diversity in the minds of the managers of change, the higher the involvement of the inhabitants will be.

People are living longer, and we can expect that life expectancy will continue to increase. The real issue is how to live better. Medicine and technology are contributing significantly, but that is not enough. The essential task is to deal with the challenge of a new configuration of society and how the elders will be integrated in it. Cities will have to increase the general population's solidarity with the aging population. The elderly must not be segregated; they have the right to enjoy the city in its totality.

To integrate the aging populations in the urban fabric is of the utmost importance. Cities need to understand that the aging population is not a burden, but a valuable asset. Retirees who have saved throughout their working lives now may be more inclined to spend. And the higher their income, the more they can spur the economy. The money they spend from retirement funds and pensions can now recirculate to propel economic activity. Also, jobs in the future will target the needs of the aging population. As this will take place particularly in cities, there will have to be higher integration between urban functions—such as housing, work, leisure, and mobility—and the needs and desires of the aging population.

THE DESIGN OF THE CITY: A STRUCTURE FOR LIFE AND WORK

Each city has its particular design, though it may be hidden under the layers of the natural and built environments. It is a fascinating archeology that connects in time ancient paths and all that was historically important to the city's life and gives them new content, inducing or consolidating its growth through mass transportation and land use. It is a combined structure of life and work. This structure is articulated through a network of streets (even in rural settlements), which are the basic spatial references.

A city without design is simply a metastasis of unchecked, irregular growth. It is a city without clear priorities.

A city must be a diverse mixture of functions, of income levels, and of age groups. The greater the mix, the more human the city will be.

Just as in the natural environment, isolated fragments, however diverse, cannot create the synergy that comes from interaction.

Mobility

The future of urban mobility is on the surface. Entire generations should not have to wait for construction of a subway line when in less than two years a complete network of on-surface transportation can be established.

Entire subway systems—in London, Paris, Moscow, New York—were built over a hundred years ago, when the cost to work underground was much cheaper.

The future of transportation is in the combination and integration of all systems—subway, bus, taxi, cars, and bikes. However, these systems cannot compete in the same space.

People will select the most convenient combination according to their own needs and travel with a mobility card, and all operators of the different transportation modes will be partners in the system.

In the city of Curitiba, Brazil, priority was given to public transportation via the bus. This priority was translated into the construction of a physical infrastructure. What is now the Integrated Transportation Network started in 1974 with the implementation of the North-South axis, transporting about twenty-five thousand passengers a day on express buses in dedicated lanes. Among the key tenets of this network was operating without subsidies: a coresponsibility equation was established, involving public planning and private operation.

As a transportation network expands, it should be accessible to all the citizens virtually everywhere in the city, and once passengers embark, they should be able to reach any point within the network. This was realized in the Integrated Transportation Network. Today, it transports about two million passengers each day on a metropolitan scale with a single fare. There are five axes of express buses in exclusive lanes, plus the direct lines—*ligeirinhos*—that stop at integration terminals and tube stations with prepaid and on-level boarding, in addition to several other hierarchically organized lines.

Sustainability

The debate about sustainability has raised diverse opinions and some frustration. The frustration derives from the inertia of not knowing how to face the issue. The solution lies in focusing on what we know about the problem instead of on what we don't know—and, above all, to transfer this knowledge to the children, who will then teach their parents.

Although the use of basic construction materials such as cement, metal, glass, wood, and plastic in the most sustainable possible manner can help us attain sustainability, it is in the conception of cities that the most significant contribution to a more sustainable society can be forged.

Simple functions from the day-to-day routine of cities can be shown and explained to children; for instance, how each of us can help by

- Reducing the use of the automobile

- Separating the garbage

- Living closer to work or bringing work closer to home

- Assigning multiple functions throughout the twenty-four hours of the day to urban equipment

- Saving as much as possible

- Wasting as little as possible

The Open University for the Environment in Curitiba is an example of translating and sharing this knowledge about sustainability on a daily basis to a wide, diverse public—teachers, industry managers, taxi drivers, bus drivers, janitors, barbers, journalists—people who then can help spread this awareness. Playing "sustainability games" is another strategy. Children can get to know their city by drawing it. With the Lixo que não é Lixo program, children were taught to separate organic waste from recyclables in every school, and also the meaning of reusing paper, metal, glass, and plastic.

Sustainability is an equation between what is saved and what is wasted. Waste, in its several forms, is the most abundant potential source of energy (currently almost 80 percent of all generated energy is wasted).Therefore, if sustainability $=$ saving/wasting, when wasting reaches zero, sustainability can be infinite.

To be sustainable, a city cannot afford the luxury of leaving districts and streets with good infrastructure and services vacant. Its downtown area cannot remain idle during significant portions of the day. It is necessary to use it around the clock. The twenty-four-hour city and multiple-use equipment are essential to sustainability.

Identity

Identity, self-esteem, a feeling of belonging: all of these are closely connected to the points of reference people have for their own city. Identity is a major factor of quality of life; it represents the synthesis of the relationship between the individual and his/her city.

Most cities throughout the world lost their human content when they began to modify three of their fundamental elements—the river, the street, and the square.

Common points of reference in a city are not necessarily architectural heritage, and before tearing a building down it is necessary to consider new possibilities of use. Recycling can provide the building with a new cultural content.

The frame concept is useful in this context: if one gets used to seeing what is beautiful, what should be preserved, one already has the image of what one would like to keep. From that point onward, as with any print or painting, it will be surrounded by a matt and then framed. The frame protects and highlights its content. In the city, landscapes, areas, streets, neighborhoods can also be framed, therefore preserving and enhancing their beauty, scale, character, and identity. Likewise, the mold of the form can provide an alternative when dealing with the restoration of architectural heritage, by working with the void left by the missing form.

Rivers are important reference points; instead of hiding them from view or burying them in concrete, a city's riverbanks should be valued and preserved. If we respect the natural drainage characteristics, the preserved areas can provide the necessary episodic flooding relief channels and still be used most of the time for leisure, sports, entertainment, and contemplation in an economic and environmentally friendly way. A similar logic works with parks: these provide areas that people can relate to and interact with, celebrating the diversity of the city, and restoring degraded landscapes.

Last but not least, historical districts are major reference points, preserving the life of the city since its inception. However, these areas often suffer a process of devaluation and degradation. Finding ways to keep these districts alive by connecting identity elements, recycling outdated uses, and hosting a mix of functions is key.

MAKING IT HAPPEN

To make things happen is to propose a scenario: an idea that the majority of the people consider desirable and therefore will help to realize. There can be a scenario for a city, there can be a scenario for a state, and there can be a scenario for a country.

Once the proposal is set, strategic punctual interventions create a new energy and help to consolidate it. This is "urban acupuncture": it revitalizes a sick or worn-out area and its surroundings through a simple touch on a key point. Just as in a medical approach, this intervention releases positive energy flow, creating a chain reaction that helps to enhance and cure the whole system.

Many cities today need urban acupuncture because they have neglected their cultural identities; others need it because they have neglected their relationship with the natural environment; and still others because they have turned their backs on the wounds left by economic activities. These neglected areas, these scars are precisely the target points for acupuncture treatment. With the right attention, these frogs can be turned into princes.

In every scenario conception, one must not forget that the future is just around the corner and that it will require new ways of thinking. The future requires a commitment to constant innovation.

Tendency is not destiny, as Pulitzer Prize-winning author René Dubos has said. Detecting an undesired tendency does not mean a doomsday situation: now is the right time for positive action.

Future generations will deal with future problems. It is our responsibility not to burden them with the problems we have created in our own time.

Finally, things should happen quickly. To accomplish this, it is necessary to avoid a triple trap: to avoid our own bureaucracy, to avoid our own political problems, and to avoid our own insecurities.

To innovate is to begin! One cannot be so arrogant as to expect to have all the answers beforehand. From origin to destination, the course can always be adjusted.

THE FORMAL AND THE INFORMAL

We must understand that a large portion of today's city is informal. Integration of the formal and informal sectors is a must. Sometimes, when the solution is not in space, it can be in time. The formal and informal can share the same space at different times for everyone's benefit. The key word is coexistence.

It is necessary to give dignity to the informal sector, to raise its self-esteem so it can feel part of the city. Some solutions can come through good design, others by embracing the ephemeral.

A CENTURY OF CITIES

A city is a structure of change, even more than it is a model of planning, an instrument of economic policies, or a nucleus of social polarization. The soul of a city—the strength that makes it breathe, exist, progress—resides in each one of its citizens, in each person that introduces into it and exhausts the meaning of a life.

Cities are the refuge of individuality and solidarity. They can be our safeguards from the inhumane consequences of the globalization process—the destruction of regional and local character and sense of place, the soulless sameness that replaces them.

The fiercest wars are happening in cities, in their marginalized peripheries, in the clash between the wealthy enclaves and the deprived ghettos. The heaviest environmental burdens are being generated there because of our lack of empathy for present and future generations. And one of the most telling measures of quality of life can be seen in the care we give (or fail to give) to our elders, which is revealed most obviously in our cities. This is exactly why it is in our cities where we can make the most progress toward a more peaceful, healthy, and balanced planet. A more generous view of the potential of cities means a more optimistic outlook on human beings and all their potential.

CHAPTER

CREATING A HEALTHY ENVIRONMENT FOR AGING POPULATIONS

GLORIA M. GUTMAN

Around the world, when elders are asked about their three greatest concerns, the answers generally fall into three broad categories: health, income, and housing. The three are obviously related: persons with high income have the wherewithal to purchase superior housing and health care and have been shown in many studies to enjoy better physical and mental health than their less-affluent age peers. However, traditionally health, wealth, and housing have been considered separately at the organizational, policy, and program levels. Ministries of housing, of health, and of finance exist as separate entities in the governmental structures of most countries.

Although federal agencies such as the Canada Mortgage and Housing Corporation and the U.S. Department of Housing and Urban Development were created explicitly to ensure an adequate supply of affordable housing for the population, it is only in recent years that the three-way relationship between the built environment, wealth, and health has become of central interest to urban and regional planners, housing policy makers, and housing researchers. In large measure this is a result of the advent of the population health movement and the crossover of some of its ideas from public health to other disciplines.

The assumptions underlying the population health movement approach are as follows

a) Health is determined by the complex interactions between individual characteristics, social and economic factors, and physical environments.

b) Strategies to improve population health must address the entire range of factors that determine health.

c) Important health gains can be achieved by focusing interventions on the health of the entire population (or significant sub-populations) rather than individuals.

d) Improving health is a shared responsibility that requires the development of healthy public policies in areas outside the traditional health system.

e) The health of a population is closely linked to the distribution of wealth across the population [Visions Centre of Innovation, 2003].

The central argument of this chapter, and its reason for inclusion in this book, is that if we are serious about wishing to create healthy environments for the older populations of the world, then older adults themselves, and their supporters and advocates, must also adopt a population health approach. That is, as in the World Health Organization's (2002) Active Ageing policy framework, they and we must recognize that at any time and any stage in the human life course, one's health is the product of a confluence of factors that have impinged on one over time. Some of these factors or determinants of health are intrinsic to the individual; others are extrinsic. The latter category includes the "big picture" items: the policies and programs of the community, state, country, or geopolitical region in which one resides, which determine the range of health care, housing, income support, education, human rights protection, and the like, and the extent of their availability to all segments of the population. The former category includes one's biological and genetic endowment as well as such individual-level variables over which one has some choice and control as lifestyle and personal coping strategies.

As well, the active aging approach draws attention to the need to consider the two cross-cutting variables of culture and gender. The environment that is conducive to the health and well-being of males cannot automatically be assumed to convey the same benefits to females. In many parts of the world gender inequity is unfortunately the rule rather than the exception; older women may experience double or triple jeopardy as they attempt to access shelter and services from a position of poverty. Their social exclusion may be compounded by discrimination resulting from the racial or religious or cultural group into which they were born.

But when we talk of "the older population," how many are we referring to? Where do they live? What progress has been made in identifying and meeting their needs? To provide context for discussion, it is important to establish at the outset that older persons now constitute a significant subpopulation in all parts of the world. It is important to draw attention to the fact that population aging is occurring at different rates in the more and less developed regions of the world. Attention should also to be drawn to two landmark events convened by the United Nations: the 1982 and 2002 World Assemblies on Ageing. In particular, the recommendations deriving from the Second World Assembly on Ageing are important in defining the key issues and in framing discussion of environments and older persons.

THE AGED AS A SIGNIFICANT SUBPOPULATION

Using the United Nations' standard of age sixty as the threshold for entry into the category of "older persons," statistics show that in 2005 there were approximately 244.5 million persons aged sixty and over in the more developed regions of the world, where they constituted 20.1 percent of the population, and 428.3 million in the less developed regions (8.1 percent of the population). By 2020 the population of those aged sixty and over is projected to increase worldwide to 1.04 billion, with 69.3 percent living in the least developed regions (United Nations Department of Economic and Social Affairs, 2007).

GEOGRAPHIC DIFFERENCES IN THE RATE OF POPULATION AGING

Currently, very rapid population aging is a hallmark of the developing world—brought about by the three simultaneous trends of more and more persons living to be old, a dramatic decrease in the birthrate, and high rates of mortality in the young adult population as a result of recurrent warfare and the HIV/AIDS epidemic. In the Introduction to the Political Declaration and Madrid International Plan of Action on Ageing (United Nations, 2003), the key document to result from the Second World Assembly on Ageing, Kofi Annan—then secretary-general of the UN—noted that the world had changed "almost beyond recognition" in the twenty years since the first World Assembly on Ageing. Much of the change was due to the unanticipated pace and magnitude with which population aging had occurred in the developing world.

POPULATION AGING, POVERTY, AND HEALTH

Alex Kalache, chief of the World Health Organization's Ageing and Life Course Programme, cogently notes, "Industrialized countries became rich before they became old, while developing countries will become old before they become rich" (Kalache, Barreto, and Keller, 2005, p. 37). A number of the ways in which poverty, health, and aging are linked are described in section 1.6 of the report of the Valencia Forum, a gathering of experts in the field of aging convened immediately before the 2nd World Assembly on Ageing under the auspices of the International Association of Gerontology and Geriatrics (Andrews, Gray, and Sykes, 2002). The most important document to examine, however, is the Madrid International Plan of Action on Ageing and its three priority directions (introduced in Chapter One). To recap, the first is concerned with older persons and development, the second focuses on advancing health and well-being into old age, and the third addresses ensuring enabling and supportive environments. Under Priority Direction III, four issues are identified:

- Housing and the living environment

- Care and support for caregivers

- Neglect, abuse, and violence

- Images of aging

Each of these issues is accompanied by a set of objectives and recommended actions. The discussion that follows highlights and elaborates on some of these recommendations.

THE SIX A'S OF HOUSING FOR SENIORS

In the subsection of the Madrid Plan dealing with housing and living arrangements, one finds reference to what are known as the "Six A's of Housing for Seniors": it must be Accessible, Affordable, Appropriate, Attractive, and Acceptable, and there should be Alternatives for people to choose from.

Accessibility Isn't Just for Wheelchair Users

As most environmental gerontologists will be quick to point out, the issue of accessibility goes far beyond simply ensuring that elderly wheelchair users have easy entrance to and egress from the building or living unit or rooms within. Accessible construction also allows these users to safely transfer from wheelchair to bed, chair, toilet, and bath, and helps enable all elderly residents to perform independently, to the extent possible, such ADLs as bathing, dressing, grooming, meal preparation, and housekeeping. Ensuring this may entail the purchase and installation of such relatively low-cost items as grab bars in the bathroom, or it may require extensive structural renovation to add an elevator to a single-family detached dwelling or a bedroom for a live-in caregiver, or to reconfigure a kitchen so that an elderly person can age in place in a familiar environment.

As well as accommodating wheelchair and electric scooter users (and the needs of others with mobility impairments who use canes or walkers), the unit must also be able to compensate for sensory fading. There are many design guides on ways to make living units more elder-friendly for people with diminished eyesight, hearing, taste, touch, and smell—the "normal" age-related changes that most people experience. Other design guides address ways of ensuring the safety and maintaining and enhancing the quality of life of people with cognitive impairment, whether living at home, in assisted living, or in institutional settings. However, the guides' recommendations are not universally adhered to, perhaps because they are not as well known beyond the design-for-aging community as they should be, because of cost considerations, or because some developers fear that including these could "scare away" the healthy, wealthy young-old seniors (those aged fifty-five to seventy-four) they would most like to attract as residents.

Worldwide, seniors and their advocates need to lobby to ensure that these guidelines are followed in new construction specifically designated for occupancy by older persons, whether built by the public sector, NGOs, or the private sector. More widespread application of universal and transgenerational design principles in public buildings and spaces is also desirable. As well, funding must be available in the form of low-interest loans or outright grants so that individuals and landlords in the lower socioeconomic strata can retrofit dwellings to make them more elder-friendly.

Consideration must also be given to ensuring the elder-friendliness of street architecture in the surrounding neighborhood, and to ways in which seniors can move beyond the confines of their dwelling unit and the area immediately surrounding it. Providing effective, readily available transportation alternatives has long been recognized as a key component in maintaining the health and well-being of rural elders. Left behind when younger family members migrate to urban centers in search of better work opportunities, when elders are no longer able to drive they may be unable to travel even short distances to access food, health care, and other necessities. Recently we have recognized that similar constraints apply to seniors aging in place in the suburbs. Designed for young families who have their own transport, many suburbs lack adequate public transportation systems—or indeed any at all. Seniors and their advocates must speak out about this aspect of accessibility.

Housing Affordability: An Issue That Cuts Across Jurisdictions

With respect to housing affordability, the Madrid Plan draws special attention to the plight of seniors in developing countries and countries in transition, where rapid population aging is taking place in a context of continuing urbanization. But the lack of affordable housing and services for impoverished urban seniors and its affect on health is a problem that cuts across jurisdictions. It is important to recognize that currently in Canada and in other parts of the developed world, the majority (75 percent) of older persons live in cities. Although countries such as China and India presently have largely rural populations (60 percent and 71 percent, respectively), both are urbanizing rapidly. The same holds true for countries such as Jamaica, whose urban population is already a slight majority (52 percent), and Tunisia, where 64 percent of the population now live in urban areas.

It is also important to recognize that a number of developing countries in which rapid population aging is under way are already highly urbanized—examples include Brazil (84 percent urban), Chile (88 percent), Colombia (78 percent), and Singapore (100 percent). Yet a recent literature review and study commissioned by the Canada Mortgage and Housing Corporation (2005a, 2005b) indicates that few urban centers in Canada or elsewhere are planning for population aging. This seems particularly shortsighted given that, as documented in the UN-Habitat publication *The State of the World's Cities 2004/2005: Globalization and Urban Culture* (2005), poverty is increasing in many cities.

In the urban context, poverty and slums are closely related. Of the three billion people worldwide who live in urban settings, an estimated one billion live in slums (World Health Organization, 2006). Urban slums—defined as residential areas that lack adequate water and sanitation and security of tenure and have housing of poor structural quality and insufficient living area—are most prevalent in sub-Saharan Africa, where they are home to an estimated 72 percent of the urban population. Southeast Asia comes second, with 57 percent of its urban population living in slums (United Nations Human Settlements Programme, UN-Habitat, 2005). The UN-Habitat (2005) report shows that malnutrition rates among children in countries such as Ethiopia, Uganda, India, Pakistan and Guatemala are as high among those living in urban slums as in rural areas. Although the report draws attention to the plight of children, it should be noted that slums are also home to millions of older persons. Their difficult living conditions are poignantly described in the summary report of the surveys and focus groups conducted in 1999 in twelve major world cities under the aegis of UN-Habitat (Tibaijuka and May, 2006). Scharf, Phillipson, and Smith (2006) also report on older persons living in "socially deprived neighborhoods." Although they emphasize the resilience of older persons, their data show higher proportions with chronic health problems among those living in inner city neighborhoods compared with the general population of older persons in Great Britain, andgreater fear of crime.

A particularly dramatic image evoked by these authors concerns emergency situations. They note that in the heat wave that struck France in 2003, there were 14,800 unnecessary deaths. Of these, 82 percent occurred among people aged seventy-five and over, most of whom lived in densely populated metropolitan areas. They suggest that, as in the Chicago heat wave of 1995, many older persons may have placed themselves at risk by staying in overheated dwellings rather than risk being the victim of a street crime, or by not opening doors or windows lest an intruder enter.

Appropriate Means a Good Person-Environment Fit

In the preamble to Priority Direction III, the Madrid Plan states that "Whatever the circumstances of older persons, all are entitled to live in an environment that enhances their capabilities" (United Nations, 2003, p. 39). The Plan goes on to remind us of the heterogeneity of the older population—some need a high level of physical support and care, whereas others are healthy, active, independent individuals who are willing and able to serve as resources for their family, community and country. In the aging and environment literature, one of the most important theoretical concepts is that of person-environment fit (P-E fit). Good P-E fit enables individuals to age in place in their familiar surroundings in the community; poor fit can propel them into an institutional setting.

Underpinning P-E fit theory is the Environmental Docility Hypothesis (Lawton and Simon, 1968), which addresses the relationship between the competencies that individuals bring to the environment and the degree of "press," or demand, the environment places on them. As shown in Figure 26.1, although some mismatch can be tolerated, once outside of a zone of comfort, if press exceeds competency, then negative

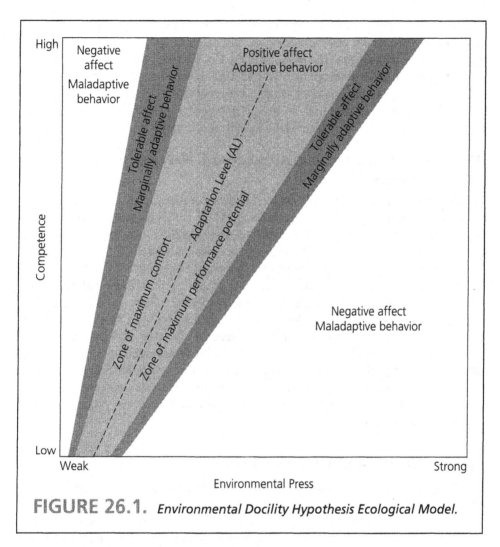

FIGURE 26.1. *Environmental Docility Hypothesis Ecological Model.*

Source: Lawton, 1980; Lawton and Nahemow, 1973.

affect (stress) is experienced. Negative affect also is experienced in situations where competency greatly exceeds press. The figure also shows that the width of the zone of comfort narrows as competency decreases. What this means is that as an individual ages and becomes more frail (that is, less competent), he or she is less able to deal with the demands of the environment and more at its mercy.

Key elements in rebalancing P-E fit include the availability of technology and rehabilitation services designed to support independent living. Several laboratories and research consortia around the world are exploring ways in which miniaturized sensors worn on the body and integrated into homes can unobtrusively and continuously monitor the health and well-being of frail elders and raise an alarm if the data indicate significant changes. The BT Care in the Community Virtual Center, a collaboration between British Telecom and several UK universities (Sixsmith, and others, 2007), is one example. In another example, a team of researchers from the University of Toronto and affiliated hospitals is using computer vision to assist institutionalized persons with dementia to perform ADLs (Mihailidis, Carmichael, and Boger, 2004).

Alternatives, Aesthetics, and Acceptance of New Housing Forms by Seniors

Sometimes bringing help into the familiar residence or retrofitting it is not the best nor the desired solution. Also key to maximizing P-E fit is the availability of alternative housing forms and tenure options. Oswald and Rowles (2006) note that today increasing numbers of older persons are moving into purpose-built dwellings, variously called "continuing care retirement communities," "supportive housing," or "assisted living." These fall somewhere between the independent dwelling unit at one end of the shelter-care continuum and the skilled nursing home at the others. They also include some residential facilities specifically designed for demented persons. Most of these new housing forms provide some supportive services and are designed and marketed to project a noninstitutional image. The rationale for implementation of home-like décor and interior design is to cue and maintain independent functioning and to enhance quality of life. Since most are provided by the private sector, their marketability would appear to attest to their acceptance by seniors. Their cost, however, precludes access by low-income individuals.

CARE AND SUPPORT OF CAREGIVERS

The Madrid Plan contains a number of recommendations designed to create an environment in which family caregivers can continue to maintain their loved ones in the community. This includes providing access to respite care, which may be delivered by sending someone into the home to relieve the family caregiver of some of the tasks of providing personal care to a frail elder, such as bathing. Alternatively, it may involve placement of the care recipient for several days or weeks in an alternate location so that the caregiver can take a holiday or have some time to rest and attend to his or her own health needs. Support for caregivers also has a psychological dimension that involves recognizing the value of the service that is provided. Most commonly, the caregiver is an older woman who may or may not get the respect (and tangible resources) that she deserves from other family members or the formal health-care system.

The Madrid Plan gives special mention to the social support needs of older women in developing countries caring for their children with HIV/AIDS and later for their orphaned grandchildren. Grandparents' parenting of their grandchildren is growing more common around the world because of increased divorce rates and substance abuse rates and the spread of HIV/AIDS. Attention needs to be given to the determinants of health of the caregiver and the care recipient(s), including the physical environment in which care is provided.

In assessing the care setting, the Canada Mortgage and Housing Corporation's concept of "core housing need" may be useful. CMHC defines acceptable housing as housing that is adequate in condition, suitable in size, and affordable. Adequate dwelling units are those reported by their occupants as not requiring major repairs; suitable dwelling units have enough bedrooms for the size and make-up of resident households according to National Occupancy Standard requirements; affordable dwelling units cost less than 30 percent of before-tax household income. Households living in housing below one or more of the adequacy, suitability, or affordability standards are considered to be in core housing need. This definition is based on the belief that "Dwelling units that are well maintained and suited to the needs of the occupants contribute to general health, well-being, and social interaction. Housing that is affordable leaves households with sufficient financial resources to participate fully in the community at large. Households unable to access good housing are potentially at a disadvantage from a variety of perspectives" (Engeland and Lewis, 2004, p. 27).

Data from Canada and elsewhere show elderly renters to be more disadvantaged homeowners. For example, the 2001 Census of Canada showed 43.0 percent of senior renter households to be in core housing need, compared with 12.2 percent of senior owner households. Living alone and renting compounded the risk for core housing need among both seniors (53.3 percent) and nonseniors (32.6 percent).

NEGLECT, ABUSE, AND VIOLENCE

Since the late 1980s, there have been two major approaches to the issue of elder abuse and neglect. The first places it in the context of family violence, recognizing that some of the same dynamics that cause family violence at other points in the life course also apply to old age. The second considers it a health issue. The WHO Programme on Ageing and the Life Course and the International Network for Prevention of Elder Abuse have been vocal in drawing attention to the fact that older persons cannot enjoy health and well-being in situations where they live in fear of or experience abuse or neglect. Both the Active Ageing document and the Madrid Plan recommend a multisectoral and cross-disciplinary approach to the problem, involving justice officials, law enforcement officers, health and social service professionals, governments, and civil society.

Although much of the work on violence and abuse suffered by older persons has focused on the family setting, it cannot be separated from consideration of the broader experience of people in later life. As a result, discussions of developing legislation, policy, and practice to deal with family abuse situations almost inevitably lead to discussions about human rights violations, negative attitudes, and stereotypes. In Canada, the United States, and other developed countries, progress has been made in developing services that help individual older people. Societies have been less willing to address systemic factors, such as poverty, that increase the potential for elder abuse and neglect to occur. Elder abuse occurs in all sections and segments of society. It can happen to the richest, it can happen to the poorest—but the probability of being the victim of elder abuse, particularly physical violence, is higher if one's income is low (Mouton and others, 2004).

Societies have also been much less active than they should be in taking action to shift values that perpetuate gender inequities and ageist attitudes. Far too often elderly persons are portrayed as a drain on the economy. As the Madrid Plan notes, "Older women are particularly affected by misleading and negative stereotypes: instead of being portrayed in ways that reflect their contributions, strengths, resourcefulness and humanity, they are often depicted as weak and dependent. This reinforces exclusionary practices at the local and national levels" (pp. 44–45).

SUMMARY AND CONCLUSION

This chapter began by drawing attention to the interconnectedness of health, wealth, and housing. The horizon was quickly expanded to suggest that an approach that embraces determinants of individual and population health—such as the approach presented in the World Health Organization publication *Active Ageing: A Policy Framework* (2002)—is needed to create healthy environments for older populations. To make the case, I highlighted and elaborated on selected subsections of the Madrid Plan. These subsections—all part of Priority Direction III, for ensuring enabling and supportive environments—focused on four issues: the housing and living environment; care and support for caregivers; neglect, abuse, and violence; and images of aging. I chose these four issues to frame discussion for two reasons. First because, by their nature and diversity, they broaden the concept of environment far beyond bricks and mortar, community planning principles, and even the five-point taxonomy articulated by Lawton (1980) in his groundbreaking book *Environment and Aging*. Second, I hope that the reader may be motivated to work toward implementation of the recommendations attached to each issue.

As the Madrid Plan notes, implementation requires sustained action at all levels, both in responding to the demographic changes that have resulted in population aging and are projected to continue for the foreseeable future, and to mobilize and engage the skills and energies of older persons. Although national governments have primary responsibility for implementing the plan's recommendation, progress will require cooperation and collaboration among the public sector, the private sector, and civil society—group to which all of us, young and old, weak and strong, belong.

REFERENCES

Andrews, G., Gray, J., and Sykes, J. *A Report on Outcomes of a Meeting of Gerontological Researchers, Educators and Providers, Providing an Evidence Base in Support of the International Plan of Action on Ageing 2002.* International Association of Gerontology, Valencia, Spain, April 1–4, 2002. [iagg.com.br/pdf/ValenciaForum.pdf]. Accessed April 29, 2007.

Canada Mortgage and Housing Corporation. "Aging, Communities, and Planning for the Future: A CMHC Literature Review." Toronto: SPR Associates Ltd., April 2005. [https://www.surveycentral.ca/cmhc-aging/literaturereview.pdf]. Accessed February 8, 2007.

Canada Mortgage and Housing Corporation. *Determining the Implications of Population Aging for Housing and Residential Communities: Discussion Paper #2: Validating and Extending What Was Learned from the Initial Literature Review (Through Expert and Practitioner Views).* Toronto: SPR Associates Ltd., June 2005. [https://www.surveycentral.ca/cmhc-aging/expertviews.pdf]. Accessed February 8, 2007.

Engeland, J., and Lewis, R. "Exclusion from Acceptable Housing: Canadians in Core Housing Need." *Horizons,* 2004, *7*(2), 27–39.

Lawton, M. P. *Environment and Aging.* Monterey, Calif.: Brooks/Cole, 1980.

Lawton, M. P., and Nahemow, L. "Ecology and the Aging Process." In C. Eisdorfer and M. P. Lawton (eds.), *Psychology of Adult Development and Aging.* Washington, D.C.: American Psychological Association, 1973.

Lawton, M. P., and Simon, B. "The Ecology of Social Relationships in Housing for the Elderly." *The Gerontologist,* 1968, 8, 108–115.

Kalache, A., Barreto, S. M., and Keller, I. "Global Ageing: The Demographic Revolution in all Cultures and Societies. In M. L. Johnson (ed), *The Cambridge Handbook of Age and Ageing,* pp. 30–46. Cambridge, UK: Cambridge University Press, 2005.

Mihailidis, A., Carmichael, B., and Boger, J. "The Use of Computer Vision in an Intelligent Environment to Support Aging-In-Place, Safety and Independence in the Home." *IEEE Transactions on Information Technology in Biomedicine,* 2004, *8*(3), 1–11.

Mouton, C. P., and others. "Prevalence and 3-Year Incidence of Abuse Among Postmenopausal Women." *American Journal of Public Health,* 2004, *94*(4), 605–612.

Oswald, F., and Rowles, G. D. "Beyond the Relocation Trauma in Old Age: New Trends in Elders' Residential Decisions." In H.-W. Wahl, C. Tesch-Romr, and A. Hoff (eds.), *New Dynamics in Old Age: Individual, Environmental, and Social Perspectives,* 127–152. Amityville, N.Y.: Baywood, 2006.

Scharf, T., Phillipson, C. and Smith, A. "Aging in a Difficult Place: Assessing the Impact of Urban Deprivation on Older People." In H.-W. Wahl, C. Tesch-Romr, and A. Hoff (eds.), *New Dynamics in Old Age: Individual, Environmental, and Social Perspectives,* 153–173. Amityville, N.Y.: Baywood, 2006.

Sixsmith, A., and others. "Monitoring the Well-Being of Older People." *Topics in Geriatric Rehabilitation,* 2007, *23*(1), 9–23.

Tibaijuka, A. K., and May, R. *Living Conditions of Low-Income Older Persons in Human Settlements. Summary of Final Report.* Handout at UN World Forum III side event, Vancouver, Canada, June 20, 2006.

United Nations Department of Economic and Social Affairs. "World Population Prospects: The 2006 Revision, Population Database." [http://esa.un.org/unpp]. Accessed April 29, 2007.

United Nations Human Settlements Programme (UN-Habitat). *The State of the World's Cities 2004/2005: Globalization and Urban Culture.* London: Earthscan, 2005.

United Nations*Political Declaration and Madrid International Plan of Action on Ageing.* New York: United Nations Department of Public Information, 2003.

Visions Centre of Innovation. Health Canada's Determinants of Health. [http://www.visions.ab.ca/content/healthdeter.asp]. 2003. Accessed April 30, 2007.

World Health Organization. *Active Ageing: A Policy Framework.* Geneva: World Health Organization Ageing and Life Course Program, 2002.

World Health Organization. *Optimizing the Impact of Social Determinants of Health on Exposed Populations in Urban Settings.* Kobe, Japan: The Core Project of the World Health Organization Centre for Health Development, 2006.

CHAPTER

27

HOW GOVERNMENT, BUSINESS, AND SOCIAL SECTOR PARTNERSHIPS CAN FINANCE PROGRAMS FOR THE AGING

A. JAMES FORBES, JR.

My personal experience, earned by working with or in over 120 countries, has affirmed that financial synergy can be enhanced if the financial resources applied to healthy aging are thoroughly defined and are then deployed through a well-thought-out plan that incorporates the business, government, and social sectors.

There are no absolute numbers on financing programs for the aged on a global basis, but glimpses of certain of the statistics help frame a picture. Among them, the United States' Administration on Aging begins to clarify the dimensions when it reports that "In 2000, the number of persons aged 60 years or older (globally) was estimated at 605 million. That number is projected to grow to almost 2 billion by 2050, when the population of older persons will be larger than the population of children (0–14 years) for the first time in history." In the United States alone, the assets of the top one hundred companies set aside for pension liabilities are in excess of $1.3 trillion dollars. And this is only the tip of the iceberg in just one well-developed country.

When we address the issues of healthy aging from a global perspective, today's missed opportunities become tomorrow's ever-growing challenge, as the statistics in the previous quote are dynamic and exponentially growing, particularly in developing countries with accelerated population growth. Time is of the essence.

Early intervention is essential at the childhood level of the health care continuum. This is especially important in developing countries and regions such as Latin America and Africa, where population growth is fast approaching 3 percent per annum, coupled with life expectancies that within developing Latin America (including the Caribbean) range from 52.9 years in Haiti to 69.1 years in Guatemala—due to humanmade and natural disasters, inadequate health care systems, and poverty—and within developing Africa range from only 33.2 years in Swaziland to 52.7 years in Mauritania, due to all these factors plus the epidemic of HIV/AIDS. Early intervention is not only sound health practice, but also prudent economics, because as a direct consequence of even reasonably competent medical care—whether center-based or community-based—with an early intervention component, fewer people will end up needing to use the health care system and to cope with expensive critical health care issues along the continuum of life.

On the positive side of health care's daunting statistics, there are opportunities to better marshal our global financial resources to aid all in meeting the challenge. This effort begins at the social sector organization level, which directly serves the developing countries in need.

This chapter focuses on the marshaling of the financial resources of social sector organizations into a financial footing (much like the support for physical structures) that, in turn, supports vertical pillars under the healthy aging platform. For this chapter, we shall refer to the combined elements as the *healthy-aging structure*. The healthy-aging structure is directed at those organizations that serve as a resource for healthy aging—whether they are in a country such as the United States, with a GDP of over $10,500 per capita, or a barely subsisting country such as Haiti, with $800 GDP per capita.

All planning and activities must center on this operating principle: *Being able to understand and optimize the interplay of the stakeholders and the assets they control or are able to marshal is critical in the healthy-aging paradigm.*

The primer outlined by this chapter should help generate new ideas and bring increased awareness about solving problems that healthy-aging stakeholders experience. This chapter has been written principally for the social-sector partner who is, more often than not, the accountable stakeholder in the healthy-aging model.

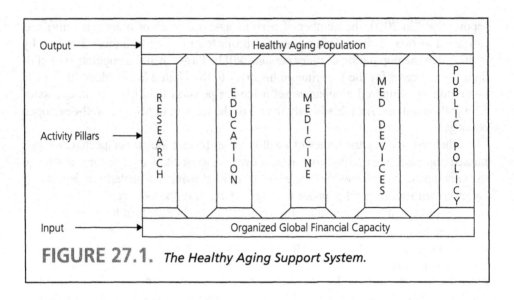

FIGURE 27.1. *The Healthy Aging Support System.*

THE HEALTHY-AGING STRUCTURE

When financial capacity (the input into the structure) is released and allocated in a coordinated fashion, the pillars (activities) are strengthened. These pillars, or activities, are, at a minimum, research, education, advocacy, medicine, medical devices, and public policy. Pictorially, the healthy-aging structure could look like Figure 27.1.

Financial capacity is generally defined as the ability of an organization to sustain itself via a suitable financial model. *Applied financial capacity* may be a clearer descriptor for this healthy-aging analysis: a pool of globally suited financial resources sourced from governments, businesses, and social sector organizations that, when taken together, provide direct or indirect financial resources applied to create measurable outcomes. In this case, they are applied to the global healthy-aging model.

WHAT ARE THE FINANCIAL RESOURCES?

Financial resources can take many forms—and not all are currency. These include the following:

Direct monetary infusion at a particular point within the health-care financial continuum. The applied resources may be sourced from any of the stakeholder partners or from a third party; for example, a grant-making organization. Of course, there are other modalities to infuse funds. One of the most interesting is the venture philanthropy model, which mimics deal structures similar to those in the for-profit business world. How the gift is structured is quite often a deciding factor for the organization.

One cannot place a price tag on good health, nor can one readily compute the return on the investment. But suffice to say, one dollar invested in solving a child's health problem will reap benefits all along the continuum—especially in the adult and senior adult portions of the continuum, when the initial investment in good health may avoid a call on the financial resources to deal with a more complex problem. Invested well, it may also allow for a longer income stream back into society.

Monetary capacity as a driver of influence. Often we learn of issues being addressed by governments and business because an institution of substantial financial means (capacity) has shown only a preliminary interest in a cause. The Gates Foundation is an interesting model in this regard. Without having disbursed a single dollar, their mere attention to a matter, albeit preliminary, becomes a catalyst for a resource allocation or a call on financial capacity by others. So unapplied financial capacity by certain substantial organizations is often a driver for global attention and a basis for considering their influence as a kind of financial capacity.

Strategically distributed gifts-in-kind. Financial capacity is not just pecuniary or bank balances. Healthy aging also requires products, whether it be medicines, devices, or food. It also includes volunteer services. Although there is no single franchise on the sourcing and distribution of goods, the social sector is often the driver for creating such resources in coordination with business and government stakeholders.

Having been involved in the relief response to some of the world's worst natural and manmade disasters, I have witnessed a sea change in the delivery of relief goods in recent years. There are substantially fewer instances of "cut and run"—that is, dropping goods into a program and then leaving them for others to manage. Responses to the initial emergency more often become sustainable programs. In particular, I think of mother-and-child programs in Central America for which immediate attention was raised during disasters—such as the decimating earthquake in El Salvador in 2000—and then actions were taken to build longer-term programs (more about that example later). These sustainable programs do challenge the business, social, and government sectors to continue the flow of goods driven by a continuing financial capacity.

Governments. The government sector is at once a stakeholder and a financial capacity to social sector organizations. It can also be the "good news" and, in certain limited cases, the "bad news" resource unless the stakeholders are careful in their planning. In the "good news" side of the relationship, there are highly effective resources created and administered by governments. Close to home, one example is the well-known programs of the United States Agency for International Development (USAID), which is often both a financial capacity and a partner.

In some developing countries, blockages are created when foreign governments go awry, so much so that worthwhile programs directed at healthy aging—and equally often at saving lives—are aborted or nearly aborted through in-country "toll gates" to aid: customs duties on products in emergencies, "allocations" to those who really don't require the product or funds, and unjustifiable seizure into government warehouses, to name a few. That said, there are those global health-focused programs that are a testimony to partnership with government stakeholders. In project planning, one must consider all aspects of government cooperation.

It is essential to any social sector organization that it attract government partners and also maintain the ability to be a qualified government partner when and as needed.

Being a qualified preferred partner is a kind of indirect financial capacity that is central to being an effective deliverer of health care along the aging continuum.

Business sector. The ability to garner products and services as required is necessary for effective leadership in healthy-aging initiatives. It is essential that the social sector implementer have a sound organizational relationship with businesses that can supply products or services at no or low cost. As the social sector works diligently to maintain a pristine image, so must the business partner, as in recent years these have often been subjected to extraordinarily close scrutiny when global funds are involved in the partnership.

Equally as important as all of the above factors, the social sector partner must have a healthy financial balance sheet (not to be confused with wealth) as well as a lean operating structure to discharge its responsibilities. This is a necessary element in financial capacity that allows for both the execution of the model and staying power for the long term.

Financial capacity to deliver comes in many forms. Knowing how to grow each and blend as needed toward an effective healthy-aging program is financial capacity at its best.

ROLES AND RESPONSIBILITIES

Figure 27.2 depicts the flow of funds and products in a well-managed endeavor to optimize financial capacity while delivering optimum program effectiveness.

Several points about the chart flows should be highlighted:

■ Although there may be several operating partners, there is only one point of accountability for the healthy-aging project. Customarily, it is the social service sector partner.

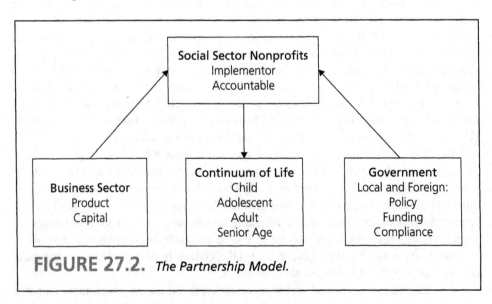

FIGURE 27.2. *The Partnership Model.*

■ Government and business gain the benefit of a multiplier when working through the social sector partner. An analogy might be that they "hired" the social sector partner to apply skills and experience they do not have. This arrangement allows for the application for even larger financial critical mass (more partners). Financial capacity is enhanced through the skills of the social sector partner, who often has greater contact at the field level. There are fewer wasted resources for the government and business than if they attempt to develop and operate a program on their own.

■ The model is expandable to meet a particular need. Quite often, the business partner will consist of a small consortium of businesses, or the U.S. and foreign partners join together for the initiative. Again, this is an opportunity for critical mass and enhanced financial capacities.

NOT ALL ORGANIZATIONS CAN BE PARTNERS

From my experience, there are at least several guidelines that must be considered in bringing together business, government, and the social sectors, especially in a project with a long continuum such as healthy aging.

■ Although it may seem intuitive, it is not always grasped by all that there must be mission alignment among all the partners to optimize financial capacities and outcomes. For example, just because a business partner manufactures a healthy-aging product, it is not necessarily aligned with where and how it should be distributed. Not to take away from corporate good intentions, but products to be distributed within a certain country for a special need may not yet be part of their marketing strategy. Yes, marketing and philanthropy do intertwine at certain levels. That said, however, it can also work in reverse.

■ All the partners' roles and responsibilities must be clarified prior to commencing the program. Open issues not resolved before inception most certainly can cause severe project damage and create a strain on the project's financial and operating viability.

■ There must be common agreement to follow global health's best practices—the standards set by many global agencies.

■ Particularly when the parties are coming together on global health matters, special attention must be paid to the credentials and reputations of the business, government, and social sector organizations. It is too late to manage these issues once they are in the headlines. Some of the questions to answer: Have partners failed in previous attempts with this particular kind of program? Any controversy with a partner doing business in any location previously? Are the products socially acceptable?

■ Define up front how the project will measure success. I have had business partners
  declare success to be the sum of money they disbursed on the project, with little
  sensitivity to the human outcome. I learned that financial capacity, if not intelli-
  gently disbursed, can drive a very undesirable outcome.

A MODEL CASE STUDY

There is a continuing need in Central America, as well as many other places on the
globe, for mother-and-child clinics. An organization I was affiliated with was tasked
with expending a $5 million grant from USAID to develop a model for mother-and-
child clinics in certain countries and then operate them. That model was also to be
replicable and sustainable. The roles of the partners were clear: USAID funded the project
and my organization was tasked with all of the inputs into and outputs from the
projects. It was *the* accountable partner. We also enjoyed partnership with one of
the United States' largest manufacturers of medical equipment. All the partners were
in place with set roles. There was agreement on the metrics or outcomes: number
of people to be served, reduction in manifestations of a particular disease, costs to see
patients, and many others.

As the accountable partner—the one to whom the funds were disbursed—we had
to build the case regarding locations to be served, services of those locations, unit
designs, and setting the measurable standards (metrics) to measure program inputs and
outputs. There was periodic accounting to USAID, and we assured USAID that all
subcontractors complied with the same level of financial stewardship.

Although there were funds available to build the clinics, the financial viability of
the partners to deliver had to be verified. Each partner had to have financial strength
not only to execute the initial development, but also to operate it on an ongoing basis.
Financial capacity of the combined partners was central to the awarding of the grant.

FACTORS TO BE CONSIDERED IN OPTIMIZING
FINANCIAL CAPACITY

There are at least three core elements that are common and necessary components of
most healthy-aging partnerships.

Alliances

I have stated that some nonprofits may have trouble forming alliances to engage in
projects, either as a matter of principle or for some other reason. Financial viability or
capacity may at times be secured only through partners, alliances, and ventures. The
ability to come together is often necessary to develop the required financial capacity
for a project at any point along the health care continuum. This ability to form
partnerships for projects is often a missed opportunity.

Estimated Impacts

To deliver a project in a high-cost program, such as healthy aging, organizations must have a clear picture of the effects they wish to have on those being served and the costs to achieve those effects. I have noted that when this has not been adequately considered, there are insufficient funds—or financial capacity—to deliver the desired outputs; in fact, financial capacity has been wasted. In calculating costs, especially in health care, overhead is one of the chief weak points. Thus the next principle: know your organization's cost of doing business. One is often loath to acknowledge the high cost of doing business—or, in the case of some non-profits, to run it like a business (with a heart). But it is this kind of thinking and culture that rapidly dilutes financial capacity.

Measure Outputs with a Rational and Pertinent Plan of Metrics Management

Social and health impacts are in the forefront of all successful projects from the outset. But all too often, measurement of progress with some initially agreed-to metrics will doom the project to failure and waste scarce financial resources. The metrics should reflect not only financial metrics but also programmatic metrics. This means common metrics: people served during a period; cost per patient encounter; vital signs achieved (for example, the average patient's glucose tolerance changed xx percent after four months, the average life span of the target audience was extended by xx years), and so on. An active and realistic metrics model will preserve financial capacity.

CONCLUSION

On a stand-alone basis, most social sector organizations are impeded by insufficient financial capacity to advance projects to the degree and direction that could make a meaningful difference. Although there are many global resources that help programs to finance healthy aging, the potential for combining those of the business, government, and social sectors is real and available. However, for many, the potential remains untapped until the opportunities are examined in light of the principles discussed here.

Central to multiplying financial capacity directed toward healthy aging is knowing the social sector organization's financial capacity and then strengthening it through an intelligent alignment of business and government partners as necessary to answer this most vital call to action. And that call to action is addressing healthy aging not only at the senior age level, but also along the continuum of life toward healthy aging.

CHAPTER

28

POLICIES AND PRACTICES AFFECTING HEALTH AND LONGEVITY OF PEOPLE WITH DISABILITIES: LESSONS FROM THE UNITED KINGDOM

HECTOR MEDORA AND ANGELA HASSIOTIS

"A historic achievement for the 650 million people with disabilities around the world" said United Nations Secretary-General Kofi Annan. On August 26, 2006, this statement signaled the agreement reached on the text of a treaty to protect the rights of people with disabilities, creating a "paradigm shift in the way that governments think about disabilities . . . a real and concrete difference. . . ." according to New Zealand's Ambassador to the UN Don MacKay, who chaired the sessions (United Nations News Centre, 2006).

The convention does not create new rights; however, it does take a clear stand that people with disabilities should not be discriminated against in any part of their lives, such as their civil rights, access to justice, and the right to health and education.

BACKGROUND

At the heart of all health and social care legislation in the United Kingdom for the past six decades is an attempt to ensure that people do not experience avoidable hardship and discrimination, but are able to lead as near an ordinary life as possible. This has been underpinned by the strongest possible belief that each and every citizen is entitled to enjoy a fulfilling and rewarding life.

Of particular importance are the steps taken by the state to support those who are most at risk of being vulnerable or devalued in their social roles. Therefore, legislation and social policy aims at "the application of what science can tell us about the enablement, establishment, enhancement, maintenance, and/or defence of valued social roles for people" (Flynn and Lemay, 1999, p. 125).

The underpinning of the United Kingdom's social administration was established as early as the fourteenth century with the introduction of the poor laws, evolving into the Old Poor Law (Act for the Relief of the Poor, 1601) and the New Poor Law (Poor Law Amendment Act, 1834) (http://users.ox.ac.uk/). The poor laws heralded a shift in the attitudes toward poverty, from its being inevitable to its being a condition that could change with social support and provision of opportunities.

The *welfare state*, a term believed to have been coined by Archbishop William Temple during the Second World War, was applied to the gradual process of developing widely ranging schemes for poverty relief, which began in the nineteenth century. However, not all systems of social protection fall under the term *welfare state;* according to British sociologist T. H. Marshall (1950), the *welfare state* is a distinct combination of democracy, welfare, and capitalism. Particularly after the Second World War, many countries that had initially offered partial coverage of social care to specific sections of the community extended this to almost all of the population.

Today, the activities of present-day welfare states extend to the provision of both cash welfare benefits (such as old-age pensions or unemployment benefits) and in-kind welfare services (such as health or child-care services). Through these provisions, welfare states can affect the prevalence of well-being and personal autonomy among their citizens, as well as influence how their citizens consume and how they spend their time (Rice, Goodin, and Parpo, 2006; Esping-Andersen, 1999). Despite the controversial nature of the concept, there are compelling humanitarian, ethical, economic, and cultural justifications for the existence of a welfare state.

The culmination, in the UK, of far-reaching national social policy was the inauguration of the National Health Service (NHS) in 1948, based on proposals embedded originally in the Beveridge Report (1942). The NHS, although it has undergone several major reforms over the years, still has at its core the provision of health care services to all, "free at the point of delivery." Other systems of social welfare worldwide include social security, which was identified in the Universal Declaration of Human Rights (1948).

Welfare provision is generally available in developed countries but quite limited in developing ones with weak economies. Welfare expenditure across the globe ranges from over a quarter of the national gross domestic product to less than a tenth (United Nations Development Programme, 2003).

AGING AND HEALTH

This process of demographic aging is not only unfolding globally, it is unfolding in an increasingly globalized world—a world shaped by ever greater flows of goods, capital, and people across national boundaries. Globalization has indeed become an essential feature of the policy environment in which aging societies try to understand and deal with the challenges and opportunities of demographic change (Oxford Institute of Ageing, 2006). Significant implications are associated with the demographic challenges of an older population. For example, there are currently sixty-six million people over age eighty worldwide, with 135,000 over one hundred. In fifty years, it is predicted that 13.7 percent of the world's population will be aged sixty and over. Europe, for instance, is already made up of mature societies with more old people in their populations than children. Asia and America appear to be following a similar pattern.

Such longevity is attributable to better health care and medical advances, decline in birth rates, control of infectious diseases, and better living conditions.

Today, 20 percent of the population in England is over sixty, compared with 16.5 percent in the USA. Between 1995 and 2025 the number of people over eighty is projected to increase by almost 50 percent, and the number of those over ninety will double (Department of Health, UK, 2001). By 2040 the life expectancy for both men and women will rise by two years per decade.

Any legislation or social policy should therefore aim to optimize life circumstances as well as enhance opportunities for its older citizens, especially in addressing the impact on individuals as they realize the potential of life spans, which may take them beyond the ninth or even tenth decade. This has implications for the entire life course, as individuals consider how to balance work, education, reproduction, and leisure within these ever-increasing life spans. In addition, the belief that it may be possible to manipulate the basic biology of aging to radically extend the human life span is beginning to claim serious attention as a policy issue (Oxford Institute of Ageing, 2003–2004).

"Successful aging" refers to the concept of being free of disease, being active and involved, and contributing to society in older age. Older people are, and will continue to be, healthier and more educated than their predecessors, but there is low expectation that families will be able to absorb all the older people who will need care at home (Janicki, 2006). Those with disabilities, either lifelong or acquired in later life, will continue to need increasing health and social care.

DISABILITY AND AGING

"People with early onset disabilities are said to 'age with disability' while those with mid- or-late-life onsets are said to have 'disability with ageing'" (Verbrugge and Yang, 2002).

Disability can be a function of lifelong impairment—for example, from conditions present at birth or acquired in childhood, such as cognitive disabilities, intellectual disabilities, sensory impairments and so on—or it can result from a late-life impairment. The latter may be the result of injury, disease, or decline. It is predictable that physical and other changes will occur in older people. In adults with motor, neurological, and other significant conditions, the impact of aging is likely to be experienced more adversely.

Currently, there is no universally agreed definition of disability or single method of identification, thereby making any comparison difficult.

It is estimated that disability affects 15 to 20 percent of every country's population— this translates to at least 610 million people worldwide. The causes vary: in industrialized countries it is closely linked to aging; in countries with developing economies it is linked with conflict and poverty (Employers' Forum on Disability).

In 2001 injuries and violence caused more than five million deaths worldwide, and injuries and violence have also led to an increase in disabilities. Traffic crashes are the largest single cause of serious injuries worldwide, and these will rapidly increase as the numbers of motor vehicles escalate in developing countries (Disease Control Priorities Project, n.d.).

The incidence of disability varies from continent to continent; in Europe it is estimated that more than forty-five million citizens aged between sixteen and sixty-four years have some form of long-term disability (European Parliament, n.d.); the United Kingdom has the second largest prevalence (27.2 percent); estimates in Australia, New Zealand, and the United States range between 18 and 20 percent.

The European Association of Service Providers for Persons with Disabilities estimate that "over 15 million people in the European Union 25 in addition to today's figures, will be confronted with severe functional limitations and disabling conditions" as a direct effect of aging, and will need appropriate support (European Association of Service Providers for Persons with Disabilities, n.d.).

As the financial and emotional burden of health problems in older people is considerable, preventive strategies are paramount in combating treatable health problems such as cardiovascular disorders or lifestyle-related disabilities. Physical exercise (particularly weight-bearing exercise for women), healthy nutrition, social and cognitive engagement, and mental agility can reverse or slow physical and mental decline.

INTELLECTUAL DISABILITIES AND AGING

The umbrella term *intellectual disabilities* is used to describe a combination of intelligence quotient (IQ) below 70, lifelong disabilities caused by mental or physical impairments (or both) manifested during the developmental period, and an impairment of daily functioning in two or more of the following areas:

- Capacity for independent living
- Economic self-sufficiency
- Learning
- Mobility
- Receptive and expressive language
- Self-care
- Self-direction

Other terms for intellectual disabilities include *mental retardation* and *learning disability*.

Major barriers to people with intellectual disabilities receiving health care are difficulties in communication, which impede articulation of health needs, and health professionals' lack of awareness of the increased risk of ill health in people with intellectual disabilities.

Common problems for people with intellectual disabilities are epilepsy, sensory impairments, obesity, poor dental health, common mental disorders, and psychosis. Life expectancy is estimated at twenty years less than the average for their peers without intellectual disabilities (International Association for the Scientific Study of Intellectual Disabilities, 2002). However, advances in social and health provision—such as deinstitutionalization, improved community living, improved medical care, public policy attention, and legislation—have all contributed to increasing longevity in people with intellectual disabilities.

Debilitating and progressive diseases such as dementia occur more commonly in older people with intellectual disabilities, although those with intellectual disabilities due to Down Syndrome appear to develop the disorder at an earlier age, typically in the fourth and fifth decades of life.

A UNITED KINGDOM PERSPECTIVE

In the United Kingdom, the National Health Services spent £65.4 billion on health care in 2002–2003. In 2002, the Labour Government committed itself to matching the

European average on health spending (8 percent of the GDP). In the same year, 1.2 percent of GDP was spent on health care from private sources such as personal medical insurance ("NHS Finance 2002—2003 . . . ," 2002). By 2005–2006 NHS spending rose to £85 billion, with a deficit of £750 million, and it is projected to reach £92 billion in 2007–2008 (Department of Health, 2006a).

The recent reforms in the NHS have meant that that there is more emphasis on health services that are consumer-led and delivering to a high standard of care. Several government publications, legislation, and guidance have led to improved standards of care in care homes (National Standards Care Commission), extended access to services (such as free NHS sight test for those over sixty and extension of the breast screening program to women over seventy), fairer funding of long-term care (free nursing care for those in nursing homes as of 2001), initiatives to maintain independence (Promoting Independence Grant, Supporting People), and public health programs to help older people stay healthy (such as free influenza vaccinations, increased access to dentistry, and the Keep Warm, Keep Well campaign).

The Department of Health published the National Service Framework (NSF) for Older People in 2001. "It is a programme of action and reform to address these problems and deliver higher quality services for older people. There will be more consultants, nurses and therapists working for older people and better access to high-tech surgery and community equipment . . ." (Department of Health, 2001a, p. ii).

Other relevant NSF programs for older people are the NSF for Mental Health (1999), Coronary Heart Disease (2000), the NHS Cancer Plan (2000), and NSFs for Diabetes (2001), Renal Services (2002), and Chronic Conditions (2005). These all set standards for improving diagnosis, assessment, and treatment of the various disorders as well as coordination of provision. These documents attempt to provide general guidelines of good practice based on research evidence; however, these can be open to local resources and interpretation. Nonetheless, the standards set are "to root out age discrimination, to provide person-centered care, to promote older people's health and independence and most importantly to fit services around people's needs" (Department of Health, 2001a, p. 13).

Aside from specific health legislation, other organizations—such as the British Council of Disabled People (http://www.bcodp.org.uk/), set up in 1981, and the Disability Rights Commission (http://www.drc.org.uk/)—are trying to address discrimination in accessing employment or health care in cases of people who have disabilities, including older people.

Another important group of service users is that of older people from minority racial and ethnic groups. A report by the Inspection of Community Care Services investigated whether social services departments provide services that meet the needs of elderly people from ethnic minorities (Murray, 1998). "Research has shown that this group has suffered as a result of racism, low incomes, poor housing, isolation and comparatively poor health. Studies have also shown that over a third of Asian older people receive neither a pension nor state benefits because they have not qualified for these" (p. 1).

The inspection was carried out in eight local authorities with significant numbers of black and Asian elders. The report concluded that although efforts are being made to provide appropriate services, choice tends to be limited, and ethnic minority elders still face difficulty in having their needs met.

Recommendations on good practice are presented for six key areas: policy and planning, communication and information, assessment and care management, service delivery, protection from abuse, and equality of opportunity. Alongside the NSFs, the government published a strategic document, "Valuing People" (Department of Health, 2001c) to consider the needs of people with intellectual disabilities. The white paper is wide-ranging, encompassing both social and health aspects of the lives of people with intellectual disabilities across the life span and from all ethnic groups.

As the life expectancy of people with intellectual disabilities was increasing, so was awareness of a new cohort of individuals who would be older and in the community for the first time. Therefore, a number of projects were developed to deal with issues that are relevant to those older service users with intellectual disabilities as well as to their elderly relatives. A prime example of such work is the Getting Older with Learning Disabilities (GOLD) programme. The 2002 report, which included the results of research projects and consultation with service users and their caregivers from 1998 to 2002, contains the following key themes:

- A charter of rights for older people with learning disabilities and for older family caregivers

- Sharing the views and voices of older people with learning disabilities and their families

- Supporting and disseminating innovative practice in this field to positively influence future service developments

- Underlining the need for service providers to think about how they will meet people's age-related changing needs and support them as they get older, using person-centered planning

- A series of recommendations for policy makers and planners, service planners, commissioners, and providers

Projections of population changes estimate that there will be up to a 36 percent increase in older people with intellectual disabilities by 2021. In the United States, it is estimated that there will be $44.1 billion of lifetime additional costs for the care of people with intellectual disabilities (Cooper, 2006). For the extended lifetimes of older people with intellectual disabilities , their health and support needs are related to having both learning disabilities and aging. Their health care is already compromised by the current service delivery, which includes inflexible appointment systems, short appointment times, reliance on ability to read, reactive delivery of health care, physical barriers, and poor coordination of information between services and agencies.

Other barriers are related to current medical practice and a social system that does not include people with intellectual disabilities. Examples are inexperience in intellectual disabilities, low contact level, lack of confidence, fear, feeling unskilled in working with this population group, attribution of additional health needs to intellectual disabilities, inappropriate stereotypes and negative assumptions about patients' ability to maintain quality of life, and lack of recognition of family caregivers' contribution.

Recently, primary care physicians (also called general practitioners or GPs) have been collaborating with Primary Care Trusts in creating ways in which people with intellectual disabilities, including those of older age, can have their health care needs managed. Limited locally enhanced schemes have been set up in some areas where GPs are remunerated for offering regular check-ups and participating in the development of the Health Care Plan (HAP) for each individual with intellectual disabilities registered with those surgeries. HAPs, health facilitation, and Person-Centered Thinking are some of the core features of improved care for people with intellectual disabilities found in the "Valuing People" white paper. But so far there has been no clear evidence that they work, and given the limited finances in the NHS as well as the inevitable rationing of health care resources, they may well remain an initiative too far.

LEGISLATIVE FRAMEWORK OF THE WELFARE STATE

Traditionally, religious and voluntary organizations have played a major role in shaping the welfare state. Often they led the way and encouraged governments to fulfill their duty to their citizens. The concept of small like-minded groups of people with a common cause getting together and forming pressure groups is common around the world; such groups play an increasingly major and significant role in determining how services are shaped and delivered. In the United Kingdom, nineteenth-century social reformers such as Barnardo, Booth, Fry, and Shaftesbury were visionary in their approach to shaping the way in which Victorian Britain cared for its vulnerable citizens.

The origins of organizations such as the National Society for Mental Handicap (now Royal MENCAP) have roots in parent organizations getting together to develop services that they believe should be in place and to which their relatives have a right. Today in the United Kingdom voluntary organizations such as Royal MENCAP, Age Concern, and SCOPE play a major role in the provision of health and social services. Increasingly they are developing into businesses, delivering services that are purchased by public health and social care agencies, who are encouraged to move away from being both commissioners and providers and act more as "brokers" of services, pointing potential customers in the right direction, and thereby empowering users and offering them "more choice and a louder voice" (Department of Health, 2006b).

Caregivers play an essential role in the health and social care system. There are approximately six million caregivers caring for aged relatives or those with a long-term illness. A study concluded that by 2037 the aging population in Britain, coupled with current community care policy, would require an extra 3.7 million caregivers to cope with an estimated increase of three million people aged seventy-five and over in need of care (George, 2001). In the past a small but significant number of caregivers have formed themselves into voluntary organizations; they continue to do so and have taken on the responsibility of lobbying for an improvement in services. Increasingly they also deliver a range of local and community-based services.

Today many of these voluntary organizations, which continue to have charitable status, are major players in the provision of services to vulnerable people and their families in the community.

Every constitution upholds the human rights of the individual. The practice may differ somewhat from country to country. Introducing the draft treaty to protect the rights of disabled people, New Zealand's ambassador to the United Nations, Don MacKay, warned "the reality is that persons with disabilities are often deprived of those rights" ("Disabled Treaty to Reverse Years of Neglect," 2006).

A study undertaken by the Joseph Rowntree Foundation (2001) found that

> *legally, people either have the capacity to make a decision or they do not, but the decision frequently goes untested in law. The process of decision-making for and by vulnerable adults in England is currently under the spotlight. The Mental Capacity Act 2005 aims to improve and clarify the decision-making process for those unable to make decisions for themselves. The act is underpinned by a set of five key principles, namely the presumption of capacity, the rights of the individual to be supported to make his or her own decision, the right to make what might be seen as "eccentric" or "unwise" decisions, best interests and least restrictive interventions (Department of Constitutional Affairs, 2004). How whatever is ultimately agreed will assist or hinder the use of supported-decision-making models is critical [Medora and Ledger, 2005, p. 154].*

THE DEBATE

So, do positive health policies on aging and disability have an effect on the well-being and the quality of life of citizens? Clearly they do, but not in isolation. Good health policies are interrelated to policies in social care, education, environment, leisure and recreation, and so on; they cannot be developed in isolation.

This was the emphasis of the Ottawa Charter for Health Promotion (World Health Organization, 1986), capitalizing on the growing interest in and understanding of universal health promotion that is focused on the way in which societies might improve the health and well-being of their citizens. The Charter stated that "health promotion is not just the responsibility of the health sector but goes beyond healthy life-styles to well-being" (World Health Organization, 1986).

The Charter advocated a holistic focus to bring about improvements in the quality of people's lives, an approach since echoed in a variety of ways to establish communities with high-quality lifestyles for their citizens. It identified a number of prerequisites, fundamental conditions, and resources for a healthy lifestyle: peace, shelter, education, food, income, a stable ecosystem, sustainable resources, social justice, and equity.

The STEPS (Structures Toward Emancipation, Participation and Solidarity) Project (2002–2004) and other research projects, examining local and national systems and arrangements for people with intellectual disabilities in Europe, found that, at a national level, there remain significant differences in the way policies (specialist versus generic) are formulated and implemented. For the most part, the same principles also apply to people with other disabilities. In some other countries there is a tendency to use a specialist approach to deliver health and social care services (for example, in Spain, Greece, and Italy), whereas in the United Kingdom—because its constitution is largely unwritten—and in Germany, a more generic approach has been adopted. The Scandinavian countries have adopted fully integrated, often constitutionally enforceable models. At local levels, however, central policies can be subject to differences in implementation.

Research in the United Kingdom suggested that in the population of people with intellectual disabilities there continues to be a significantly higher prevalence of various disorders, such as epilepsy (22 percent compared to 1 percent of the population) and mental health disorders (50 percent compared to 25 percent of the population) (Department of Health, 2001c).

The challenge for successive administrations in the United Kingdom and elsewhere has been to develop equitable and inclusive health and social care services for people who, for whatever reason, are less able to articulate their needs. Successive pieces of legislation in the United Kingdom have focused on the need to "mainstream" and avoid specialist services; the "Valuing People" white paper (Department of Health, 2001c) advocates that specialist services should be offered only where they are of real benefit to service users and their caregivers and relatives.

In the United Kingdom, the health and welfare agenda has become increasingly politicized. It is frequently an electioneering issue, of concern to citizens, especially those aged fifty and over, who are worried about the care they will receive when ill and in old age—a view shaped by culture and attitude.

Social changes and consumer attitudes have forced changes in the public sector providing health and social care services. The Labour Government in 1997 was elected in part because of its promises to reform and retain the National Health Service and make it accessible to all. Ten years on, the promises have been difficult to fulfill for a variety of reasons—some of the government's making, others because of global developments. Huge advances in health and social care for people with disabilities and in old age have resulted in an increasing demand for the state to provide its citizens, nationally and locally, with a broad range of services. Increasingly the reality has to be different; efforts to persuade and educate the public to change attitudes are under way.

There is now also an increased expectation that health and social services will offer choice and promote independence. This is partially available, but only to younger disabled people; older people still receive little choice in health provision and much of it continues to be about maintenance. There are increased expectations from disabled people, who as citizens rightly believe that they too have every right to demand and receive the level and quality of services available to the rest of the population. Increasingly these expectations are being voiced by a vocal and growing lobby of older people who also are no longer content to be shunted off to a care home to spend their last years in quiet and solitude. The biggest fear of people confronted by a long-term illness, disability, or old age is that they will lose their independence and rights as individuals.

The demand for health services continues to grow, with a significant increase in the demand for care in the community; for example, nursing and residential homes, and individuals taking control of their care. The shifting attitudes of the public have shaped legislation and in turn focused the attention of the public and private sectors. Public and private health sector providers now recognize that the future lies in improving and developing community provisions.

In the past, there was a tendency to provide services and expect that they would be acceptable and appreciated, without any real consideration of user choice or what the users might have thought they needed. The increasing use of Direct Payments (personal budgets), especially among younger disabled people, has empowered them to be uncompromising about their needs, wishes, and aspirations. Direct Payments create more flexibility in the provision of social services. Giving money in place of social care services means people have greater choice and control over their lives and are able to make their own decisions about how their care is delivered (Department of Health, n.d.). Further, concepts such as "person-centered services" and "person-centered planning" have become part of the vocabulary of health and care agencies in the UK, and there is at very least an attempt to speak the language, even if the reality is not all that the terms suggest.

CONCLUSION

We all want access to affordable and good health services, safe and accessible communities, good housing, accessible transport systems, recreation and leisure facilities, and the opportunity to work. For vulnerable adults—particularly those coping with mental health disorders, disabilities, and old age—the provision of institutional health and social care has been the norm. In the United Kingdom the future is going to look different. Legislation and central and local policies are beginning to make a difference.

There is a growing mixed economy delivering health and social care services, and no longer a reliance on "monopolistic" public institutions to provide a "one size fits all" approach. The attitude that the state has to provide everything is changing. Although there will always be a section of the community that will need the support of the state to receive appropriate services, increasingly there is a willingness to accept that this is an exception. These changes and the growth in assistive technology and housing, which can continue to be adapted to enable people with disabilities and older people to remain independent for as long as possible in the community, have led to significant increases in consumer choice.

Old age and disability can no longer be ignored or confer stigma to individuals. In the long term, policies and practices will have to adapt to ever changing ideas about what is possible and the need of all individuals to aspire to a continuing participation in society.

REFERENCES

Ageing Horizons: Policies for Ageing Societies. The Oxford Institute of Ageing.http://www.ageing.ox.ac.uk/ageinghorizons/index.htm (accessed November 2006).

Beveridge Report. Social Insurance and Allied Services, 1942.

Cambridge, P., and Ernst, A. (eds.). STEPS (Structures Toward Emancipation, Participation and Solidarity): The Experience of the STEPS Anti-discrimination Project, Working Documents, August 2004.

Cooper, A. "Services for Older People with Learning Disabilities." Conference Presentation, Coventry, UK, 2006.

Department of Health. Coronary Heart Disease: National Service Framework for Coronary Heart Disease: Modern Standards and Service Models. London: Her Majesty's Stationery Office, 2000a.

Department of Health. The NHS Cancer Plan: A Plan for Investment, A Plan for Reform. London: Her Majesty's Stationery Office, 2000b.

Department of Health. National Service Framework for Older People. London: Her Majesty's Stationery Office, 2001a.

Department of Health. National Service Framework for Diabetes. London: Her Majesty's Stationery Office, 2001b.

Department of Health. "Valuing People: A New Strategy for Learning Disability for the 21st Century. A White Paper." London: Her Majesty's Stationery Office, 2001c.

Department of Health. Chronic Conditions. London: Her Majesty's Stationery Office, 2005. [http://www.dh.gov.uk/PolicyAndGuidance/HealthAndSocialCareTopics/LongTermConditions/fs/en]. Accessed November 2006.

Department of Health. National Health Services Expenditure. London: Her Majesty's Stationery Office, 2006a.

Department of Health. Our Health, Our Care, Our Say. London: Her Majesty's Stationery Office, 2006b.

Department of Health. Direct Payments. London: Her Majesty's Stationery Office, n.d. [http://www.dh.gov.uk/en/Policyandguidance/Organisationpolicy/Financeandplanning/Directpayments/index.htm]. Accessed April 2007.

"Disabled Treaty to Reverse Years of Neglect." United Nations, August 29, 2006. [www.ipsnews.net]. Accessed November 2006.

Disease Control Priorities Project, n.d. [www.dcp2.org]. Accessed November 2006.

Employers' Forum on Disability. [www.realising-potential.org]. Accessed November 2006.

Esping-Andersen, G. Social Foundations of Post-industrial Economies. Oxford: Oxford University Press, 1999.

European Association of Service Providers for Persons with Disabilities, n.d. [www.easpd.org]. Accessed November 2006.

European Parliament, n.d. [www.europarl.europa.eu/facts4_8_8en.htm]. Accessed November 2006.

Flynn, R. J., and Lemay, R. A. (eds.). A Quarter-Century of Normalization and Social Role Valorization: Evolution and Impact. Ottawa, Ontario: University of Ottawa Press, 1999.

George, M. It Could Be You: A Report on the Chances of Becoming a Carer. London: Carers UK, 2001.

International Association for the Scientific Study of Intellectual Disabilities. Health Guidelines for Adults with an Intellectual Disability. Cardiff, Wales: International Association for the Scientific Study of Intellectual

Disabilities, 2002. [http://www.intellectualdisability.info/mental_phys_health/health_guide_adlt.htm]. Accessed April 2007.

Janicki, M. "Older People with Intellectual Disabilities." Conference presentation, Coventry, UK, 2006.

Marshall, T. H. *Citizenship and Social Class and Other Essays*. Cambridge, UK: Cambridge University Press, 1950.

Medora, H., and Ledger, S. "Implementing and Reviewing Person Centred Planning: Links with Care Management, Clinical Support and Commissioning." In P. Cambridge and S. Carnaby (eds.), *Person Centred Planning and Care Management with People with Learning Disabilities*. London: JKP Publishers, 2005.

Murray, U. "They Look After Their Own, Don't They? Inspection of Community Care Services for Black and Ethnic Minority Older People." London: Department of Health and Social Services Inspectorate, 1998. [http://www.dh.gov.uk/assetRoot/04/08/42/86/04084286.pdf]. Accessed November 2006.

"NHS Finance 2002–2003: The Issue Explained." *Guardian*, April 26, 2002.

Oxford Institute of Ageing. Annual Report. Oxford: University of Oxford, 2003–2004. [http://www.ageing.ox.ac.uk/ageinghorizons/index.htm]. Accessed September 2006.

Rice, J.M., Goodin, R. E., and Parpo, A. "The Temporal Welfare State: A Crossnational Comparison." *Journal of Public Policy*, 2006, *26*, 195–228.

United Nations Development Programme (UNDP). "Human Development Indicators: Human Development Report." New York: Oxford University Press for the UNDP, 2003.

"Annan Hails Agreement on Treaty Protecting Rights of Persons with Disabilities." United Nations News Centre, August 28, 2006. [http://www.un.org/apps/news/story.asp?NewsID=19641&Cr=disab&Cr1=].

"Universal Declaration of Human Rights." Office of the High Commissioner for Human Rights, December 10, 1948. [http://www.unhchr.ch/udhr/]. Accessed September 2006.

Verbrugge, L. M., and Yang, L. "Ageing with Disability and Disability with Ageing." *Journal of Disability Policy Studies*, March 1, 2002, *12*(4).

World Health Organization. Ottawa Charter for Health Promotion: First International Conference on Health Promotion, November 21, 1986.

CHAPTER

KEEPING PEOPLE ACTIVE: CONTINUING EDUCATION PROGRAMS THAT WORK

JULIA PREECE AND BRIAN FINDSEN

This chapter is organized in two parts. First, it takes a critical look at the social construction of older adulthood: how this construction impacts generally on the nature of educational opportunities for older adults and potentially on the nature of participation by older adults in education. We argue that older adults prefer to contribute to their own learning in a multiplicity of ways and that health, whether as an educational process or outcome, is frequently an integral aspect or by-product of a range of activities involving both formal and informal learning.

In the second part of the chapter we address more specifically the underresearched relationship between learning and health, and the World Health Organization's concept of active aging—focusing on both empirical evidence of the general impact of learning on health and the impact of targeted health programs on quality of life for older adults. We conclude with some suggestions for further research. Our perspectives draw primarily on the UK, but we also include other OECD countries such as New Zealand and the United States.

OLDER ADULTHOOD IN CONTEXT

Older adults, whatever the context, do not constitute a uniform group. In the UK the diversity of people in older adulthood is great, arguably greater than in many countries (given considerable immigration from around the world), thus refuting the notion of a homogeneous group in society. The myth of homogeneity is one of several surrounding the realities of later life. In addition, the medical profession has tended to focus on older people's frailties and physiological inadequacies, thus characterizing many older people as dependent on society, as consumers of social services who tend to live a passive existence. This myth of decrepitude has been largely challenged by critical educators who emphasize instead the collective wisdom of seniors, their active contributions to society (such as through volunteering), and their capacity to be self-sufficient (or at least interdependent with others such as family members). In the contemporary perspective of later adulthood, adult development theorists (for example, Fisher, 1993) have argued for a distinctive period of later life that has accompanying periods of task achievement, including adaptation to declining physical capacities and possible loss of good health.

In educational terms, the work of Peter Laslett in the UK has been seminal in the positive depiction of later adulthood and associated learning opportunities. In *A Fresh Map of Life,* published by Weidenfeld and Nicolson in 1989, he draws attention to four main phases of the life course. The first phase involves dependency, as a child becomes socialized into the prevailing norms and patterns of behavior in particular cultural groups, primarily through the family. The second is concerned with the mature adult, who typically focuses on parenting, career advancement, financial security, and heightened responsibility toward others. The third age, that associated with later adulthood, is characterized by a presumed enhanced freedom to be creative and fuller autonomy (given that the constraints of earning a living and childrearing presumably have been lifted). The fourth age is short; in it the adult once again becomes largely dependent on others in preparation for death. This characterization of major ages in life has been much criticized, as it tends to be overly romantic and based primarily on a white male view of the life course. Yet the notion of the third age has gained increased acceptance in social policy and accords with an emergent idea of the "learning society" in which lifelong learning is an important ingredient (as exemplified by John Field's book *Lifelong Learning and The New Educational Order*, published by Trentham Books in 2002).

It is important to acknowledge the consistency of the third age of learning in a lifelong learning framework. The fundamental issue is that people have the right to equal access to education at any point of their lives, older people included.

PARTICIPATION IN CONTINUING EDUCATION

Continuing education covers a wide range of offerings, ranging from formal (institutionalized, hierarchically graded modes of study prevalent in further and higher education in the UK), to nonformal (organized systematic learning outside education institutions), to informal (incidental learning closely associated with daily living). (*Further education* colleges in the UK originated as day-release technical education colleges for industrial workers. Their catchments are local—unlike universities—and they offer post-compulsory education in vocational and nonvocational subjects. Traditionally they did not offer undergraduate/degree programs, though many of them now offer undergraduate level courses and sometimes full degrees.) The question of who gets to access particular forms of knowledge has been a preoccupation of adult educators around the world. The trend internationally is for those who have most benefited from formal education (such as schooling) to continue to prosper in later life (as in continuing education for the professions)—hence, the level of prior education is a powerful predictor of future education. In the depiction of who misses out in the equal opportunity stakes, older adults as a category tend to be identified in all societies. However, this observation is indeed flawed, as many older adults are very capable of looking after their learning needs and require minimal assistance to achieve their goals (Findsen, 2006). Nevertheless, the effects of social stratification (gender, race, ethnicity, geographical location) mean that a significant proportion of older adults are left out and do not benefit from the wider participation initiatives of some educational providers.

In the UK very useful research has been conducted by the National Institute of Adult Continuing Education (NIACE) in the realm of participation, including those studies that have focused on exploring participation issues for older adults. In a major UK study of participation in adult education, for example, Naomi Sargant and associates published *The Learning Divide* through NIACE in 1997. This provided a stark analysis of those who benefit most from educational opportunities (usually white middle-class men). Indeed, considerable research internationally and in the UK has recommended focusing more attention on the marginalized of society, including a sizeable proportion of older adults, to bring them the fruits of educational opportunities (see, for example, books by this chapter's authors, such as Brian Findsen's *Learning Later*, published by Krieger in 2005, and Julia Preece's *Combatting Social Exclusion in University Adult Education*, published by Ashgate in 1999).

Consideration of why more older adults do not participate in learning opportunities is a well-researched area in the Western world. The following barriers have commonly been identified:

Situational—those related to individuals' life contexts and circumstances (for example, the need for transportation to convenient locations)

Institutional—those erected unintentionally by institutions to exclude or discourage learners (such as high fees or inappropriate pedagogy for older adults)

Informational—institutional failure to communicate information efficiently or effectively (for instance, displaying brochures where older people do not congregate)

Psychosocial—those predispositions and attitudes developed by the learners themselves about their capacities to learn (such as the belief that "you can't teach an old dog new tricks")

By far the most difficult to overcome are the psychosocial barriers, as these have been established over a comparatively long period of time and tend to be ingrained in individuals' psyches. These stereotypical beliefs about older adults' capabilities need to be challenged both by the wider society (including through the media) and by older people themselves. For instance, the stereotype of passivity in older adulthood (associated with older attitudes and the kind of retirement in which seniors withdraw from society) needs to be replaced by the notion of active citizenry in older adulthood.

Consistent analysis of research into participation highlights that providers of adult education need to collaborate with nonparticipant groups in their local communities so that they are active participants, as planners and learners, in programs of study attuned to their varied learning needs and aspirations. We will demonstrate that programs such as these have a significant impact on the health and well-being of older adults even when they were not designed solely for that purpose.

ACTIVE AGING AND CONTINUING EDUCATION

The World Health Organization (WHO) has adopted the concept of *active aging* since 1999 as an all-inclusive approach to the maintenance of health and independence, social justice and citizenship for older persons. It embraces earlier concepts such as *healthy aging*, which focused on maintenance of health through lifestyle choices and preventive measures; *successful aging*, with an emphasis on personal well-being and psychological adjustment; and *positive aging*, with the goal of countering negative perceptions of aging and retirement (Davey, 2002). Elements of active aging include "working longer, retiring later, being active after retirement, engaging in health sustaining activities, being as self-reliant and involved as possible" (Davey, 2002, p. 97). The goal of an active aging approach is to optimize "opportunities for health, participation and security in order to enhance the quality of life as people age" (World Health Organization/Europe, 2006, p. 21) through empowerment and participation in planning implementation and evaluation of services. The focus goes beyond just the labor market to include general quality of life, mental and physical well-being, and opportunity to make choices. There has therefore been a shift in emphasis over the past twenty years from a curative and social care model of health to one that advocates prevention, rehabilitation, self-reliance, and independence. This more holistic approach to aging itself is one that is reflected in recent UK initiatives for older adults.

At a national (UK) level, NIACE has produced a significant program of sustained activity under the banner of the Older and Bolder campaign. This macro-level initiative was developed in accordance with the UK Government's Better Government for Older

People (1998) policy that advocates different organizations working with others on a cooperative rather than a competitive basis. The older person is the unit of attention rather than the service or the provider. This program is holistic in approach—education is one part of a multifaceted strategy in which other social needs of older people are taken into account (for example, housing and health). More recently, the Older and Bolder movement has been aligned with the March 2005 UK governmental paper *Opportunity Age: Meeting the Challenges of Ageing in the 21st Century* (Department of Work and Pensions 2005). A strategy of public seminars by NIACE is provided for different groups of people (older people themselves, policy makers, local educational authorities, training providers, and community groups).

Some national adult education agencies have cells in different parts of the UK. For example, the University of the Third Age (U3A), particularly strong in British Commonwealth countries, operates under the control of older adults themselves, many of whom have been professional people and successful continuing education participants through their lives. The U3A is a self-sufficient organization characterized by heightened autonomy, minimal costs to members, considerable informality, a negotiated curriculum, teachers as colearners, the absence of formal assessment, and interactive teaching styles appropriate to older people's preferred learning methods. (For a recently published history of U3A in the UK, refer to Eric Midwinter's *500 Beacons: The U3A Story*, published by The Third Age Press in 2004). In short, many of the favored working principles of adult educators for effective adult learning are employed in this organization.

It is important to recognize that many continuing education programs that work for older adults do not neatly fit the education label. For instance, outside the education sphere, agencies concerned centrally with older people's issues—such as Help the Aged, the Pre-retirement Association of the UK, and Age Concern and City Councils—conduct effective programs, usually for paraprofessionals working with seniors. In addition, it is wise not to discount the plethora of programs conducted in workplaces (in which older people should have equal rights of access) and in voluntary organizations that are highly dependent on older people for their sustainability. Hence, programs exist in many nooks and crannies of society; the essential questions to continually ask are "Who benefits from continuing education programs?" and "Continuing education programs that work for whom?" In other words, we need to keep a critical eye on whether participation issues are sufficiently taken into account in these educational opportunities.

THE RELATIONSHIP BETWEEN HEALTHY LIVING AND EDUCATION FOR OLDER ADULTS

Literature on the relationship between education and health for older adults encompasses these separate perspectives in the form of (1) education per se that has the impact of increasing health and well-being, (2) preventive education for prolonging active life, and (3) education to help individuals manage health concerns. We now explore some of the research evidence and offer some examples of good educational practices that have claimed particular links to health and well-being.

The Evidence

Research into the link between education and health is surprisingly underdeveloped, though on a more general scale it has long been argued by the World Bank and similar organizations that countries whose populations have high education levels generally have lower infant mortality rates and longer life expectancy. There is also empirical evidence that positive educational experiences in early life and higher educational attainment influence health in later life and longevity (see, for example, Hammond and Feinstein, 2006; Schneider, 2003). Equally, it is now understood that older people who exercise regularly are more likely to maintain brain function into later life and that healthy aging strategies need to stress good diet and exercise (Novelli, 2005). Following the association of exercise with increased brain functioning, Schneider (2003) emphasizes that learning slows down specific aspects of aging and also that "older persons who perform aerobics have shorter reaction times, [and] higher levels of fluent intelligence" (p. 813). A report published in 2000 by Fiona Aldridge and Peter Lavender of NIACE, *The Impact of Learning on Health*, demonstrates that learning improves the general well-being of people with dementia, contributes to physical and mental health, improves self-confidence, and increases community activity and ability to cope with life events. These positions are backed up by more targeted quantitative studies such as the one by Sabates and Feinstein (2004); they argue that adult education increases the probability of women's undergoing health screening. There is less evidence, however, to tell us what education works in terms of health outcomes, in what contexts, how it works, and why.

There are some examples of quantitative impact studies that investigate the effectiveness of particular intervention programs on health behavior of older adults. In terms of preventive education, Chernoff (2001) reported on a longitudinal study that tracked the impact of a targeted diet and exercise promotion program for older adults. Changes in health behavior were identified, though the impact of the program lessened in older age. In terms of programs designed to help individuals manage their existing health conditions, McWilliam and others (1999) reported the test effects of a health promotion intervention for people over sixty-five discharged from the hospital. The intervention involved ten weekly, hour-long sessions in which a nurse facilitated critical reflection on life and health through a participatory, person-centered approach to care, based on the adult education theory of perspective transformation (Mezirow, 1981). This entailed enabling individuals to alter their expectations, beliefs, and values related to experience of illness and to improve their personal attitudes toward health, the self, and ability to control their own lives. The intervention aimed at enhancing a sense of self, self-care agency, and personal control to develop greater ability to realize aspirations, satisfy needs, and respond positively to medical challenges with less use of hospital or home care services. This group and a nonintervention control group were assessed after twenty-two weeks and again at one year. It was found that those who received the intervention were more independent and better able to manage their own health than the control group. Although the differences after one year had declined, the intervention group still scored higher on both counts.

In most studies, there is little qualitative investigation into the educational philosophies or perspectives that inform those intervention programs. Nevertheless, the majority of targeted programs have identified the practice of using informal and community-based initiatives. Green and Frankish (2002) discuss how health promotion initiatives that may in the past have focused purely on public health messages now recognize that there is a need for a more intersectoral and interdisciplinary approach to health education that is concerned with the complexity of life conditions, wider social forces, social trends, and lifestyles. Similarly, Weare (2002) illustrates that health promotion campaigns have changed from hard-hitting campaigns about altering lifestyles to emphasizing "enhancement of the individual with the knowledge, skills and motivation to make competent decisions about their health" (p. 102) in a more holistic and context-sensitive way. Weare shows how an educational model that (1) teaches generic competencies such as assertiveness, problem solving skills, communication, and decision making and (2) uses adult education principles of starting where people are at, tailoring courses for the needs of particular groups, and encouraging active engagement in the learning process is more likely to have an influence on behavior change: "We tend to choose to look after our health, according to how we feel about, for example, the level of control we have in the world" (p. 117). This is linked to the notion that high self-efficacy (the internalized perception of one's ability to achieve a desired outcome) is linked to lower health risk, even when allowing for other variables such as socioeconomic and health status.

A report in 1999 by the Alcohol and Public Health Research Unit in Auckland, called *Advice for Purchasing Strategy on Public Health Issues: Health of Older Adults* (Alcohol and Public Health Research Unit, 1999), also points out that increased knowledge about health does not necessarily translate into better health behavior. So education needs to be combined with peer support and personal health plans, often in community-based program settings, working with self-help groups, and combined with other social activities: "health cannot be imposed on a community" but programs can develop in "response to people's own perceptions of risk and priorities" (Alcohol and Public Health Research Unit, 1999, p. 26). This includes relevant guidance provision (Ford, 2005) and recognizing cultural or gender-specific issues (Torsch and Ma, 2000). An example of a gender-specific project that embraced the holistic empowerment philosophy is cited by the Alcohol and Public Health Research Unit (1999). A project to combat issues of loneliness, isolation, and grief for depressed older women started as an informal lunchtime meeting that organized a celebratory festival for older women, with workshops on health, creativity, spirituality, writing, theatre, and culture. From there, self-help support groups evolved, with support from a community center. In these examples we see that health and well-being are not addressed in isolation from other life forces.

As we have already mentioned, many continuing education programs for older adults are designed to train for a specific, non-health-related skill. The study by White and others (2002) provided an opportunity to assess the health and well-being indicators of one such course on computer skills in relation to loneliness, quality of life, and depression, as well as attitude toward computers.

At the end of the trial, 60 percent of participants were using the Internet on a weekly basis. There were trends toward decreased loneliness and depression along with more positive attitudes toward computers. Participants were using the Internet to communicate with family and friends, explore interests and hobbies, obtain consumer information, access community resources, and meet new people through chat rooms and bulletin boards.

The wider benefits included increased activity generally; some participants started their own computer interest group and began to publish a communitywide newsletter, indicating its potential to strengthen existing social ties as well as develop new social activity. The researchers admitted that the participants "appeared to gain from exposure to this technology in several ways not captured in our measures including self efficacy, mastery, and empowerment" (White and others, 2002, p. 220).

In contrast to this skills-specific project, the story of the Senior Studies Institute at the University of Strathclyde in Glasgow, Scotland demonstrates the integrated nature and potential of a responsive, participant-led educational program that combines health, skills, knowledge, and understanding with a general development approach for older adults. From a modest start of five classes in French, Spanish, computing, exercise, video-making, and health for two hundred people, the institute now has a membership of over four thousand. Participants maintained the momentum of the early classes during term breaks with their own initiatives, including organizing trips to France and volunteering for administration work in the university. Language clubs and other social activities continued, and classes expanded into other subjects, with negotiation of dedicated space and staffing along with funding support from Glasgow Development Agency. Programs now include courses for credit, participation in undergraduate courses, and outreach initiatives for less-privileged communities, ethnic minorities, and rural areas. Volunteering included retraining for work, personal development, drop-in times that enabled networking about work opportunities, and development of research activities to assess the impact of learning on older people's lives.

The director, Lesley Hart (2001), identifies some critical factors for the center's success: support from senior management; an integrated social dimension to the learning activities; integration with other university activities; the volunteering activities, which created a sense of ownership and belonging to the Institute; and the fact that the learning programs were responsive and evolving—so that standard weekly classes also became day workshops, half-day seminars, study trips abroad, and lunchtime talks, and topics developed according to demand. The informal nature of the learning environment, its accessibility, and the quality of staffing were also a contributory factor. Health and fitness classes evolved in response to student demand, rather than the other way around.

Retraining opportunities for older adults are few and far between. A Scottish Enterprise report entitled *Getting Old and Grey?* (Brown, 2001) reported on one exception. Pekham and Rye, a small chain of luxury foods and delicatessen goods, overcame high turnover among younger workers by targeting older people, believing they would offer more stability and consistency and might be looking for a higher level of job security. The firm obtained funding from Glasgow Development Agency, a training employment grant scheme, to train long-term unemployed adults over forty for a National Vocational Qualification level 2 in warehousing. Turnover was significantly reduced, resulting in greater work efficiency and accuracy, enhanced self-esteem, and more motivated teams. Business costs and absenteeism were reduced and the workforce felt motivated and valued, with consequent increased well-being among this age group.

SUMMARY AND RECOMMENDATIONS FOR FURTHER RESEARCH

This chapter has highlighted both general issues having to do with participation in education for older adults and research into health that accrues from different forms of educational opportunities. It can be seen from the examples that the qualitative gains in health and well-being are rarely assessable in isolation from wider socioeconomic benefits, as one form of achievement triggers or feeds off another. The pedagogic essence of engendering health success through education initiatives seems to be through social interaction and enablement rather than decontextualized information-giving. This aspect has also been found by Preece and Ntseane (2004) to be a critical factor in relation to HIV/AIDS education in African contexts, suggesting the global applicability of holistic and interactive health education programs. Furthermore, a key feature to encourage participation is the engagement of a collaborative approach: negotiating programs with older adults themselves, being flexible and responsive to their perceived needs.

Research into the relationship between learning and health, especially for older adults, is still in its infancy. Aldridge and Lavender (2000) emphasized the ongoing need to (1) investigate the extent of health improvement following educational participation, (2) explore the roles and relationships between health and education staff to maximize health outcomes, and (3) explore programs in which health settings are used to bring opportunities to adults who are not participating in learning programs. Other areas of research might also include investigation into

- The impact of work-related training on workforce health for older adults

- How to support older adults in work situations in which they have chronic health issues

- The health and well-being impact of education (health or otherwise) programs on different cultures of older adults, including adults who left school with few qualifications

- The effects on health of different types of educational intervention

- The effects of targeted versus nontargeted skills training programs on older adults' health and well-being

Case studies could include pilots for community learning as a preventative service, the role of guidance services in enhancing participation, and the efficacy of health promotion interventions. Finally, further research is needed into which older adults, in what environmental contexts, are more likely to benefit from internet education.

The picture of continuing education programs that work, therefore, is complex and dependent on the nature of involvement and the outcomes being measured.

REFERENCES

Alcohol and Public Health Research Unit. *Advice for Purchasing Strategy on Public Health Issues: Health of Older Adults.* Auckland: APHRU, 1999.

Aldridge, F., and Lavender, P. *The Impact of Learning on Health.* Leicester: NIACE, 2000.

Brown, R. "Getting Old and Grey? The Implications of Demographic Change and Population Ageing for the Scottish Labour Market." Futureskills Scotland Unit, Scottish Enterprise, 2001.

Chernoff, R. "Nutrition and Health Promotion in Older Adults." *The Journals of Gerontology Series A: Biological Sciences and Medical Sciences*, 2001, 56, 47–53.

Davey, J. "Active Ageing and Education in Mid and Later Life." *Ageing and Society*, 2002, 22, 95–113.

Findsen, B. "Social Institutions as Sites of Learning for Older Adults: Differential Opportunities." *Journal of Transformative Education*, 2006, 4(1), 65–81.

Fisher, J. C. "A Framework for Describing Developmental Change Among Older Adults." *Adult Education Quarterly*, 1993, 43(2), 76–89.

Ford, G. *Am I Still Needed? Guidance and Learning for Older Adults.* Derby: Centre for Guidance Studies, University of Derby, 2005.

Green, L. W., and Frankish, C. J. "Health Promotion, Health Education, and Disease Prevention." In C. Everett Koop, C. E. Pearson, and M. R. Schwarz (eds.), *Critical Issues in Global Health.* San Francisco: Jossey Bass, 2002, 321–330.

Hammond, C., and Feinstein, L. *Are Those Who Flourished at School Healthier Adults? What Role for Adult Education?* London: Centre for Research on the Wider Benefits of Learning, Institute of Education, 2006.

Hart, L. The Strathclyde Centre for Lifelong Learning: Senior Studies Institute, 2001. [http://www.cll.strath.ac.uk/ssi/intro/history.htm]. Accessed November 2006.

McWilliam, C. L., and others. "Home-Based Health Promotion for Chronically Ill Older Persons: Results of a Randomized Controlled Trial of a Critical Reflection Approach." *Health Promotion International*, 1999, 14(1), 27–41.

Mezirow, J. "A Critical Theory of Adult Learning and Education." *Adult Education*, 1981, 32(1), 3–27.

Novelli, W. D. "Managing Health, Health Care, and Aging." In W. H. Fogge, N. Daulaire, R. E. Black, and C. E. Pearson (eds.), *Global Health Leadership and Management*, pp. 37–54. San Francisco: Jossey-Bass, 2005.

Preece, J., and Ntseane, P. G. "Using Adult Education Principles for HIV/AIDS Awareness Intervention Strategies in Botswana." *International Journal of Lifelong Education*, 2004, 23(1), 5–22.

Sabates, R., and Feinstein, L. *Education, Training and The Take-up of Preventative Health Care.* London: Centre for Research on the Wider Benefits of Learning, Institute of Education, 2004.

Schneider, K. "The Significance of Learning for Aging." *Educational Gerontology*, 2003, 29(10), 809–823.

Torsch, V. L., and Ma, G. X. "Cross-cultural Comparison of Health Perceptions, Concerns, and Coping Strategies Among Asian and Pacific Islander American Elders." *Qualitative Health Research*, 2000, 10(4), 471–489.

Weare, K. "The Contribution of Education to Health Promotion." In R. Bunton and G. Macdonald (eds.), *Health Promotion: Disciplines, Diversity and Developments* (2nd ed.). London: Routledge, 2002, 102–126.

White, H., and others "A Randomized Controlled Trial of the Psychosocial Impact of Providing Internet Training and Access to Older Adults." *Aging and Mental Health*, 2002, 6(3), 213–221.

World Health Organization/Europe. "Healthy Ageing." Geneva: World Health Organization, 2006. [http://www.euro.who.int/eprise/main/WHO/Progs/HEA/Home/]. Accessed November 2006.

CHAPTER

LONGEVITY'S IMPACT ON RETIREMENT SECURITY

C. ROBERT HENRIKSON

DEMOGRAPHICS: THE FUTURE THAT CANNOT BE CHANGED

In the decade of 2006 to 2016, according to futurist Andrew Zolli (2006), the U.S. population figures will begin taking on the shape of an hourglass, with the largest number of older people in our society's history (the baby boomers) up top, and the largest generation of young people since the boomers (the millennials, or echo boomers) at the bottom. Generation-Xers will form the narrow point in the middle.

To understand the implications that this aging of the population has for retirement security, it is important to analyze the demographic trends. In the United States, during the time of the American Revolution, the average life span was less than thirty-five years; By 1920, it had risen to fifty-four years (*The Columbia Encyclopedia*, Sixth Edition, 2001–2005). In 2003 that figure reached 77.6 years (Centers for Disease Control, 2005). The U.S. Census Bureau projects that life expectancy in the United States will be in the mid-eighties by the year 2050 and will eventually level out in the low nineties. The United States currently has the greatest number of centenarians in the world, numbering over sixty-seven thousand in 2005. The Census Bureau predicts

323

that the U.S. will have 580,000 people over age one hundred by the year 2040 (U.S. Census Bureau, 2004).

In additions to these improvements in life expectancy, the number of older Americans is growing. During the boom years of 1946–64, seventy-seven million babies were born in the United States. The leading edge of the United States baby boom generation turned sixty in 2006—just five years away from the traditional retirement age of sixty-five.

GLOBAL TRENDS IN AGING AND RETIREMENT

Around the world, many countries are experiencing an age boom similar to that in the United States, with improved public health, declining birth rates, and increases in longevity having profound societal effects on government pension and health care policies. Many developed countries face even more serious retirement and aging challenges than the United States, and mature and developing economies alike will need to find new solutions to address the growing numbers of elderly who are dependent on the government or families for support in their old age (see Figure 30.1).

Of all the world's regions, Europe currently has the highest proportion of its population aged sixty-five and over—16 percent—and this is projected to almost double by 2050. According to the Manheim Institute for the Economics of Aging, birth rates declining to well below replacement levels mean that Europe's expensive social services structures will place an enormous financial strain on fewer and fewer working-age individuals (The Survey of Health, Aging, and Retirement in Europe, 2005).

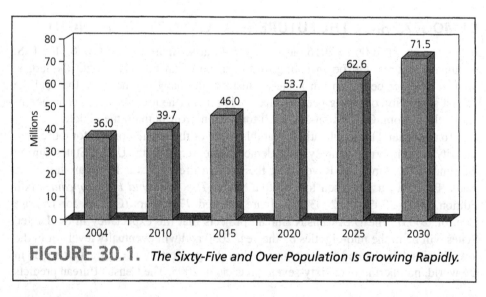

FIGURE 30.1. *The Sixty-Five and Over Population Is Growing Rapidly.*

Source: U.S. Census Bureau, 2004.

Asia's population is also aging. Japan, for example, already has a high percentage of elderly due to the long life expectancy for Japanese people coupled with a low birth rate and the minimal immigration allowed into the country. Japan's society is among the fastest-aging in the world. The proportion of the population that is elderly will effectively double from the 1995 figures of 14 percent to over 27 percent by the year 2025 (Farugee and Muhleisen, 2001). Likewise, South Korea's population is aging rapidly—according to some research, faster than any other country in the world. Only 3.3 percent of Korea's population was over age sixty-five in 1966. By 2005 the share had risen to 9.1 percent. According to current projections, it will reach 24.3 percent by 2030 and 38.2 percent by 2050 (Korea National Statistical Office, 2006). China's efforts to curb population growth have also created unintended demographic consequences. The "one child per family" policy instituted in 1979, which succeeded in reducing explosive population growth, has jeopardized labor force replacement as the society transitions from a system of total state provision of welfare for all to an emerging capitalist-socialist hybrid (Quanhe, 1988).

RETIREMENT SECURITY AT RISK WORLDWIDE

These population trends point to the difficulties that both developed and developing economies will have in sustaining and supporting their elderly and their pensioners of the future. The mature welfare states have been providing lifetime retirement income as well as health coverage to pensioners for many decades. However, with fewer younger workers available to support the growing number of retirees, and more public money needed to pay for pensions and health care, these countries will not be able to sustain the same level of support in the decades ahead. As the vast majority of older citizens of these nations have counted on the government to provide for them in their retirement, they have not needed to concern themselves about financial security in retirement and are not adequately prepared for an old age in which their governments may no longer be able to deliver on their former commitments (see Figure 30.2).

The developing world is not yet at as critical a juncture, but eventually it will also be impacted by the aging of the population—for different reasons. The challenge for those countries, however, is not so much how to afford the rising fiscal cost of generous government retirement promises, but how to support a rapidly growing number of elders in societies in which most of the population has no formal retirement protection at all. These countries in the early phases of their economic development lack the resources to provide health coverage or pensions to the vast majority. The family continues to be the traditional support network, providing informal care for old and young alike. But as these countries become more developed, family support networks are coming under increasing pressure. As younger people are likely to leave their villages to seek employment in the cities, the elderly are often left behind. Along with "modernization," the traditional ethic of "filial piety" that required the young to care for the old is also being eroded. Meanwhile, falling fertility and declining family size mean that tomorrow's elders will have fewer children to share the caregiving burden.

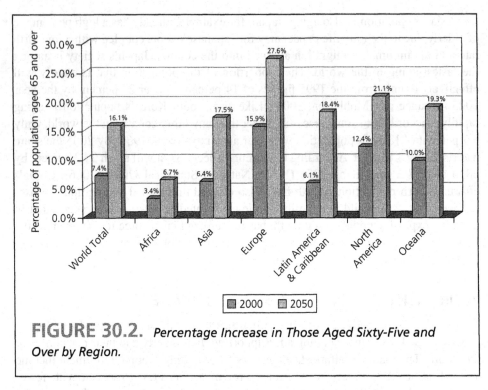

FIGURE 30.2. *Percentage Increase in Those Aged Sixty-Five and Over by Region.*

Source: United Nations Population Division, 2005.

These trends raise serious questions about retirement policy worldwide. It is clear that governments alone cannot solve these problems with their existing systems and resources.

AMERICA'S FINANCIAL BURDEN SHIFT

In the United States, as in other developed countries, changing demographics have resulted in seismic shifts in our society in the last few decades with regard to private pensions, Social Security, and health care. As a result, for the first time since the Great Depression individuals are increasingly being called on to fund and finance the risks that had previously been managed, in large part, by the government or employers. And, given that many retirees may live up to forty years in retirement, individuals need to build a nest egg large enough, and manage it well enough, to sustain them for a retirement that may be as long as their working lives.

The United States is quickly moving toward an "era of personal responsibility," and individuals are now aware that the retirement burden has been shifted to their shoulders. However, many are not prepared to act. It may seem an insurmountable challenge to dedicate the time and energy to figure out—on their own—how to manage the risks they face. Unfortunately, most individuals are not equipped to manage these risks on their own.

For many older people, Social Security is their main source of income. However, many individuals have relied on the investments in their retirement portfolio to supplement their public pension (Social Security). Investments, however, while a powerful tool for helping consumers grow their wealth, may not, by themselves, adequately fund and finance the cost of caring for their own or a loved one's long-term illness. Nor can they adequately ensure that an individual won't run out of money if he or she lives a long and healthy life. With the erosion of government and employer benefits, insurance must play an increasingly important role in protecting individuals from retirement risks.

So how did we get here? Many of our parents and grandparents—the World War II generation and the Silent Generation—didn't need to worry about these issues. Take, for example, saving for retirement. They often sought out jobs with large corporations or the government that offered defined benefit pension plans. When these workers retired, their pension "paycheck" continued for as long as they lived. They felt secure that when they retired they and their families didn't run the risk of running out of money.

Over the last two decades, the number of employer-sponsored defined benefit pension plans in the United States has declined precipitously. This number reached a peak of 112,000 in the mid-1980s, with about one-third of American workers covered. According to the Pension Benefit Guaranty Corporation, today only 30,000 defined benefit pension plans remain (Belt, 2005). In recent years, many employers have chosen not to adopt defined benefit pension plans, and others, including a number of Fortune 100 companies, have chosen to terminate or freeze their existing plans in "exchange" for a larger 401(k) company match. According to Watson Wyatt Worldwide, in 2005 113 companies froze or terminated at least one defined benefit plan, compared with 71 in 2004 and 34 in 2001.

Trends are similar in other parts of the world where private pensions have a history. In the UK, the number of workers in private sector–defined benefit plans that are open to new entrants dropped by 50 percent between 2000 and 2005 (Capretta, 2007).

PREPARING FOR AND LIVING IN RETIREMENT

It becomes clear that growing numbers of individuals who are approaching retirement in the United States, as well as those in other mature economies, will not be adequately prepared.

In 2003, the MetLife Mature Market Institute created the Retirement Income IQ test. Twelve hundred men and women between fifty-six and sixty-five years of age and within five years of retiring were asked fifteen questions to assess their level of retirement preparedness. Ninety-five percent of the respondents scored 60 percent or less; the average score was 33 on a grading scale of 100 points (MetLife, 2003). It is likely that individuals in other developed countries would also score low on the quiz.

Respondents misunderstood how long people will likely live. A sixty-five-year-old man has a 50 percent chance of living beyond his average life expectancy. ("Life expectancy" means that half the population will live beyond that point and the other half will not). But the majority of respondents thought there was only a 25 percent or less likelihood of living beyond the average life expectancy. Only 16 percent of respondents replied correctly that for a couple, both aged sixty-five, there is a 25 percent chance that one of them will live beyond age ninety-seven (Society of Actuaries, 2006).

The findings from the Retirement Income IQ are corroborated by many other industry studies. In April 2006, the Employee Benefits Research Institute (EBRI) released its sixteenth annual Retirement Confidence Survey (RCS), a survey of 1,252 individuals in the United States aged twenty-five and over. The RCS found that 52 percent of workers saving for retirement report total savings and investments (not including the value of their primary residence or any defined-benefit plans) of less than $50,000. The large majority of workers who have not put money aside for retirement have little at all in savings; 75 percent of these workers say their assets total less than $10,000 (Employee Benefit Research Institute, 2006).

Americans' personal savings rate dipped into negative territory—minus 0.5 percent—in 2005 for the first time since the Great Depression. This means that they not only spent all of their after-tax income but also had to either dip into previous savings or increase borrowing.

UNDERSTANDING RETIREMENT RISKS

Retirement increases the impact of some familiar risks and presents some new ones. The three primary risks that an individual will face in retirement are inflation, market volatility, and longevity, including the risk of outliving retirement savings or being afflicted with a chronic illness. The effects of inflation are substantial. Income must double over a twenty-year period just to stay even with average rates of inflation (Society of Actuaries, 2006).

Market volatility is another risk that can have a devastating impact on retirees, especially if market downturns occur early in their retirement years. Too often people rely on averages and base their planning (if any) on the assumption that their account will return the average. They research the historical market returns, plan to withdraw an amount less than the historical average return, and then feel confident their money will last them well into their retirement years. Often, however, retirees simply do not have time to recover from serious stock market losses. Using average returns while planning can be dangerous because the market does not earn averages in any given year and once you withdraw in a down market, you realize losses never to be recovered.

While inflation and market risk can have a tremendous impact, longevity is, in my opinion, the biggest risk facing retirees because it is the only risk individuals cannot manage on their own, no matter how financially literate they are (see Figure 30.3).

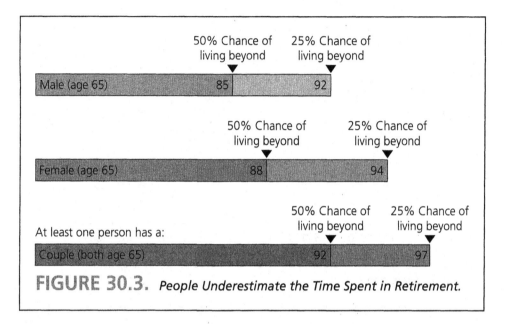

FIGURE 30.3. *People Underestimate the Time Spent in Retirement.*

Source: Society of Actuaries, 2006.

The longevity risk faced by an individual retiree is comparable in magnitude, but not in nature, to the inflation or investment risks that he or she faces at retirement. Market risk can be alleviated somewhat through asset allocation, and inflation risk can be addressed by investing in growth equities. But longevity risk only serves to exacerbate these other two risks by increasing the length of time an individual is exposed to them.

MANAGING LONGEVITY RISK

As governments and employers worldwide roll back pension promises, individuals will increasingly be required to take responsibility for their financial security in retirement. Many who have counted on a pension for their sole income in retirement will find that it will not be sufficient. Education about the risks of retirement is essential in order to ensure a decent standard of living in the future. One tool that individuals should consider is turning to mortality pooling to convert their retirement savings into guaranteed income that they cannot outlive.

The use of pooled risk is still an individual's best and most cost-effective defense, because when a group is assembled and mortality experience is pooled, monumental efficiencies are realized. An average retiree, for example, would need to have saved about one-third more to attempt to replicate the power of a mortality pool and even then could still risk running out of money (see Figure 30.4).

The pooling concept is a powerful one that's at the heart of all insurance products (as well as public pensions such as Social Security). Individuals cannot self-insure for

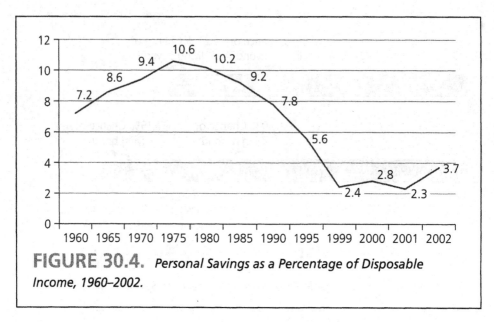

FIGURE 30.4. *Personal Savings as a Percentage of Disposable Income, 1960–2002.*

Source: United States Department of Commerce, 2003.

the risk of outliving their money because they cannot accurately predict how long they will live. Longevity creates a much smaller risk for large defined-benefit pension plan sponsors because the "law of large numbers" permits them to fund for the average life expectancy of the entire group of retirees. When a large group of retirees are pooled together, the retiree who lives a long time is offset by the retiree who dies early.

One of the biggest challenges faced by preretirees is the ability to calculate—and generate—the income they will need to comfortably live twenty, thirty, or more years in retirement. Individuals with suitable asset and income levels can consider managing this risk by converting a portion of their savings into an annuity. Annuities use the averaging effect created by pooling together the mortality experience of a large number of annuitants. An income annuity, also known as an immediate or payout annuity, is an insurance product that converts a sum of money into a stream of income that is guaranteed to last throughout the lifetime of the policyholder. It is, in effect, a personal pension plan that pools the lives of many individuals.

MANAGING HEALTH AND LONG-TERM CARE RISKS

Longevity and health are also intertwined. The question is whether, as life spans rise, health spans will rise as well. Will we age in relatively good health, or will poor health increase due to longevity? There is some good news to report. Research indicates that rates of disability among the elderly, as measured by limitations on Activities of Daily Living (ADLs), have declined over the past twenty-five years. In other words, the ability of the elderly to function and live independently is improving. But the good news is tempered by some bad news. Some studies of the underlying incidence of chronic health conditions among the elderly find that rates of morbidity are actually flat or rising. A Census Bureau study commissioned by the National Institute on Aging points out that about 80 percent of older Americans have at least one chronic health condition and 50 percent have at least two. Approximately 105 million Americans had chronic conditions in 2000, and that number is projected to increase to 158 million by 2040. It is also estimated that by age eighty-five one of every two people will develop Alzheimer's disease or another type of dementia. Costs associated with chronic conditions could double in the first half of the twenty-first century, from $470 billion in 1995 to as high as $864 billion in 2040 (Robert Wood Johnson Foundation, 1996).

OECD research finds that long-term care costs have risen steadily in recent years. They now account for some 7 percent of GDP across the OECD countries and could nearly double by the year 2050 (Organisation for Economic Co-operation and Development, 2006).

In the United States, individuals must finance their own long-term care costs unless they do not have sufficient assets and meet the eligibility requirements for Medicaid, a means-tested public benefit program. Many individuals thus find themselves paying for long-term care services out of their hard-earned savings. Nursing home care in the United States is costly: according to the MetLife Market Survey of Nursing Home and Home Care Costs, the average annual rate in 2006 for a private room was $75,190. For the average stay of 2.4 years, an individual would spend $180,456 for care. Most people prefer to remain in their homes as long as possible, but home care costs can be expensive too, averaging $19 per hour (MetLife Mature Market Institute, 2006).

Those individuals with suitable asset and income levels can protect against long-term care risks through products such as long-term care insurance. This type of insurance is widely available in the United States and is likely to become more commonplace in other developed countries as population aging puts pressure on public budgets and access to public coverage is restricted. In the United States, according to America's Health Insurance Plans (AHIP), the number of Americans who have purchased long-term care insurance has grown significantly in recent years, going from 1.9 million in 1990 to approximately 10 million in 2004. The number of employers offering it as an employee benefit jumped from 135 in 1990 to over 6,600 in 2004 (American Health Insurance Plans, 2004). Yet despite these trends, a study using Census data and information compiled for use by the Medicaid program shows that more than eight out of every ten Americans over the age of forty-five (85 percent) who have annual incomes of $20,000 or more are unprotected against the costs of long-term care by virtue of having neither public nor private insurance coverage (Long Term Care Financing Group, 2005).

Many other countries depend on a mix of publicly funded and mandated privately-funded long-term care insurance. In Japan, Germany, and Sweden, employers are required to fund some part of long-term care insurance for their workers, while the governments create safety nets for the unemployed. Canada and the UK, countries with nationalized health care systems, also use some form of insurance coverage outside their general healthcare funding system to fund the long-term care needs of their citizens. Without these safety nets, the financial burdens on their retirees would be significantly greater.

Some retirees will look to meet the financial demands of retirement and long-term care by tapping their largest asset—the equity in their primary residence. A reverse mortgage, which allows homeowners to draw periodic payments from the equity in their homes, can provide a stream of income without the need to sell and relocate. To qualify, a homeowner must be at least age sixty-two. However, according to AARP, the older the individual is, the more money he or she can receive from the reverse mortgage. And understandably, the more the home is worth, the more cash the individual can get. The transaction is a form of loan, but it is a loan that does not have to be repaid until the homeowner sells the home or dies. With a conventional or "forward" mortgage, the outstanding loan balance decreases as the homeowner makes periodic payments; with a reverse mortgage, the outstanding balance of the loan actually increases with each payment the homeowner receives.

This retirement funding option is growing in popularity. According to the National Reverse Mortgage Lenders Association, the number of federally insured reverse mortgages jumped 77 percent in 2006, from 43,131 the prior year to 76,351 (National Reverse Mortgage Lenders Association, 2006). It is likely that there will be increasing reliance on reverse mortgages as the baby boomers age, as many lack adequate retirement savings and will need to find another source of income and protection to enable them to live comfortably in their later years. Similar products are growing in popularity in markets like Japan and the UK.

IMPACT ON GOVERNMENTAL FINANCES

The aging of the population is putting a significant amount of pressure on governments worldwide. As noted earlier, Europe and Asia are experiencing a strain on government programs due to birth rates declining to well below replacement levels. These trends are similar in the United States. By 2012, according to the U.S. Government Accountability Office, Social Security's annual tax revenues may be insufficient to cover its benefits payments. In 1950, there were sixteen workers paying into the system for each beneficiary. By 2030 there will be just two workers per beneficiary.

The growth in Medicare, the public health insurance program for individuals aged sixty-five and over or disabled, is also a concern. Medicare already costs four times as much as it did in 1970, measured as a percentage of the nation's gross domestic product. It currently accounts for 13 percent of federal spending. The Congressional Budget Office projects it will consume nearly a quarter of the budget by 2030 (Congressional Budget Office, 2003).

State governments in the United States are also facing a major financing crisis in health and long-term care. The Centers for Medicare and Medicaid Services (CMS) estimates that expenditures for Medicaid—which is financed jointly by the federal and state governments and provides health and long-term care services to low-income families, the elderly, and those with a disability—have increased at a rate exceeding overall health care spending over the past decade. Spending on Medicaid has increased faster than any other category for states. Medicaid has risen from 19.5 percent of total state spending in 1999 to an estimated 21.9 percent in 2004, and it now surpasses spending on elementary and secondary education as the top spending category for states. Although more children than elderly individuals are enrolled in Medicaid, the elderly incur higher annual expenses, and the largest category of expenditures is for nursing home costs, representing 20 percent of total expenditures in 2004 (U.S. Department of Health and Human Services, 2006).

IMPACT ON THE WORKPLACE

As the population ages, it is projected that the workforce will age as well, and employers will be faced with both challenges and opportunities. In the United States, these issues include rising health care costs and increasing pension fund liabilities. There are also higher incidences of workplace disabilities among an older workforce due to serious illness and chronic disease.

Employers are also affected by their employees who are providing care to an aging parent or other loved one. Currently, in the United States there are caregivers in one out of every five households, and well over half are employed. Employees who must juggle work and family responsibilities often spend time on the job making care-related phone calls, are absent from work to provide care, transition from full-time to part-time work, or leave the workforce altogether. Research indicates that employers lose up to $33 billion in lost productivity due to caregiving (MetLife Mature Market Institute, 2005).

The major challenge, however, is the potential "brain drain" of talented, knowledgeable workers. Countries that experienced a baby boom in the early postwar decades have large numbers of workers eligible to retire in the next ten years. They will need to develop strategies to ensure that the knowledge and experience these workers bring will be retained. In Japan many employers already offer a post-retirement position to retirees at lower pay levels and diminished work hours. But despite these steps, Japan is likely to see a decline in its workforce of over 30 percent by 2050 (Organisation for Economic Co-operation and Development, Directorate of Employment, Labour, and Social Affairs, 2006).

Many workers will wish to remain in the workforce well past the traditional retirement age for two primary reasons: the need for income to supplement shortfalls in retirement savings and the desire to remain mentally and physically active. Research in the United States indicates that individuals in midlife want to continue to work, and they want meaningful work (David DeLong & Associates and Zogby International, 2006).

Civic Ventures, a national nonprofit organization dedicated to expanding the contributions of older Americans to society, collaborated with the MetLife Foundation on the New Face of Work Survey, which identifies opportunities for combining employment with community service among older adults. Among the key findings of the survey, half of Americans aged fifty to seventy want work that helps others. Second careers in the retirement years are often about people, purpose, and community. Many think it won't be easy to find second careers doing good work, and they strongly support public policy changes to remove obstacles (MetLife Foundation/Civic Ventures New Face of Work Survey, 2005).

What does this mean for the future of the workforce? With individuals working longer, the good news is that many companies will be able to retain a critical resource of talent, knowledge, and experience. More than one-third of employers in the United States—and nearly half of the companies with twenty-five thousand or more workers—agree that the aging workforce will have a significant impact on their company. The manufacturing sector expects to be hardest hit, followed closely by the government, heavy industry, and financial services industries (MetLife, 2005).

Despite this concern, more than three-quarters of companies have not taken steps to accommodate older workers, but there are some notable exceptions. IBM has a program that helps near-retirees prepare for a new (or second) career as teachers. As the MetLife Foundation/Civic Ventures study indicated, boomers, in particular, are interested in second careers and in working in the social services or education fields. These two areas already face labor shortages in some areas of the country, and as the population continues to age, the need for teachers and social service workers will grow even larger. Monsanto has implemented a creative program to engage retirees and former employees. The company's "Resource Re-Entry Center" matches interested Monsanto retirees and former employees with current temporary jobs in functional areas such as engineering, finance, law, information technology, research and development, and human resources.

These forward-thinking companies are paving the way for the future with innovative ideas. I also believe that in the decades ahead many more companies will need to identify strategies for attracting and retaining trained and experienced workers, such as innovations in phased retirement.

The many issues brought about by the aging population—caregiving, potential to outlive assets, the reallocation of resources from other age groups, and people leaving the workforce in key fields due to retirement—must be addressed now and creative solutions developed. The traditional meaning of words such as *work*, *retirement*, *volunteer*, and all the language related to aging (such as *seniors*) oversimplify a complex reality and will serve as barriers until the definitions change. Retirement is no longer a fixed date—it is a transition period as individuals move into a new stage of their life.

EDUCATION AND PLANNING: INTEGRAL TO IMPROVING RETIREMENT SECURITY

With continued increases in life expectancy, coupled with the erosion of public and private pensions, workers are entering a period of great risk with regard to retirement security. There is a tremendous challenge to individuals, as they are being asked—many for the first time—to determine, largely on their own, how much to save, how to invest that money wisely, how to prepare for their future health and long-term care needs, and how to prudently save and then draw down those savings so they are not depleted prematurely.

Many workers have not been in a position to save for retirement and will need to rely on government safety nets to sustain them. Those workers with sufficient assets, however, will need to manage their money to ensure that it will last a lifetime. Education and sensible interventions will be necessary to ensure they are up for the challenge.

There is no panacea for ensuring retirement security, but there are some important steps that can be taken today that can lead to financial security in the future. First, individuals must receive better retirement planning education. A logical place for better retirement education and advice to be provided is at the workplace. Governments also have an opportunity—and perhaps a responsibility—to provide education, tools, and incentives to help their citizens understand their retirement risks and how they can adequately finance their retirement. Organizations such as the Employee Benefit Research Institute (EBRI) (a private, nonprofit research institute that focuses on health, savings, retirement, and economic security issues) and the Women's Institute for a Secure Retirement (a nonprofit organization devoted to educating women about retirement and financial security issues) can also play an important role in helping to bring about change.

Individuals also need to start saving for retirement as early as possible. By turning to a financial professional, they can identify the investment strategies and insurance products that can help them grow and protect their retirement savings. This requires a delicate balancing act between income and expenses—choosing the right investments, getting protection against retirement risks, and choosing a level of spending that will allow assets to last a lifetime. By building a secure plan for their future, individuals can help ensure that their retirement savings will last as long as they do.

REFERENCES

American Health Insurance Plans. LTC Market Survey. Washington, D.C.: American Health Insurance Plans, 2004.

Belt, B. D. Executive Director, Pension Benefit Guaranty Corporation. Testimony Before the Committee on Education and the Workforce, United States House of Representatives, March 2, 2005.

Capretta, J. C. Global Aging and the Sustainability of Public Pension Systems: An Assessment of the Reforms of Twelve Developed Countries. Washington, D.C.: Center for Strategic and International Studies, January 2007.

Centers for Disease Control (CDC), National Center for Health Statistics (NCHS). "Deaths Preliminary Data for 2003." *National Vital Statistics Reports* (NVSS), February 28, 2005, *53*(15).

The Columbia Encyclopedia (6th ed.). New York: Columbia University Press. [http://sss.encyclopedia.com/doc1E1-longevit.html].

Congressional Budget Office. The Long-Term Budget Outlook. Washington, D.C.: Congressional Budget Office, December 2003.

David DeLong & Associates and Zogby International. *Living Longer, Working Longer: The Changing Landscape of the Aging Workforce.* MetLife Mature Market Institute, April 2006.

Employee Benefit Research Institute. Retirement Confidence Survey. Washington, D.C.: Employee Benefit Research Institute, April 2006.

Farugee, H., and Muhleisen, M. *Population Aging in Japan: Demographic Shock and Fiscal Sustainability.* Washington, D.C.: International Monetary Fund, April 2001.

Korea National Statistical Office. Population Projections for Korea (2005–2050) (in Korean). Daejeon, Republic of Korea: Korea National Statistical Office, 2006.

Long Term Care Financing Group. Index of the Uninsured. Washington, D.C.: Long Term Care Financing Group, 2005.

MetLife. MetLife 2005 Employee Benefit Trends Study.

MetLife. Retirement Income IQ Test. Westport, Conn.: MetLife Mature Market Institute, 2003.

MetLife Foundation/Civic Ventures. New Face of Work Survey. San Francisco, Calif.: MetLife Foundation, 2005.

MetLife Mature Market Institute. MetLife Caregiving Cost Study: Productivity Losses to U.S. Business. Westport, Conn.: MetLife Mature Market Institute, July 2005.

MetLife Mature Market Institute. MetLife Survey of Nursing Home and Home Care Costs. Westport, Conn.: MetLife Mature Market Institute, 2006.

National Reverse Mortgage Lenders Association. Washington, D.C., October 2006.

Organisation for Economic Co-operation and Development. "Future Budget Pressures Arising from Spending on Health and Long-Term Care." *OECD Economic Outlook,* May 27, 2006, *79,* 145.

Organisation for Economic Co-operation and Development (OECD), Directorate of Employment, Labour, and Social Affairs (DELSA). "Older Workers: Living Longer and Working Longer." *DELSA Newsletter,* January 2006, *2.* [www.oecd.org/els].

Quanhe, Y. "The Aging of China's Population: Perspectives and Implications." *Asia Pacific Populations Journal,* 1988, *3*(1).

Robert Wood Johnson Foundation. *Chronic Care in America: A 21st Century Challenge.* Princeton, N.J.: Robert Wood Johnson Foundation, 1996.

Society of Actuaries. *Longevity: The Underlying Driver of Retirement Risk, 2005 Risks and Process of Retirement Survey Report.* Schaumburg, IL: Society of Actuaries, July 2006.

Survey of Health, Aging, and Retirement in Europe. Manheim Institute for the Economics of Aging, April 2005.

Transactions of the Society of Actuaries, *Annuity 2000 Table for Males and Females.*

United Nations Population Division. *World Population Prospects, 2004 Revision, Volume III.* New York: United Nations Population Division, Department of Economic and Social Affairs, 2005.

U.S. Census Bureau. U.S. Interim Projections by Age, Sex, Race, and Hispanic Origin. Washington, D.C.: U.S. Census Bureau, 2004.

U.S. Department of Commerce. Bureau of Economic Analysis, June 2003.

U.S. Department of Health and Human Services. Assistant Secretary for Planning and Evaluation (ASPE), Historical and Projected Trends in Medicaid. Washington, D.C.: Department of Health and Human Services, October 2006.

Zolli, A. "Demographics: The Population Hourglass." *Fast Company,* March 1, 2006.

CHAPTER

31

IMPROVING HEALTH CARE IN AMERICA: LESSONS LEARNED FROM THE GLOBAL VILLAGE

WILLIAM D. NOVELLI

When Marshall McLuhan told us in 1964 that we were living in a "global village," not everyone grasped the significance of his observation. But with the arrivals, over the years, of inexpensive long-distance phone service and expanded air travel, the rise of the Internet and methods of moving capital across borders with virtually no effort, the idea of globalization came home to everyone. More interesting still, people throughout the world have grown more comfortable thinking and acting globally, especially with regard to health and aging issues.

When I was appointed to lead AARP (see box) in 2001, I stated three great goals for our association:

1. AARP will be the most successful and acknowledged organization in America for positive social change.

2. We will deliver on our promise to each member to help them make their own choices, reach their goals and dreams, and make the most of life after fifty.

3. AARP will be a leader in global aging.

ABOUT AARP AARP is a nonprofit, nonpartisan membership organization that helps people aged fifty and over have independence, choice, and control in ways that are beneficial and affordable to them and society as a whole. We produce *AARP The Magazine,* published bimonthly; *AARP Bulletin,* our monthly newspaper; *AARP Segunda Juventud,* our bimonthly magazine in Spanish and English; *NRTA Live & Learn,* our quarterly newsletter for fifty-plus educators; and our website, AARP.org. AARP Foundation is an affiliated charity that provides security, protection, and empowerment to older persons in need, with support from thousands of volunteers, donors, and sponsors. We have staffed offices in all fifty states, the District of Columbia, Puerto Rico, and the U.S. Virgin Islands.

The third of those goals is perhaps the most significant in the present context. Our interest in aging had never stopped at the shoreline. AARP has had an international outlook since our founding in 1958. Our founder, Dr. Ethel Percy Andrus, was a dedicated internationalist, launching the Association of Retired Persons International in the early 1960s. Later, AARP Executive Director Bernard Nash was instrumental in founding the International Federation on Ageing in 1973. And AARP has continued to be involved in global aging issues since that time.

By 2001, the time had come to take our commitment to a new level, so I elevated international aging issues to be one of our three goals—and for good reason. The global aging phenomenon, as thoroughly detailed in the previous chapters of this book, was beginning to affect nearly every sector of public life and demanding the attention of governments, academe, business, nonprofits, and the public.

But we and others believe that global aging also presents substantial opportunities to the economy and to society. The over-fifty population of the world is both a *production* power as an employee force and a *purchasing* power as a consumer force. If we seize the opportunity now, these forces combined can yield economic growth, rather than the stagnation that some predict.

Although there are certainly differences among nations, the reality is that we have much in common. We're all wrestling with the same aging issues in different ways and at different points on the aging curve. The questions around aging are being asked not just in the United States, and so, we reason, the answers will be found not just here at home. We believe that countries have much to teach and learn from one another as we share experiences with aging issues in the workplace, in health care, in pension systems, and in other areas.

Our mission at AARP is to improve life for people as they get older—both in the United States and abroad—so they can live long, healthy, secure, and productive lives. Aging populations offer opportunities as well as challenges. And by elevating AARP's international goal to become a leading voice in global aging, we are increasing our commitment to tackle both. We strive to be *a* global leader—one among many—but not *the* leader. To do this, we are reaching beyond our borders to engage leaders in other countries to address policy challenges and to help find solutions. We can learn much from the experiences of other countries, and there is a lot we can share with them as well. Nowhere has this been more evident than in the area of health and health care.

GLOBAL QUESTIONS OF HEALTH AND AGING

Increased longevity is one of the great success stories of our time, but it also presents us with challenges. An increasingly older population will mean more people using more medical services for a longer period of time. This puts pressures on all nations' economies, especially those with a tradition of legislated health care. This is not a future problem; it's here now, and it will become more dramatic as the world's older population continues to grow.

There is no single model anywhere that we can borrow right off the shelf and apply to fix our health care system in the United States. There are some answers to questions that might work, for example, in France, but for reasons of economics and culture would probably not work well here. The European Union is as fragmented in policy on aging and health as any two unconnected or unaligned nations. The Health Consumer Powerhouse in Brussels, in a study of twenty-six European national health systems (Hjertqvist, 2006), found no uniformity in matters as ordinary but important as the right to review medical records, consumer influence in choice of medications, or availability of no-fault medical insurance. (No-fault medical insurance is viewed as a leading alternative for resolving medical injuries. Under no-fault, claims for compensation are decided administratively instead of in the courts, and the injured party does not have to prove negligence. Proponents contend that this approach can compensate more injured patients more fairly and with less administrative overhead than the tort system.)

Clearly, no one is getting the answer to the conundrum of aging and health completely right. It is encouraging, though, that no one is getting it completely wrong, either. What we have is a robust marketplace of ideas and practices concerning health and aging—a global marketplace without borders. Our view at AARP is that we need to test and evaluate the various ideas and practices of others to see if we can find the best practices that will work for us while offering our best practices in hopes they will work for others.

Whether looking for ideas at home or abroad, we must engage the broad spectrum of the marketplace, public and private, as well. Federal, state, and local government all have an important role to play in confronting health and aging issues. But the private sector and nongovernmental organizations also have much to contribute to the pursuit of ideas and best practices, as do individuals with no particular affiliation. No one—no single person, no single organization, no single country, and no single sector—has a monopoly on good ideas. As such, we must collaborate with other organizations concerned with global aging and health.

Before turning to what we are learning from other countries, however, it is instructive to look at some of the problems in our health-care system in the United States that we believe require fixing.

AMERICA'S NONSYSTEM OF HEALTH CARE DELIVERY

"First, do no harm." We all know that line from the Hippocratic Oath. But here in the United States, we also know that hospitals that perform the least well or actually harm their patients are often better rewarded by Medicare and private insurers than those that do right by their patients. For example, a patient goes into a hospital for heart surgery and acquires an infection. The patient is readmitted or kept in the hospital to treat the infection—and the hospital gets paid for performing the surgery *and* treating the infection for which it is responsible. The better hospital gets paid *only* for the surgery. Health care providers should not benefit from medical errors.

This is only one example of how the American health care system needs to be fixed. The following are seven areas of health care in America that need vast improvement.

First, we need to wring more out of information technology. Some 80 to 90 percent of all medical records—charts, prescriptions, physicians' notes, and so forth—are on pieces of paper. The Bush administration announced an initiative to create a Nationwide Health Information Network in 2004; so far the Department of Health and Human Services has awarded contracts of only about $19 million to four groups to develop prototypes of network architecture. (More information on the Nationwide Health Information Network is available at http://nhinwatch.com. The *Nationwide* Health Information Network should not be confused with the *National* Health Information Network, a private organization providing services to pharmacies.) Many hospitals and practices have excellent internal information technology, but they cannot communicate outside their own networks, so if you're from Washington and get seriously ill in Dallas, the hospital or physician treating you will have no idea of your medical history or, if you are unable to tell them your doctor's name, how to get vital information. It appears that we have taken only one step toward a national medical infrastructure: the Medicare Modernization Act requires e-prescribing, so that drug prescriptions will be legible, easily stored on the computers at the pharmacy and the computers of others treating the patient, and, theoretically, screened for inaccurate dosage instructions or harmful interactions. A very small step—and we need twenty-league boots.

Second, and this is related to the previous point, we need to reduce medical errors. Errors lead to as many as ninety-eight thousand deaths a year and many readmissions to hospitals. This number comes from Lucian Leape, a physician who teaches at Harvard and has been the pioneer in researching medical error (see www.hsph.harvard. edu/faculty/LucianLeape.html). This situation is both harmful and costly. Moreover, admitting to a medical mistake should not open up the practitioner to a lawsuit. We need national standards of care and better performance review of practitioners and hospitals. Medical practice reform must precede medical malpractice reform.

Third, we need to promote good health from infancy onward. At the National Institute of Child Health and Human Development they say that "Osteoporosis is a pediatric disease with geriatric consequences." If you don't consume enough calcium in your teens, you can wind up with fragile bones when you're older. The same is true of an unhealthy diet, smoking, and being a couch potato.

Fourth, and this is related to the previous point, we need a better focus on what health care does. Our spending is focused on acute and episodic care. We need more focus on lifestyle and equal focus on chronic conditions, like diabetes and asthma, which are more common and disabling than acute problems. The new Medicare law has added management—in addition to treatment—of chronic conditions. All to the good, but not everyone with a chronic condition is on Medicare.

Fifth, and this too is related, we need to highlight the importance of prevention, which we at AARP are doing through our alliance with the Centers for Disease Control and Prevention. And it is very important that we increase the funding of the National Institutes of Health, which has gone flat after years of generous and wise increases.

Sixth, we need to control—or even reduce—the costs of prescription drugs. Evidence-based research, generic drugs, negotiated prices, prescription of drugs only when needed, and scrupulously managed drug importation all could help and would not be costly.

Finally, we have to make sure that everyone has health insurance. Some forty-five million of our fellow citizens have no insurance. Many are working people whose employers don't offer it or offer it only at rates beyond the means of these people. This exposes them to dangers that they could avoid by having regular medical care. It also turns out to be costly for the rest of us because the uninsured often wait to get treatment, letting a minor problem become major, and often seek their treatment in an emergency room, the most expensive place to get care. Hospitals typically shift the very high costs of uncompensated care to those who pay through insurance or out of their own pockets. We save nothing—and we offend equity—when these people are uninsured.

This list, of course, could be longer, but these are the points AARP thinks most important and compelling. They also provide the context in which we are looking for better ways to provide health care—to turn our patchwork nonsystem into a real system that delivers health care to all equitably and at an affordable price.

With this context and our global outlook in mind, several of my AARP colleagues and I traveled to Europe in summer 2006. We learned a great deal.

SOME IDEAS FROM EUROPE

Our trip to Europe enlightened all of us as to what other countries were doing in terms of health care policies and practices. We published our findings in the AARP European Leadership Study (the four studies are available online at www.aarp.org/research/international/report/leadershipstudy_reports.html). The study addresses four critical areas of the health care conundrum: containing medical costs, health information technology, long-term care, and the costs of prescription drugs. AARP's leaders interviewed knowledgeable members of government, the private sector, and nongovernmental organizations in France, the Netherlands, Norway, and the United Kingdom. Not surprisingly, there is no model in any of these areas that appears to be the solution to any of these puzzles. Europeans are wrestling as much as we are with these daunting problems. But their fighting techniques are different, and that is where we may learn some lessons. Here are some instructive samples of findings in the four areas.

Cost Containment

In France, the government pays 75 percent of all health spending, with the national parliament setting annual spending limits. In Norway, the government funds 85 percent of health care, with the contribution rates and grants set by parliament. The United Kingdom sets health budgets every three years and provides 83 percent of the total expenses. In all three countries, the balance comes from comparatively low payments by patients and almost always (except in the UK) from supplemental insurance.

The Netherlands is an exception. In 2006, it began a kind of regulated competition in the medical insurance market, which requires everyone aged eighteen and over to buy a private insurance policy; the prices range from around $1,400 to $1,700 a year, with about 60 percent of the population getting a government subsidy to buy a policy. However, on a second look the Dutch system is not a very radical departure from the others. The net effect of the mandatory insurance policies is similar to the taxes citizens of the other three countries pay to fund national health care. Moreover, government overseers in the Netherlands can estimate reasonably well what the total spent on private insurance will be. Thus, all four systems are, in one way or another, budgeted in advance.

Budgeting like this appears to have an impact on containing costs. In the United States, we spend 15.3 percent of GDP on health, whereas the four countries AARP studied range from 8.3 percent to 10.5 percent. According to *OECD Health Data 2006*

(2006), per capita expense in the United States as of 2004 was $6,100, whereas the average in the four study countries was slightly less than $3,200. Some of this substantial difference, however, may arise from our having a higher GDP per capita—in other words, we have more to spend. And as the same report explains, spending more seems to produce results. France, where patients have more choice of doctors and no delays in getting appointments or elective surgery, spends the most of the three—10.5 percent of GDP. The UK's National Health Service, which is plagued by inefficiencies and long waits for treatment, spends the least—8.3 percent. This suggests that budgeting for health care—rather than keeping an open checkbook—can help contain costs, but more money still buys more and better care.

Even so, centralized budgets for health seem to save substantially on administrative costs: we spend nearly 7 percent of our total health outlay for administration, whereas the countries we studied go from a low of just under 2 percent in France to a high of 4.4 percent in the Netherlands, where regulated competition has decentralized payment.

As a separate issue, three of the countries have used rewards for quality and safety to cut down on medical errors—which, in addition to the harm they cause, drive up costs. In France, private hospitals are paid for meeting defined standards of quality and safety. In the Netherlands, hospital payments are based on similar performance standards. In the UK, physicians can increase their incomes by as much as a third if they do well on an "evidence-based" scorecard. Moreover, physicians in the UK are required to report "adverse events and near misses." This, as I suggested earlier in this chapter, seems very good practice: better to admit the mistake and learn from it than to ignore it and endanger patients.

Health Information Technology

It seems strangely old-fashioned these days to have to make a case for information technology (IT). Our computers, of course, but also our phones with streaming video, our cars with GPS, and even our toys and games demonstrate daily and constantly the value of IT. Yet in American health care it is still a subject of debate. The future existence—let alone the success—of the Nationwide Health Information Network that I mentioned earlier is not assured. Skeptics question both the high costs and the actual benefits to practitioners. The costs will be high, but the real question is how patients will benefit.

In the UK, the National Programme for Information Technology is a work in progress. It has been bedeviled by cost overruns and delays. When it is completed, however, it will provide a medical electronic infrastructure that will deliver information where and when it is needed most.

Thus, a patient's complete records will be available on a doctor's or hospital's computers, and a summary record of essential medical information (prescriptions, allergies, diagnoses) will be held on a national database. The system will allow electronic referrals to specialists and enable a physician to book an appointment for the patient being referred. The system will enable electronic prescriptions. It will store and transmit images such as x-rays and MRIs. And it will support payments to physicians.

Interestingly, no one in the UK appears to support this system because of the potential savings, though it may deliver them. The idea is simply to improve the quality and safety of medical care.

France may be behind the UK, but it is building out a system that today is based on smart cards, which for the time being are used primarily for payment. France plans to increase the functionality of the smart cards by allowing doctors and hospitals to get access to a patient's electronic medical records from any computer anywhere, with a double card-reading system to protect privacy and confidentiality.

The French estimate saving as much as €7 billion annually by banishing paper, duplication of effort, errors, and strayed information. The deficits in the French health care system, however, have cooled the government's enthusiasm for the next stages of investment.

The Norwegian Health Network provides electronic communication among various practitioners and between practitioners and their patients. Its physical network is up and running and has adequate capacity and coverage. The system, however, is still not completely integrated and thus there are gaps in connectivity among hospitals, physicians, and pharmacies.

Not one of these systems is perfect, but at least all three (the study did not include the Netherlands) have medical IT that is working or in the works. There are two inseparable reasons that these other countries are so far ahead of the United States. First, all three have universal health coverage; second (and related), everyone in each country has a medical identifier. Thus, two barriers to building and adopting a national IT infrastructure have been removed.

Another perceived barrier that must be removed is the notion that the investment in an IT infrastructure will benefit only payers. It is clear that providers also will benefit from having better information, from making fewer errors, and from not wasting time with bits and pieces of paper. And patients certainly will benefit from better care.

To put this in different terms, the various stakeholders in health care in America need to agree that they are collaborators, not antagonists. Convincing them of this is no small task: the fragmentation of our system has made them at least suspicious of one another and at worst full competitors. I am optimistic enough to believe that getting agreement on a medical electronic infrastructure might be the beginning of fixing the rest of health care delivery in America.

Long-Term Care

If we are looking for new ideas about long-term care that appear to work well, we would do best to concentrate on Norway and the Netherlands. The UK has stringent means testing for personal and nonmedical care, and France requires steep copayments based on income; in other words, their approaches are not very different from long-term care financing in America.

In Norway, most of the cost of long-term care is covered by municipalities: the focus is local. People in need of long-term institutional care pay about three-quarters of their public pension, which is universal in Norway, and 85 percent of any other after-tax income. Fees, however, exclude savings and property, so those in need of care do not have to spend down all their assets as they must to be eligible for Medicaid in the United States.

Residential care is funded by government and individuals, but out-of-pocket expense is only about 5 percent of the total, and individual expense for medical care is limited to about $250 a year. Home nursing, care for activities of daily life, and respite care are all free. There is virtually no long-term care insurance.

The Dutch finance long-term care with a substantial payroll tax: 13.45 percent in 2005, up to a wage threshold, and the employer does not contribute. There is very little private long-term care insurance. The Netherlands also offers a broad range of home and community services, especially to those who have no formal caregivers but rely mainly on relatives. For home care, individuals can choose between receiving services from an agency or from a consumer-directed "personal budget" with a given amount of cash; those in need of care may combine services and cash. Budgets average around €12,000 a year and allow those needing care to hire family and neighbors. This is an important feature because although care workers in the Netherlands are unionized and are entitled to benefits usually unavailable to their American counterparts, home-care workers are in short supply. Norway also has an inadequate number of care workers, and turnover in urban areas especially is very high. Lacking the Dutch safety valve of personal budgets, Norway has been experiencing a shortage of nursing-home and home-care workers.

In both Norway and the Netherlands, long-term care financing and programs are managed locally, and in both this has at times led to uneven distribution of services and substantial variations in service from one municipality to another.

Perhaps the most important lesson we can learn from these two examples is that no amount of planning and financing can make a long-term care system work without professional care workers. We face the same shortages and rates of turnover in America as the Dutch and the Norwegians do. If we want long-term care to work, especially at home rather than in institutions, we need to look for ways to find, train, qualify, and compensate care workers—including relatives. No system, however funded (through taxation, insurance, or a combination) will ever work without the human touch and human competency. That, it seems to me, is the first problem to explore and solve.

Prescription Drug Pricing

The methods used by France, Norway, and the UK (the Netherlands was not included in this part of the study) to control prices of drugs may be a bitter pill for the pharmaceutical companies to swallow.

In France, where nearly two-thirds of prescriptions are paid for with public funds, the government imposes direct price controls on drugs. This can take two forms, internal or external. Internal control requires the manufacturer of a drug to justify the price relative to costs of research and development, the drug's therapeutic benefit, projected sales, and economic impact, among other criteria. The external control examines the prices of the same or similar drugs in other countries; if no similar drugs exist, the new drug is compared to a basket of drugs with the same therapeutic uses.

To qualify for insurance or reimbursement, drugs must be accepted on a national formulary that covers about 4,500 drugs. To be included in the formulary, a drug must either represent an improvement in comparison to other drugs in its class or decrease the cost of treatment.

To control costs (the French spend more on drugs than other Europeans), the government has promoted the use of generic drugs and has mandatory treatment guidelines for physicians—that is, best practices.

Norway regulates the costs of drugs with no competition from other branded products. This method, called reference pricing, limits the price of the drug to the average of the three lowest prices for a market-basket of drugs from nine European Union countries. This is the reference price that qualifies for reimbursement; any charge above the reference price is paid by the consumer or by supplemental insurance. Pharmaceutical companies are free to sell their drugs at any price.

Norway encourages the use of generics by sharing the savings with pharmacies when a generic is dispensed instead of a name-brand drug. Norway also uses "step pricing," a method that gradually lowers the price of a branded drug once its patent has expired. This offers incentives to manufacturers, pharmacies, and consumers.

The UK controls prices by negotiating the profits of pharmaceutical companies; profits may be defined, for example, as return on capital or negotiated profit margins for each company. Manufacturers are free to price drugs as they please, but they must return excess profits to the government or lower prices if they exceed their negotiated rate of profit.

Most prescription drugs are eligible for reimbursement by the National Health Service (NHS), though there are some blacklisted drugs that are not covered—for example, certain sedatives, and some so-called "graylisted" drugs that may or may not be covered, depending on circumstances.

About three-quarters of all prescriptions in the UK are written as generics even if there is no generic on the market. The NHS also monitors physicians' prescribing patterns monthly, comparing them to a theoretical but demographically similar group of patients.

This last idea sounds very helpful. A physician's prescribing patterns may vary from the norm for good reasons: the physician's patients may be more ill or have more uncommon problems than most. A physician can also prescribe carelessly. In either case, monitoring informs the physician and promotes improvement where necessary. We have no data on what monitoring costs; these would be helpful to have. If monitoring can be done at modest cost, it could save a great deal in unnecessary prescriptions and avoid harm in some circumstances.

Controlling price, through law or negotiation, is the bitter pill I referred to. Yet we already have a model in the United States: the Veterans Administration negotiates drug prices. But the Medicare Modernization Act (MMA) that created the Part D drug insurance program expressly prohibits the U.S. Secretary of Health and Human Services or a designee from negotiating drug prices for the Medicare program. Although AARP did not agree with this, the benefit of the MMA far outweighed the negatives, and so we supported its passage. We are now working to get that prohibition removed from the law.

Skeptics say that regulating price will stifle research and innovation. I am not convinced that is true. The government, through the National Institutes of Health and other agencies, spends over $30 billion a year on basic, clinical, and targeted research from which pharmaceutical companies benefit, at no cost to themselves. In this sense, the drug companies are already getting a subsidy. The UK model, which negotiates on the basis of cost *and* profit, is worth consideration.

LESSONS LEARNED

Different readers will draw different conclusions and learn different lessons from this sampling of ideas and practices I have presented. But I think there are some that are worthy of serious consideration as possibilities or inspirations, not necessarily models to copy outright.

It is impossible to miss the obvious: all four countries we looked at have national, universal health care coverage of one kind or another. It helps to rationalize delivery of care, though local administration could defeat the intentions of equitable coverage. The Dutch idea of regulated competition is probably the most palatable to American economic thought and behavior, and it is worthy of serious analysis since we already have a sophisticated private health-insurance industry.

Budgeting health care expenses seems to save substantial amounts of money by reducing administrative costs and keeping costs lower, both per capita and as a percentage of GDP. Traditional Medicare's administrative costs have held steady around 2 percent, but those of Medicare HMO (or privatized Medicare) are running about 9 percent as of this writing (see, for example, www.medicarerights.org).

Rewarding improvements in quality and safety, requiring reporting of adverse events, and monitoring prescribing patterns all would make the system less likely to cause harm and less adversarial, and this too is something we should consider.

Europe has a way to go in medical IT, but the countries in the study are far ahead of the United States. We need to put more effort into defining what kind of IT infrastructure we want, then proceed toward building it as quickly as possible.

Long-term care is nearly as problematic in Europe as it is in the United States: very costly and with an inadequate cadre of care workers. The Dutch "personal budget," allowing payments to relatives, may not be visionary, but it is practical and lets those needing care live at home where most, in this country anyway, prefer to be.

Although regulating drug costs by fiat would be a nonstarter in the United States, negotiating prices nationally with a healthy respect for profit is worth serious analysis. This will require diligent economic modeling and cannot be done on the back of an envelope. Our goal must be to make prescription drugs affordable to all, without thwarting the drug industry's ability to bring new life-saving drugs to market.

These lessons—and the more exhaustively detailed ones in the full AARP European Leadership Study—do not solve the puzzle of global health and aging in a graying world with ever-increasing medical costs. But they do offer some solid evidence that there are ideas we ought to explore and steps we then can take. The puzzle has so many pieces that clearly there is no comprehensive solution, rather an imperative to look at each area of health-care delivery and apply what remedies we have faith in, after rigorous analysis of benefits, costs, and—most significant—improvement in the quality of life.

When addressing important issues of global aging and global health, AARP's position is not to believe in a single cure or a magic potion, but to explore what appears to work, to test it, to adapt it to our needs and culture, and finally to apply it equitably— and not just for the benefit of one generation at high cost to another. We recognize that this approach will not succeed overnight, but I believe we will succeed if we open our minds to the ideas and practices of others, collaborate with other like-minded organizations, and always remember that we are working for the present generation of older persons globally and also for the generations that will follow them.

REFERENCES

Hjertqvist, J. "Can Consumers Drive the Future of Care?" AARP Global Report on Aging, Summer 2006. [http://www.aarp.org/research/international/gra/summer_2006/].

Organisation for Economic Co-operation and Development. *OECD Health Data 2006*. Paris, France: Organisation for Economic Co-operation and Development, June 2006.

PART

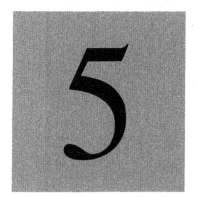

EPILOGUE:
THE ROAD AHEAD

CHAPTER

32

EPILOGUE:
THE ROAD AHEAD

ERIK OLSEN

A century ago, Rudyard Kipling wrote that "East is East and West is West and never the twain shall meet." But Kipling wrote before the age of the Internet. He did not live to see a time when nations around the world would begin to converge on a common destiny of longevity. Today, East and West must meet and meet again. Above all, we must listen to each other and learn from one another. True, not all countries have received the blessing of longevity. And among those that have moved further along the path of population aging, new challenges have arisen. Yet the message of this book is that we all have so much to learn from each other and that this task of learning will take more than the lifetime of any individual. Our learning, like our destiny, will be collective, and such learning has barely begun.

Global health and aging is an international development demanding a new international perspective, as contributors to this volume have richly demonstrated. We need to draw important lessons from the global tapestry of experience documented in this book. Despite vast demographic research, international bodies have inadequately reflected the profound importance of chronic diseases in the aging process. For example, the same institutional arrangements are in place today as were devised during the decades after the Second World War. Yet leadership today increasingly comes from non-state players such as foundations and NGOs, as well as private corporations. The burden of chronic disease is not a matter of concern only for advanced industrialized countries. As several authors in this volume suggest, the problem is that developing countries are getting old before they get rich. The hope is that dichotomies of "North and South" can now give way to mutual interest. The current trend toward greater prevalence of chronic disease calls for new attention to healthy aging, including approaches such as home-based care, self-management, and an enhanced role for nurses.

The global demography of age shows dramatic differences between different regions. Europe currently has the highest proportion of population aged sixty-five and over, and that proportion is projected nearly to double by mid-century, largely because of declining birth rates long below replacement level. But Europe is not alone. Asia's population is also aging, both in Japan—now the world's oldest country in terms of population—and in China, which is now reaping the consequences of successful efforts to slow population growth. In both East and West, financing arrangements for old age are at risk. For example, the number of defined-benefit pension plans has declined precipitously, and in the United States personal savings rates are below zero. How will we find innovative solutions for the future?

Some solutions have been proposed. The ideal of active aging, promoted by international groups such as the World Health Organization and the UN, remains a promising strategic goal. What Fries (2005) defined as "compression of morbidity" is a major theme here. A positive example of this theme is the experience of the National Health Service in the UK. The NHS has been a major force in improving the health enjoyed by Britons. Yet the NHS now faces new challenges in meeting the long-term care needs of an aging population. As in the United States, Britons have in the past two decades seen a surge in working hours and dual-income households, along with worrisome patterns of obesity and poor nutrition. In both the UK and the European Union, steps to eliminate age discrimination have been slow. There is now consideration of whether a fixed retirement age of sixty-five should be abandoned entirely.

As we think about aging and health, we must resist any temptation to think of older people as inhabiting a foreign territory of human experience. Older people are simply our future selves. Most age-related diseases are related to modifiable risk factors, so we can truly say that it is never too soon or too late for prevention. This life-course perspective is well expressed in the formulation that "osteoporosis is a pediatric disease with geriatric consequences." The positive correlations of health, life expectancy, and income per capita is well established. But these very correlations temper easygoing optimism about the future. On the one hand, there is the importance of vascular risk factors, obesity, smoking, and so on. We can and must take steps to improve health and longevity. Yet we also must confront enduring inequalities of class and education, which are much harder to change.

Even under favorable conditions, problems persist. For example, half the population in the Netherlands is now overweight and there has been no reduction in smoking among young people—both ominous trends for the future. A similar trend is evident in Denmark, which ranks among countries with the highest smoking rates. Even in Sweden, a country with one of the oldest populations, type 2 diabetes is one of the most rapidly increasing diseases, with obesity a major factor. Even wealthy, socially progressive countries such as the Netherlands and Sweden face the challenge of creating new institutions and service provision to ensure genuine quality of life in old age.

Many societies around the world are rethinking the concept of dependency, which has many meanings: for example, the dependency ratio (the number of workers divided by the number of those outside the labor force) as well as dependency related to long-term care needs. One notable contribution to policy innovation in this area is the creation of the National Dependency System by the Spanish government, which aims to coordinate a wide-ranging social services network in Spain. A contrasting example is provided by the approach of Australia, where the government is actively promoting positive dimensions of age, including healthy and productive aging.

This analysis of dependency assumes particular importance when we look at the meaning of *disability* with a global perspective. There is no general, agreed-upon definition of disability or any single method of identification, thus making cross-national comparison difficult. Still, today there is increased expectation that health care and social service providers will offer choice and promote independence. This expectation is reinforced by the acknowledgment of the rights of groups, such as the disabled, who might not have been viewed in this fashion in the not-so-distant past. This sociopolitical shift must be seen in the context of changing longevity. Increasingly, young people with physical or mental disabilities are living to older ages, while elders are experiencing the late onset of disabling conditions. There are calls in the UK for common policy responses, such as deinstitutionalization or community-based care. In the Netherlands there are proposals for small-scale housing and alternatives to nursing homes. Clearly, a "one size fits all" approach will need rethinking.

How do we think about aging, then? Does later life require more focus on dependency? Or, by contrast, on positive dimensions of productivity? We should not have to choose between these two; rather, we should recognize that each type of policy could be appropriate in addressing subgroups of the aging population. We also need to acknowledge the ways in which older adulthood is socially constructed. For example, we have long known that educational attainment affects health and longevity; two supporting studies are the Nun Study in the United States and the Whitehall Study in the UK. But we still do not know why this correlation exists. One intriguing possibility is that education, at least in some forms, can promote an attitude of high self-efficacy; that is, belief in one's ability to achieve desired outcomes. This emphasis on locus of control and individual agency has far-reaching implications for the design of health care services across wide sectors of society, in countries both rich and poor.

Issues of aging and global health have a dramatically different shape in different countries and continents. For example, sub-Saharan Africa ended the millennium poorer than it was in 1990. Moreover, the region has been devastated by the HIV/AID epidemic: more than two-thirds of the world total of those who are afflicted live in Africa. As a result, grandparents have moved into new roles as caregivers for children orphaned by AIDS, now estimated at twelve million. Because of this unprecedented social and economic crisis, traditional social welfare systems can no longer be counted on to provide elders with the social support enjoyed under traditions of filial responsibility. Along with disease, urbanization and migration trends have left elders behind in rural Africa, while eroding traditional family support systems for frail elderly. For Africa, this pattern raises a profound question about how to build intergenerational support in ways that avoid further marginalizing older people, especially older women. Will new forms of mutual aid or other policy innovations help address these challenges? How can international interventions take account of both the needs and contributions of all generations?

Attention to sub-Saharan Africa implicitly recognizes historical and cultural differences between the northern and southern parts of this vast continent. It is difference, not sameness, that should command our attention. In northern parts of Africa there has been a devastating impact of war on the well-being of elders in countries such as Somalia and Sudan. Looking to the Arab world, the socioeconomic situation in Egypt or Morocco is very different from wealthier countries such as Kuwait and the Gulf States. This dramatic heterogeneity means that countries should not be too quickly grouped under a broad label like "developing nations."

The experience of Africa reminds us that increasing longevity is not a universal destination for humankind. Indeed, the contrasting phenomenon is what Robert Butler, president and CEO of the International Longevity Center—and author of the foreword of this book—has called *shortgevity*, as shown in Russia (International Longevity Center, 2002). On the one hand, these phenomena point to the demographic and epidemiological transitions that define the new reality of population aging. On the other hand, they acknowledge that the graying of Russia's population is not being matched by improvements in health or life expectancy. On the contrary, as the General Assembly of the Russian Academy of Medical Sciences has stated, the medico-demographic processes in Russia have taken a catastrophic turn in recent decades (see Chapter Twenty-One). Adverse trends in mortality and morbidity were evident in the last years of the Soviet Union. Since the collapse of the Soviet system, the disease prevention system has also collapsed.

Latin America and the Caribbean constitute another important region where population aging is creating dramatic changes, because the demographic transition in that region has occurred very rapidly. A major characteristic of Latin America's aging process is diversity; for example, 15 percent of the population in Cuba and Argentina is over age sixty, whereas in Bolivia and Guatemala the figure is only 6 percent. The 2002 Madrid International Plan of Action on Ageing has been a significant milestone in awareness of and attention to global aging. But there is a clear need for adequate monitoring of implementation of the Madrid Plan and, equally, of efforts by the Intergovernmental Regional Conference on Ageing to focus in a regional way on population aging in Latin America.

Another significant demographic dimension of global health and aging is the role of immigration. In the United States, most workers providing care direct to older people are immigrants. Similar patterns are evident in Western Europe except that direct care workers there are from India or Pakistan; in the United States, most are from Mexico or the Caribbean. Immigration is also reshaping the face of America's aging population. By 2020, nearly a quarter of the elderly population in the United States will be members of ethnic or racial minority groups. That proportion will grow to 36 percent by 2050, with the biggest increase coming from Hispanics. This ethnic diversity necessitates looking more carefully at health disparities among subpopulations in the United States For example, there is a twenty-one-year spread in life expectancy separating Asian American women from black men living in high-risk urban areas (Murray and others, 2007). Research on health disparities suggests more careful targeting of preventive interventions using culturally appropriate means to reach specific subpopulations. As with disability policy in the UK, a "one size fits all" approach will simply not work.

There are some, like Pete Peterson and Lawrence Kotlikoff in the United States, who view population aging as a disaster and a cause for alarm. Yet the Finnish experience gives a very different picture. Relatively simple changes in lifestyles can dramatically reduce chronic disease and promote greater health, as called for in the WHO report of 2002 on reducing risk and promoting health (cited in Chapter Eight). Fear of population aging goes back to the nineteenth century in France, when observers worried that the country's low fertility rate would lead it to become "too old" and thus fall behind its rivals. Some might point to French exceptionalism, but we can recognize universal patterns of population aging found on a global basis. One of these is the so-called "female advantage" in life expectancy. Another is the paradoxical trend of increasing disability due to the aging of the population counterbalanced by a decrease in disability at each age. There is also a persistent inequality in life expectancy in different countries: for example, people in Western Europe can expect to live six years longer than those in central Europe and ten years longer than residents of the former Soviet Union. Within countries, too, socioeconomic levels account for further inequalities in longevity.

When it comes to longevity, there is much to be learned by studying the most favorable examples. Examples of exceptional longevity are not to be found in fabled exotic locations like the Caucasus or the Himalayas (the fables have actually never been proven), but rather among Seventh Day Adventists in America, a group whose life expectancy is ten years greater than that of other Americans. We note too the female advantage and can find fascinating gender differences involving hormones, chromosomal structure, and mitochondrial metabolism.

One conclusion from centenarian studies is that there is no silver bullet for exceptional longevity. While more research goes on, we ought to remember to take the standard advice: eat your vegetables, exercise, get a good night's sleep, and don't smoke. We may not live to be one hundred, but we can avoid wasting our money on unproven "anti-aging" remedies and have a longer and healthier old age.

As each of us looks at population aging from a global perspective, we see aging through different eyes depending on our cultural presuppositions. The role of cultural diversity is of enormous importance here because of our tendency to think of aging in terms that some have called the *deficit model*. Our thinking is too often dominated by narrow definitions, failing to acknowledge the role of culture in shaping the meaning of categories like disability or chronic illness. The idea of dependency, so prominent in the discourse of Western gerontology, takes on an entirely different meaning in non-Western cultures, where interdependency and intergenerational helping relationships have long-established cultural meanings.

The cultural dimensions of longevity become prominent when we look at historically influential traditions very different from those of the West. Thus a global view of health and aging would be incomplete without attention to China and India.

The growth rate of the aged in India is astonishing. From 82 million in 2004, it will rise to 177 million by 2025 and 324 million by 2040. Moreover, the oldest old are growing more rapidly than the young-old, with significant consequences such as the feminization of aging, rural poverty, and inadequate health insurance and social security. Yet along with negative trends there are developments that draw on unique cultural resources of Indian tradition: for example, the persistence of ayurvedic medicine and the link between spirituality and longevity, as illustrated in the Bhaghavad Gita, with its vision of later life as a time for spiritual fulfillment.

China is the world's most populous country and also a nation now aging faster than any other country on earth, as it experiences the unanticipated effects of its one-child family policy. Yet the demographic consequences are far from uniform across the country: for example, rural areas face problems much greater than urban areas. Early in the twentieth century, two-thirds of households in China were three-generational, but today only around one-fifth of families live in such multigenerational households. As a result of declining fertility, new cohorts of elders may not receive a level of benefits comparable to what earlier cohorts received. Yet China can draw on a vast cultural reservoir of values and attitudes favoring old age, values historically associated with Confucian tradition. Ancient traditions can furnish insights on the new realities of population aging. On this point, China, like Western countries, is developing a promising idea that British historian Peter Laslett has called "the third age" (see Chapter Eighteen). China already has an astounding seventeen thousand schools and 1.5 million students who are part of the "gray universities" that Laslett, in his *A Fresh Map of Life*, called for in the "universities of the third age" that have proven so exciting in Europe. Here we recognize a remarkable parallel between lifelong learning in Western societies and Confucian-inspired traditions of the East. Far from being locked in the old paradigm of "East is East and West is West," we see, once more, one of the many ways in which all nations of the world are learning from one another as we confront the challenges and opportunities of an aging world.

REFERENCES

International Longevity Center. *Aging on the World Stage: Perspectives for the Media on Longevity With World Experts on Population Aging*. Madrid, Spain: April 5–8, 2002, p. 12. [www.ilcusa.org/_lib/pdf/madrid2002.pdf]. Accessed May 1, 2007.

Fries, J. F. "Frailty, Heart Disease, and Stroke: The Compression of Morbidity Paradigm." *American Journal of Preventive Medicine*, Dec. 2005, *29*(5 Suppl 1), 164–8.

Murray, C. I. L., and others. "Eight Americans: Investigating Mortality Disparities Across Races, Counties, and Race-Counties in the United States." *PLoS Medicine*, *3*(9), e260.

INDEX

Page numbers in italics refer to Tables and Figures